Anthology
on Caring

Anthology on Caring

Edited by Peggy L. Chinn, PhD, RN, FAAN

Professor and Associate Dean for Academic Affairs
Center for Human Caring
School of Nursing
University of Colorado

National League for Nursing Press • New York
Pub. No. 15-2392

ISBN 0-88737-516-2

The views expressed in this publication represent the views of the authors and do not necessarily reflect the official views of the National League for Nursing.

This book was set in Palatino and Garamond by Ampersand Publisher Services, Inc. Rachel Schaperow was the editor and designer. United Book Press was the printer and binder. The cover was designed by Lillian Welsh.

Printed in the United States of America

Contents

Contributors

Andrea M. Barsevick, DNSc, RN
Assistant Professor, Nursing
University of Pennsylvania
Philadelphia, Pennsylvania

Linda Bergstrom, MA, CNM, RN
PhD Candidate
School of Nursing
University of Colorado Health Sciences Center
Denver, Colorado

Anne H. Bishop, EdD, RN
Professor of Nursing
Lynchburg College
Lynchburg, Virginia

Joan L. Bottorff, MEd, MN, RN
PhD Candidate and Research Associate
Faculty of Nursing
University of Alberta
Edmonton, Alberta, Canada

Paulette Burns, PhD, RN
Assistant Professor
College of Nursing
University of Oklahoma
Tulsa, Oklahoma

Gloria M. Clayton, EdD, RN, FAAN
Professor
School of Nursing
Medical College of Georgia
Augusta, Georgia

Carol Craig, MS, RN
PhD Candidate
School of Nursing
University of Colorado Health Sciences Center
Denver, Colorado

Carol J. Farran, DNSc, RN
Associate Professor
Rush College of Nursing
Chicago, Illinois

Sally A. Forsstrom, BA, DNE, FCNA, FCN(NSW), RN
Lecturer in Nursing
Charles Sturt University, Riverina
Wagga Wagga
New South Wales, Australia

Gary J. Foulk, PhD, EMT
Professor
Department of Philosophy
Indiana State University
Terre Haute, Indiana

Marie-Luise Friedemann, PhD, CS, RN
Assistant Professor
College of Nursing
Wayne State University
Detroit, Michigan

Joanne E. Gray, Bachelor of Health Sciences (Nursing), CM, RN
Lecturer in Nursing
Charles Sturt University, Riverina
Wagga Wagga
New South Wales, Australia

Patricia E. Greene, MSN, RN, FAAN
Vice President for Nursing
American Cancer Society
Atlanta, Georgia

Carol Green-Hernandez, PhD, FNS, RNC
Associate Professor, Graduate Program in Nursing
School of Nursing
University of Vermont
Burlington, Vermont

Nancy P. Greenleaf, DNSc, RN
Associate Professor of Nursing
University of Southern Maine
Portland, Maine

Sharon D. Horner, MSN, RN
Assistant Professor
Department of Nursing
Georgia Southern College
Statesboro, Georgia

Eleanora Keane-Hagerty, MA
Research Associate
Rush College of Nursing
Chicago, Illinois

M. Jan Keffer, PhD, CANP, RN
Lecturer
Department of Philosophy
Indiana State University
Terre Haute, Indiana

Ann M. Kolanowski, PhD, RN
Associate Professor and Chairperson
Department of Nursing
Wilkes University
Wilkes-Barre, Pennsylvania

Diane Lauver, PhD, RNC
Assistant Professor
University of Wisconsin, Madison
Madison, Wisconsin

Joan K. Magilvy, PhD, RN
Associate Professor
School of Nursing
University of Colorado Health Sciences Center
Denver, Colorado

M. Patrice McCarthy, MSN, RN
PhD Candidate
School of Nursing
University of Colorado Health Sciences Center
Denver, Colorado

Joyce P. Murray, EdD, CS, RN
Director of Accreditation
National League for Nursing
New York, New York

Christine L. Pollack-Latham, DNSc, CCRN, RN
Professor
Department of Nursing
California State University, Los Angeles
Los Angeles, California

Francelyn Reeder, RSM, PhD, CNM, RN
Assistant Professor and Associate Faculty
Center for Human Caring
School of Nursing
University of Colorado Health Sciences Center
Denver, Colorado

Lynn McCreery Schimmel, MS, RNC, NP
Perinatal Clinical Nurse Specialist Student
University of California, San Francisco
San Francisco, California

Carole Schroeder, MSN
PhD Candidate
School of Nursing
University of Colorado Health Sciences Center
Denver, Colorado
Assistant Professor
Orvis School of Nursing
University of Nevada
Reno, Nevada

John R. Scudder, Jr., EdD
Professor of Philosophy and Education
Lynchburg College
Lynchburg, Virginia

Martha N. Smith, PhD, MPH, RNC
Interim Chairperson, Department of Preventive Medicine
Director, Master of Public Health Program
Associate Professor, School of Medicine
Director, Master's Program in Community Health Nursing
Associate Professor, School of Nursing
Medical College of Virginia, Virginia Commonwealth University
Richmond, Virginia

Martha H. Stoner, PhD, RN
Associate Professor and
Assistant Director of Nursing and Research
University Hospital
School of Nursing
University of Colorado Health Sciences Center
Denver, Colorado

Phyllis Updike, DNS, RN
Associate Professor
College of Nursing
University of South Carolina
Columbia, South Carolina

Toni M. Vezeau, MS, RN
PhD Candidate
School of Nursing
University of Colorado
Denver, Colorado

Anna Frances Z. Wenger, PhD, CTN, RN
Associate Professor and Director
Transcultural and International Nursing Center
Nell Hodgson Woodruff School of Nursing
Emory University
Atlanta, Georgia

Elizabeth M. Whitley, MSN, RNC
PhD Candidate
School of Nursing
University of Colorado Health Sciences Center
Denver, Colorado

Gail M. Whitney, BA
Graduate Student, Master of Humanities Program
University of Richmond
Richmond, Virginia

Doris M. Williams, PhD, RN
Director of Nursing
Chemeketa Community College
Salem, Oregon

Preface

Caring is fundamental to human experience. Yet, for centuries knowledge concerning caring, and the methods that are required to address caring, have been largely unexamined as serious academic concerns. Even as nurses and women who are scholars, our location within the traditional scientific realm leads us to doubt our insights, and often to ask misguided questions. From the perspective that is familiar to most nurses, the questions: "To whom does caring knowledge belong?" and "Is caring fundamental or unique to nursing?" are admissible. Once we make the move into a frame of reference where caring is valued philosophically and practically, the competitive notions of ownership and uniqueness fade into insignificance, and the questions turn to:

- "Who benefits from knowledge about caring?"
- "Who benefits if we fail to develop caring knowledge?"
- "Why has knowledge about caring been devalued in the past?"
- "What perspectives do women and nurses offer in developing caring knowledge?"
- "Are there other perspectives that need to be explored as well?"
- "What might caring knowledge offer for the future of the world?"

The chapters in this anthology address these fundamental questions and more. This book represents a major contribution to the "conversation in the discipline" of nursing concerning the idea, the ideal, and the practice of caring. It also provides a significant resource for scholars in other disciplines who can join the ongoing dialogues and offer their perspectives to the conversation. The chapters herein do not provide "answers"; rather taken together they raise important questions and open windows of opportunity for the development of caring knowledge. This book provides a wide diversity of both perspective and method, providing for nursing and other caring disciplines a true anthology on caring.

The chapters in this volume were originally prepared, and refereed for consideration, for publication in *Advances in Nursing Science*, of which I am also Editor. Each of these chapters was eligible for publication in that journal based on positive recommendations by members of the Board of Review for *ANS*. Space limitations precluded inclusion in that journal of these eligible articles. The authors of these chapters have benefited from the comments of members of the *ANS* Board of Review and have integrated revisions based on the suggestions of the reviewers.

The large response to the *ANS* issue on "Caring" (Volume 13:1, September 1990) reflects the nature of the discipline's interest in caring. As might be expected, there is no one single view of this phenomenon within the discipline of nursing. Further, the scholarly explorations that continue to thrive within nursing provide abundant evidence of the importance of caring phenomena for human health and well-being. Human interests concerning phenomena so central to human experience cannot be parochial or singular. If as humans we are to shape a future where caring and related human values prevail, it is urgent that the best of creative effort be shared among scholars who are open to many paths and many perspectives. It is my hope that as a reader you will find the chapters of this book stimulating for the next stages of our collective conversation, and for the cutting-edge scholarship that will emerge from that conversation.

Peggy L. Chinn, PhD, RN, FAAN
Professor of Nursing
University of Colorado School of Nursing
Center for Human Caring

1

Caring Approaches: A Critical Examination of Origin, Balance of Power, Embodiment, Time and Space, and Intended Outcome

Toni M. Vezeau and Carole Schroeder

A solid reference to caring should always answer the question: Caring, according to whom? In nursing literature, the term "caring" is freely used and often discussed as if it has only one meaning, unique to the domain of nursing. Actually the term caring is used in many disciplines and can have multiple meanings which stem from very disparate assumptions.

It is the premise of this paper that underlying assumptions of caring approaches can be made explicit in order for caring to be better understood. Toward that goal, various approaches to caring will be presented to display the range of possibilities that can exist when one is "caring." The following caring approaches were selected not only from nursing, but from literature and philosophy that address caring.

Historically, nursing has been open to concepts from outside the discipline that show correspondence to those explored in nursing, integrating them into its unique perspective. Webster (1990) states that nursing needs to continue to draw on literary narratives and philosophy, particularly in the area of caring, in order to develop theories of human nature.

It is not within the scope of this article to address all literature on caring. Rather, the goal is to present many caring approaches that will reveal important differences in their assumptions about caring. Watson (1985, 1989) is well known in nursing literature for her approach to caring. Noddings (1984) and Mayeroff (1971) are also well known for their caring approaches, and have frequently been cited in nursing literature. We (the authors) have also included philosophical approaches that are perhaps less drawn upon in nursing, specifically, Buber (1965) and Jonas (1986). A literary narrative written by Griffin (1978) about naturalist John James Audubon is included in this article because of its eloquence in depicting the current approach to caring in many health care environments. Finally, Gadow (1984), a nurse philosopher, offers a fresh and novel approach to the discussion of caring that can enrich our current understanding of caring.

Each approach to caring will be briefly described and then examined critically by exploring the following:

What is the origin of caring?
What is the relationship of caring to power?
What is the relationship of caring to embodiment?
What is the relationship of caring to time and space?
What is the outcome of caring?

We consider these assumptions central to any approach to caring, but these assumptions are not generally made explicit in the discussions of caring. The illumination of these seven writers' assumptions on notions of motivation, power, time, embodiment, and outcome, will reveal distinct differences among the approaches to caring. Clearly, caring can be understood in divergent ways.

DESCRIPTIONS OF CARING

Milton Mayeroff

Mayerhoff describes caring as helping someone else grow toward self–actualization (1971). Caring is grounded in the worth the one caring experiences in the other, and also promotes the self–actualization of the one caring by serving to ground the person in the world:

> ... caring has a way of ordering his other values and activities
> around it ... because of the inclusiveness of his caring, there is
> a basic stability in his life; he is 'in place' in the world, instead
> of being out of place, or merely drifting or endlessly seeking his
> place [1971, p. 2].

Thus, although the purpose of caring is to help someone else grow, caring serves to ground the one caring in what Mayerhoff calls basic certainty. The one caring determines the direction of growth for the one cared for:

> I must know many things ... what his powers and limitations
> are, what his needs are, and what is conducive to his
> growth.... [1971, p. 13]

Sally Gadow

Gadow defines caring as supporting an individual's interpretation of one's own reality:

> ... the essence of nursing is the nurse's participation with the patient in determining the unique meaning which the experience of health, illness, suffering, or dying is to have for that individual [1980a, p. 81].

Gadow describes care as an end in itself and the highest form of commitment to patients. The most caring act can also be in nonaction, as determined by the other. Caring demands embodiment, or the conveyance of the professional's body as having the same subjective reality as the patient's body (1984).

Truth is contextual, encompassing subjective and objective realities into a coherent whole. Rather than literal truth, Gadow views science as metaphor: a story about what is, not unlike that of poetry or literature, no better and no worse (personal communication, 1989).

Nel Noddings

For Noddings (1984), caring is based in receptivity. The one caring "feels with" the other and "receives the other" completely (1984, pp. 30–35). This process is not cognitive, but emotive, requiring motivational shift and engrossment with the other. The situation of caring is not abstract but concrete, tied to a particular context. The nature of caring relationships can vary in intensity and may be enduring or episodic depending on the strength of felt obligation. Caring is a way of being, and may or may not involve action or verbal communication. Caring is an end in itself, complete, and is not a means to an end (1984).

In this view of caring, truth is contextual. Rules do not have priority over context. Different visions of reality are discovered only in relationship. Truth is not a primary concern within Noddings' caring framework (1984). The good is found in the process of seeking connection.

Jean Watson

Watson (1985) states that nursing is the vanguard of caring. Caring is depicted as the moral ideal of nursing, an epistemic endeavor, the starting point for nursing action, and a unique transaction between the nurse and other. Caring involves the will to care, the intent to care, and caring actions. These actions can be positive regard, support, communication, or physical interventions of the nurse. Caring is a commitment to an end, the protection, enhancement, and preservation of the dignity of the other (1985). Citing work by Gadow, Watson asserts that, in human caring, the usual relationship between cure and care is inverted (1988). Watson's emphasis on caring for the potentiation of self–healing results in the idea that care may also be a means to effect cure (1983, 1985).

Truth is determined in relationship. The transaction can involve a proposal by the nurse and a confirmation or improvement by the other (1985). Truth is personal, individual, and has many expressions.

Martin Buber

In Buber's work, caring is a form of dialogue which emerges from a readiness to be addressed by another. This dialogue may be spoken or silent, but is a state

> where each of the participants really has in mind the other or others in their present and particular being and turns to them with the intention of establishing a living mutual rela- tion . . . [1965, p. 19].

This dialogue requires unreserve, or the ability to be open to the claim of another person. Caring involves moving beyond the acts of observing and onlooking, beyond reflection, into a level of awareness in which one is absorbed by the present situation. For Buber, caring is a way of being rather than action:

> . . . it is too little to be ready, one must also be really there [p. 3].

Although Buber doesn't use the term caring, this dialogue clearly portrays what Noddings means by receptivity and what Watson describes as a transpersonal caring relationship.

Hans Jonas

For Jonas, a philosopher, all life is relatedness for encounter is all (1966). Caring arises out of the freedom to relate, and the necessity to relate in nature. The concept of metabolism is metaphor for life: the organism takes in energy and releases energy continually from the environment in order to survive. Jonas calls "transcendence of life" (p. 85) the extension of relatedness into space beyond the felt selfhood of interiorization. Relation- ship can be viewed as continual change involving the constant flux of energy between inwardness and outwardness in the life process. The process of relationship is the fundamental reality of life.

. . . in order to change matter, the living form must have matter at its disposal, and it finds it outside itself, in the foreign "world." Thereby life is turned outward and toward the world in a peculiar relatedness of dependence and possibility. Its want goes out to where its means of satisfaction lie: its self–concern, active in the acquisition of new matter, is essential openness for the encounter of outer being [p. 84].

Truth arises out of biological unity, and historically can be traced from vitalism through materialism to a synthesis Jonas calls organism. In Jonas' organism, experience is paramount. The whole is concrete and the parts abstract, and detail is valued in that it enriches the whole. To objectify is to remove the reality of being, for within ourselves we find evidence of existence as an integral part of nature. The fact of our existence is the whole object of inquiry, and to miss the existence of life would deny the concrete from which to make abstractions. Thus, truth resides in experience and subjectivity, both of which arise out of relationship.

John James Audubon

John James Audubon is known for his love of the natural state of life. We believe his idea of caring, as portrayed by Griffin (1978), to be a powerful example of a positivist approach to caring pervasive in the present–day health care and legal environment. Webster (1990) and Vitz (1990) advocate the use of literary narratives in the discussion of human nature because the use of metaphor is uniquely suited to support the complexity and mystery found in the caring situation.

The following excerpt from Griffin is a skillfully drawn depiction of Audubon's idea of caring:

For weeks upon weeks he observed the habits of this bird. . . . He could predict every moment of the bird; he knew its habits. . . . He disturbed the nest of this eagle since he knew then that the bird would stay there. . . . So the painter did not hurry as he went to find his gun, and he took his time loading it. Then he sequestered himself in weeds about the tree and aimed slowly and carefully. . . .

Now he was excited. He had a fire built and spent the next hours preparing the bird, stuffing him, mounting him. He had acquired this skill through the years of labor and experiment. He used wires to pierce and hold together the body of the bird in the posture he desired, and the result of his efforts created an effect whose grace and naturalness were later said to have rivaled life. . . .

Finally he would capture the eagle on paper by placing the body against a background ruled with division lines in squares to correspond to similar divisions on his own paper. . . . He was meticulous and painted with great accuracy even every barb on every feather, so great was his love for his subject. And in this, he preserved the birds of America [pp. 113–114].

Audubon's definition of caring would be the preservation, by any means, of what is perceived as the natural state.

This model of caring by Audubon is found in acts to promote what the one caring determines to be the natural good. Communication is not necessary, and truth is determined externally by the one caring and not in relationship with the other. This truth is scientific, often empirical, and can justify deception and even harming of the other.

Summary

These brief descriptions of caring show a range of approaches to caring. With this information as a base, the discussion will move to an examination of the assumptions that undergird these divergent notions of caring. These assumptions become explicit when the following questions are explored: What is the origin of caring? What is the relationship of caring to power? What is the relationship of caring and embodiment? What is the relation of caring to time and space, and what is the outcome of caring?

Table 2-1 outlines the position of each caring approach in relation to these questions. Brief phrases cannot capture the richness found in these caring frameworks; however, the intent of the grid is to function as a map. A dot on a map does not fully represent a town, but gives its relative position to other areas on the map. Throughout the following discussion of the assumptions found in the work of the seven authors, the table will help the reader locate each position relative to the others.

ASSUMPTIONS OF CARING

Origin of Caring

The origin of caring refers to the reason one cares. What gives rise to caring varies among the caring approaches. In Mayeroff's work, caring stems from self–obligation. Although one cares in order that another might grow, the one caring fulfills a basic need to be needed:

Table 2-1

Assumptions of Caring Approaches

Author	Description	Origin	Power	Embodiment	Time and Space	Outcome
Audubon	Preservation of the natural state	Desire for knowledge and control	Domination by the one caring	Disembodiment	Linear; emphasis on future orientation	Means to understand/preserve appearance of natural state
Buber	Dialogue based on unreserve	Feeling the address of the other	Reciprocity; mutuality	Caring occurring in concrete lived-body experience	Multidimensional; manifest in the concrete world	End in itself
Gadow	Protection, enhancement and preservation of human dignity	Incomparable worth of the individual	Mutuality; sharing of power	Embodiment as self-body unity requisite for caring	Multidimensional; continual patterns of experience	Engagement; an end in itself
Jonas	Relationship involving continual change	Freedom and necessity to relate in nature	Reciprocity	Cultivated self-body unity	Directional, linear; without concretion	Continuation of life process
Mayeroff	Helping the other grow	Self-obligation	May or may not be reciprocal or egalitarian	Separate mind and body	Linear time; absolute space; present and future orientation	Growth in the one cared for; basic certainty
Noddings	Receptivity	Primary value growing out of caring experienced in childhood	Reciprocity	Total engrossment; embodiment required for caring	Emphasis on infinite present	End in itself
Watson	Moral ideal of nursing; unique transaction	Nursing's moral responsibility to meet society's mandate	Mutuality	Integrated trinity of spirit, mind, and body	Caring transcendent of time and space	Potentiation of self-healing

The others' growth is bound up in my own sense of well–being [1971, p. 19].

In contrast, in Jonas' philosophy of organism, the origin of caring is the inseparability of the organism and environment in nature. Caring arises out of a dialectic of freedom and necessity that Jonas calls the paradox of material existence. Although relationship arises out of need for self–continuation (organic want), at the same time, the other inspires interest:

As the need–inspired interest seeks the other, so the uninvited presence of the other summons the interest [1966, p. 85].

The organism is free to be selective in its communication or outwardness. The concept of metabolism is metaphor for the life process. This synergism arises out of both the freedom to relate and the necessity to relate with others in order to survive.

For Buber, caring originates from unreserve,

. . . disposed to everything that may come . . . it is too little to be ready, one must also be really there [1965, p. 3].

This unreserve enables one to feel the claim and address of another and thus to engage in living dialogue. Buber states that "feeling the address," full receptivity or "unreserve" is central to caring relationships (1965, p. 11). For Buber caring is life, flowing out of his notion of concrete reality which is

. . . the creation that is entrusted to me and to every man [p. 13].

According to Audubon, caring originates from a desire to know and to control, in order to promote the caring one's perception of the natural good. The one caring seeks to preserve the appearance of the natural state, at any cost.

Caring, in Gadow's work, originates from the moral ideal of the incomparable worth of each person and the value of human dignity. Preservation of human dignity requires alleviating another's vulnerability. If cure is to be ethical, caring is requisite. Caring diminishes the distance between professional and patient:

The moment that mutuality is abandoned and the chasm re-opened, then power is again unilateral, and cure is unethical. [1988, p. 13]

For Noddings, caring is a primary value that grows out of the natural caring experienced in childhood during which interpersonal connection is fundamental (1984). One needs to have had the experience of being cared for, and to have had the value of caring instilled in one's past, in order for one to be capable of caring. The strength of one's motivation to care can differ according to the context, depending on the intimacy of the relationship. In a family, for example, caring arises from love; as the relationship becomes less intimate, one cares because of a natural imperative to care that is based on learned values (Noddings, 1984).

Like Noddings, Watson believes that caring can be fostered in nursing (1988, 1989). Caring originates from nursing's moral responsibility to meet society's mandate. Watson sees nursing as the "caretakers of care" for other helping professions (1985, p. 32).

As described above, caring can originate from very different motivations, variously understood as self–obligation (Mayeroff), freedom and necessity (Jonas), unreserve (Buber), desire to know and control (Audubon), moral ideal (Gadow), outgrowth of natural caring experienced in childhood (Noddings), and social mandate (Watson).

Relationship of Caring to Power

Basic to any approach to caring is the relationship of the one caring (self) to the one cared for (other). This relationship involves power, the balance of which can have many expressions. Although Mayeroff states that the one cared for is primary, he sees the other as a reflection of self.

> In caring ... I experience what I care for (a person, ideal, an idea) as an extension of myself and at the same time as something separate. [1971, p. 5]

For Mayeroff, caring has the same pattern regardless of the kind of relationship: helping the other grow. The one caring senses the need from the other and is able to determine what is required for the other to grow. Caring may or may not be reciprocal or egalitarian in Mayeroff's model of caring.

In contrast, relationship of self to other for Jonas is intrinsic and necessary, yet the organism is free to be selective and informed. Relationship involves "spatial self–transcendence" (1966, p. 84), the process whereby every living thing must transcend its boundaries and open to the environment, while at the same time the inwardness and subjectivity of felt selfhood prevails. For Jonas, the transcendence of life involves encounter; the balance of power is shared and reciprocal.

In Buber's work, mutuality and reciprocity of awareness prevail in the caring relationship. Caring involves recognizing other as truly other rather than as an extension of self; caring requires no justification. Self and other must be mutually turned toward one another (1965), for caring to occur.

In the Audubon approach to caring, the self as one caring is seen to be complete, the ultimate authority who exercises definitive power. The one caring does not realize personal enhancement in the relationship except for a sense of satisfaction. There is no mutuality or reciprocity between the self and the other, for the other is seen as an abstract, theoretical, and replaceable entity. The ones cared for are not to be regarded in their individual contexts, but are compared to the idealized notion of what is "natural." The more one knows about the other, the more the other becomes marginalized into a distinct conceptual compartment.

In contrast, Gadow's caring involves mutuality. The relationship between the self and other always involves embodiment, in which the body of the one caring assumes the same subjectivity as the body of the one cared for (1988). The relationship between a health professional and a patient involves decreasing patient vulnerability and reducing unilateral wielding of power by professional over patient.

Unlike Mayeroff, Gadow states that caring involves differing forms of reciprocity or mutuality of relationship, which Gadow calls existential advocacy. This is the

> ... philosophical foundation upon which the patient and the nurse can freely decide whether their relation shall be that of child and parent, client and counselor, friend and friend, colleague and colleague, ... through the range of possibilities [1980a, p. 81].

Similarly, Noddings' caring relationship is reciprocal; both partners have potential for enhancement through the caring relationship. The intensity differs in each situation, making the imperative to care dependent on the closeness of the bond within the relationship.

For Watson the relationship of self and other is characterized by mutuality in the power relationship. Both the nurse and the other benefit from the caring relationship, experiencing enhancement. Watson views the caring nurse as first needing to be self–aware and open to the relationship, with conscious will and intent to care. Before the caring relationship is fully realized, the nurse is external to the intensity of the reality of the other. The other may or may not be in this self–aware state, and more likely is experiencing difficulty in comprehending or expressing the predicament. The caring relationship fosters the release of what the other has been "longing to express" (1985, p. 67). This release enhances self–awareness of both persons, and leads to an openness toward self–healing in the other.

The relationship of self to other involves power, and the balance of power can have many expressions in the caring relationship. Some caring approaches stress the mutuality and reciprocity within relationship, although this does not necessarily imply equality within the relationship. Others stress the one caring as the starting point for caring, the one who leads the dance of relationship.

Relationship of Caring to Embodiment

The relationship of self to body involves concepts of separation, or unity of mind and body in caring. Mayerhoff's caring separates mind and body. Caring takes place in the mind from the ability to know another person intellectually and intuitively (1971).

Jonas subscribes to a body–self unity that, while innate, must be recovered and cultivated out of knowledge of a basic polarity of otherness and self. The living body is the only concrete experience of life, and "life means material life, . . . living body, . . . organic being" (1966, p. 24). The organism can and must change its form while at the same time, there is the "impossibility of resting with any concretion attained" (p. 84). Jonas speaks to the constant energy exchange necessary for life:

> This is the antinomy of freedom at the roots of life and in its most elementary form, that of metabolism. [p. 84]

For Buber, relationship with self–body involves undifferentiated oneness of self "without form or content" (1966, p. 25) which he calls the unity of life:

> . . . the unity of unbroken, raptureless perseverance in concreteness . . . [p. 28].

The fact of "bodily otherness" (p. 28) is not a deterrent to human dialogue; instead, one must live toward the other's concrete life or person. Caring can only take place in the lived body experience, which is life.

For Gadow, embodiment is a requirement for caring and arises from the lived body experience of subjectivity. Relationships with the body evolve through nonlinear stages, from initial primal immediacy (as in infancy when the lived body is the world and world the body), to the object body (where one recognizes the body as separate from self), to cultivated immediacy (where the unity of self and body is restored through mastery), to the subject body (a state in which the body's values have as much validity as those of the self) (1980b). Ones caring must be embodied themselves in order to be in caring relation with another (1989). Touch maintains an intersubjective stance through which caring is possible (1984).

For Audubon, the lived body of the other is not seen as the essence of the other. Appearance of the body has more value than the reality of the inhabited body. In the description that Griffin gives of Audubon, preservation of the appearance of the body takes priority over the experiencing self of the eagle.

For Noddings, caring is embodiment; caring is a way of being not necessarily involving specific actions or verbal communication. The other is taken in (1984), that is, the spirit of the other is totally received by the one caring. Sometimes this can occur quite literally, as in the situation of motherhood. Caring is based on feeling and sensitivity, involving total engrossment with the other. Noddings herself likens caring to the "I and Thou" relationship as described by Buber (1984).

Watson explains the person as an integrated trinity of spirit, mind, and body (Watson, 1985, 1989; Sarter, 1988). While many writers on caring view caring as embodiment, Watson's caring transcends the body (1985). Watson states:

> . . . one's soul possesses a body that is not confined by objective space and time. . . . As a result of this view, there is a great deal of respect, regard, and awe given to the concept of a human soul (spirit, or higher sense of self) that is greater than the physical, mental, and emotional existence of a person at any given point of time [Watson, 1985, p. 45].

Watson suggests that the spirit is more essential than the body in caring. Because the body "may be physically present in a given location or situation" (p. 46), only the spirit can transcend the here and now, guiding the whole person toward enhancement. However, in a 1989 article, Watson incorporates Gadow's idea that "subjectivity exists at the surface of the body" (p. 129), in this way touch is important in caring.

In caring, the notion of relationship of the body and the self varies from a view of the unity of the body and self (Jonas and Buber), to a united trinity in which the spirit is primary (Watson). Noddings and Gadow speak of caring as embodiment, whereas Audubon and Mayeroff view the body and self dualistically; the self is disembodied.

Relationship of Caring to Time and Space

Assumptions about time and space are critical to caring and vary from atomistic notions of time and space to postpositivist notions of multidimensional space–time. In Mayerhoff's model of caring, space is absolute, and time is directional and linear, emphasizing a present and future orientation. For the one caring, the act enables a sense of belonging and stability in the present. Because of the consideration for growth of the cared for, the future is dominant; relationship exists for the future outcome of self–actualization (Mayerhoff, 1971).

The future is also the dominant direction of life in Jonas' work, for the anticipation of imminent future is necessary for self–continuation. Time is directional and linear, and the present evolves from the past and into the future in the process of continuity. Jonas writes,

> As the here expands into the there, so the now expands into the future. [1966, p. 86]

As in Whitehead's (1967) process organism, Jonas also presents a reality in which the past becomes the future without concretion. For Jonas, space is the extension of the organism from felt selfhood into relatedness with the other in space.

Gadow discusses time and space as multidimensional, continual patterns of experience. During illness, a "limbo of the endless present" (1986, p. 3) may exist, and health professionals often attempt to change patients' orientation to time from the present to the future. However, future recovery is not always possible, and Gadow discusses a third type of time, ritual. Ritual time involves an altered view of the body, whereby one is,

> . . . neither master nor mastered by disability, but lives accommodatingly with it . . . [involving] time as the texture of experience, with patterns overlapping, interwoven, leading in all directions and through all dimensions, like movements in a dance [1986, pp. 4–5].

New patterns are created which acquire the status of ritual, or a

> . . . specially fashioned and personally meaningful pattern of experience, designed around the body's particular strengths and frailties [p. 5].

In a caring relationship, the one caring recognizes and assists the others' unique development of new relations with temporality, relations which incorporate the body's altered demands.

Buber's dialogue is accomplished outside traditionally understood boundaries of space and time, although dialogue evidences itself as factual and firmly grounded in the concrete human world.

> With all deference to the world continuum of space and time I know as a living truth only concrete world reality which is constantly, in every moment, reached out to me. I can separate

it into its component parts, I can compare them and distribute them into groups of similar phenomena, I can derive them from earlier and reduce them to simpler phenomena; and when I have done all this I have not touched my concrete world reality. Inseparable, incomparable, irreducible, now, happening once only, it gazes upon me with a horrifying look. [1965, p. 17]

The ability to be present in the moment of dialogue is essential to Buber; dialogue incorporates past, present, and future into a boundaryless space–time, manifest in the concrete world.

Time for Audubon is linear, characterized by a distinct separation of the past, present, and future. The past informs Audubon of values; the present is not important. The greatest good is oriented around the anticipated future. As described by Griffin (1978), the preservation of the species for future admiration takes priority over the present lived body of the eagle. The relationship of the future to the present is that of a predator to its prey.

Caring exists outside of linear time for Noddings (1984). Time is suspended, nondeliberational, experienced in the infinite present.

The caring approach described by Watson does not involve linear time, but exists in an infinite now (1988). Caring is multidimensional in Watson's model, for a caring occasion can consist of an encounter which transcends time and space. Space is nonabsolute in Watson's model, for human consciousness is spatially and temporally extended.

In the caring approaches described, assumptions about time and space involve very different ontologies that speak to time as an ontological framework and as phenomenological experience. These caring approaches reveal assumptions about time that range from absolute space and time which frames an objective reality, to multidimensional, continually changing patterns of experience.

Outcome of Caring

Finally, approaches to caring can be differentiated by whether caring is a means to an end, or an end in itself. When outcome is primary, the nature of the relationship is directed toward that goal, whatever it may be; caring becomes an instrument. When caring exists unrelated to outcome, the value is the relationship itself.

Caring is portrayed by some writers as an instrument to promote a separate good. For Mayeroff (1971), caring leads to growth primarily for the one cared for, although the one caring grows by enhanced self–knowledge and the ability to forego the need for surety about the world. In Watson's approach, caring potentiates self–healing (1985, 1988). In the example of Audubon, caring is a means to understand and preserve a perception of the natural state. For Jonas (1966), caring leads to continuation of the life process within the freedom to choose exercised by the organism.

In contrast, Gadow, Noddings, and Buber describe caring as an end in itself. Gadow sees caring as independent of outcome and characterizes a caring relationship as "engagement with no purpose" (personal communication, 1989). Noddings views caring as a primary value unto itself, in which the relationship is valued over outcome (1984). Buber describes dialogue as a relationship in which life is experienced fully; the outcome of the lived human dialogue is unimportant (1965).

SUMMARY

The caring approaches of Noddings, Watson, Buber, Jonas, Gadow, Mayerhoff, and Audubon offer a range of conceptualizations of caring found in nursing, philosophy, and literature. Assumptions about what gives rise to care, the relationship of the self and the other, the relationship of caring and the body, and the relationship of caring to time and to outcome are divergent in these approaches. It is the thesis here that when the notion of caring is invoked, the description of caring and its underlying assumptions need to be made explicit.

There is no one model of caring, and there is no one right model of caring. We, the authors, do not advocate that the reader choose among the models presented here. Instead, the reader is encouraged to examine personal meanings of caring, and to become aware of basic assumptions found in all approaches to caring. It is with this conceptual clarity that caring can be understood in its many forms of expression.

REFERENCES

Buber, M. (1965). *Between man and man*. New York: Macmillan.

Gadow, S. (1980a). Existential advocacy: Philosophical foundation of nursing. In S. Spicker and S. Gadow, *Nursing images and ideals*. New York: Springer.

Gadow, S. (1980b). Body and self: A dialectic. *The Journal of Medicine and Philosophy, 5*(3), 172–184.

Gadow, S. (1984). Touch and technology: Two paradigms of patient care. *Journal of Religion and Health, 23*(1), 63–69.

Gadow, S. (1986). Time and the body in geriatric rehabilitation. *Topics in Geriatric Rehabilitation, 1*(2), 1–7.

Gadow, S. (1988). Covenant without cure: Letting go and holding on in chronic illness. In J. Watson and M. Ray, *The ethics of care, and the ethics of cure: Synthesis in Chronicity.* New York: National League for Nursing.

Gadow, S. (1989). Clinical subjectivity: Advocacy with silent patients. *Nursing Clinics of North America, 24*(2), 535–541.

Griffin, S. (1978). *Woman and nature: The roaring inside her.* New York: Harper & Row.

Jonas, H. (1966). *The phenomenon of life: Toward a philosophical biology.* New York: Dell Publishing.

Mayeroff, M. (1971). *On caring.* New York: Harper & Row.

Noddings, N. (1984). *Caring: A feminine approach to ethics and moral education.* Berkeley: University of California Press.

Sarter, B. (1988). Philosophical sources of nursing theory. *Nursing Science Quartery, 1*(2), 52–59.

Vitz, P. (1990). The use of stories in moral development: New psychological reasons for an old education method. *American Psychologist, 45*(6), 709–720.

Watson, J. (1985). *Nursing: Human science and human care.* Norwalk, CT: Appleton-Century-Crofts.

Watson, J. (1988). New dimensions of human caring theory. *Nursing Science Quarterly, 1*(4), 175–181.

Watson, J. (1989). Human caring and suffering: A subjective model for health sciences. In R. Taylor and J. Watson, *They shall not hurt: Human suffering and human caring.* Boulder, CO: Associated Press.

Webster, G. (1990). Nursing and the philosophy of science. In J. McCloskey and G. Grace, *Current issues in nursing* (3rd ed.). St. Louis: C.V. Mosby.

Whitehead, A. (1967). *Science and the modern world.* Boston: Free Press.

2

Dialogical Care and Nursing Practice

Anne H. Bishop and John R. Scudder, Jr.

Any adequate treatment of nursing must concern practice, care, and the nurse–patient relationship. Nursing has long been defined as a caring practice, but is the nurse–patient relationship to be defined by traditional nursing practice or a general interpretation of personal relationships? Cooper (1988) contends that the nurse–patient relationship can be understood by subsuming it under a more general understanding of covenant relationships. She charges that we neglect the primacy of the nurse–patient relationship in contending that the in-between stance is an essential one in nursing, since it involves relationships to physicians and institutional bureaucrats, as well as patients. Fry (1989), on the other hand, contends that the relationship between nurse and patient should be one of caring. She charges that both Cooper and we (the authors) inappropriately draw our conception of the nurse–patient relationship from interpretations of the physician-patient relationship. In this article, we will consider the critiques of both Cooper and Fry to further clarify the integral relationship of practice, care, and the nurse–patient relationship.

PRACTICE, CARING, AND THE IN-BETWEEN

Cooper (1988) argues that we (Bishop & Scudder, 1987) make the in-between stance of the nurse more primary than the nurse–patient relationship. In the article she cites, we were merely making the point that the

17

in-between is a fundamental stance of nursing, especially in institutional settings, and that autonomy in nursing practice is overstressed. The in-between stance, we contended, is necessary for nurses to give day-to-day nursing care. Such care requires working with physicians, hospital bureaucrats, and patients. We have given this stance extensive treatment in our book, *The Practical, Moral and Personal Sense of Nursing* (Bishop & Scudder, 1990), and therefore will not treat it here. The book develops the thesis that the in-between is one fundamental structure of nursing practice, the other being the nurse's exercise of legitimate authority, in which the focus is primarily on the nurse–patient relationship. We believe that Benner (1984) has adequately described the nurse's legitimate authority as the competencies and excellences of nursing practice. Thus, for us, the primary structures of nursing practice consist of the legitimate authority and the in-between stance of the nurse. Cooper is right, however, in suggesting that we need to show how the in-between stance relates to the nurse–patient relationship. We have, in fact, also treated the nurse–patient relationship extensively in our recent book, and the book's stress on dialogue as well as practice indicates that we believe that the nurse–patient relationship is focal in nursing care. Rather than further developing that thesis, we will now follow Cooper's suggestion by showing how the in-between is related to the nurse–patient relationship.

We believe that the in-between, rather than being a substitute for the nurse–patient relationship, presupposes a caring relationship between nurse and patient which extends beyond that relationship to what Gilligan (1982) calls a "web of connection." She defines a caring relationship as "an activity of relationship, of seeing and responding to need, taking care of the world by sustaining the web of connection so that no one is left alone" (p. 62). This feminine image of relationships as a web contrasts sharply with the image of a hierarchy. In the image of a hierarchy, the autonomous person is at the top because he or she is in control and is truly self-directing. Viewed from the image of the web, however, the top of the hierarchy is peripheral and the center is focal. Those who follow the image of the hierarchy desire to be "alone at the top," while those who follow the image of the web "wish to be at the center of the connection" (p. 62). When relationships are "cast in the image of hierarchy," they "appear inherently unstable and morally problematic," but when transposed into an image of web, relationships change from "an order of inequality into a structure of interconnection" (p. 62). The in-between stance of the nurse is rooted in the web of connectedness. In this sense, nurses function to maintain the connection between patient, hospital, and physician. Such connection is not just feminine but is required for adequate or excellent everyday care. A nurse does not take an in-between stance in order to conform to traditional precedent, but in order to give everyday care. She or he must be able to work with the physician, patient, and hospital bureaucrat and be able to bring them together in a connected way that will foster good health care.

DIALOGUE VERSUS COVENANT

Gilligan (1982) also helps us understand why dialogue is more adequate for understanding the nurse–patient relationship than the covenant for which Cooper argues (1988). A web of relationships is inclusive rather than exclusive. A covenant is an agreement that both includes and excludes. For example, in the Judeo–Christian tradition, the people of the Covenant saw themselves as connected to each other through covenant but separate from those who were not of the Covenant. In contrast, according to Gilligan, a caring relationship involves "seeing and responding to needs" (p. 62) in a web of connection. This caring relationship draws on the feminists' position of "seeing life as dependent on connection, as sustained by activities of care, as based on a bond of attachment rather than a contract of agreement" (p. 57). In addition, the feminine ethic is all–inclusive rather than exclusive in that it is "an ethic of responsibility that stems from an awareness of interconnection: 'the stranger is still another person belonging to that group, people you are connected to by virtue of being another person'" (p. 57). As with Buber (1923/1970), for Gilligan "responsibility signifies response" (p. 38) to others rather than a designation of those in whose behalf you will act. Thus, responsibility "denotes an act of care" (p. 38). In contrast to covenant, which is a relationship based on an agreement, dialogue is purely relational and personal.

We believe that Cooper has shown that the nurse–patient relationship can productively be explored as a covenant one. However, we will show that the nurse–patient relationship can be better articulated as dialogue than as covenant by testing the adequacy of each against actual nursing experience. Cooper obviously believes that a covenant relationship brings the moral and the personal aspects of nursing care together. She states that "a responsiveness to the presence of the patient and his or her needs, an acknowledgement of the indebtedness by the caregiver to the patient for benefit of practice and engagement, and a recognition of the mutuality and reciprocity that distinguishes the relationship indicate a willingness by nurses to enter a covenantal relationship" (p. 57). Covenant implies an agreement entered into by both parties. Cooper stresses the nurse's side of that agreement to the neglect of the patient's side. For Cooper, the patient's involvement seems to be merely to trust the nurse.

In contrast to a covenant relationship in which the patient's trust of the nurse is stressed, a dialogical relationship requires mutual trust in which both nurse and patient share their understanding. The nurse knows more about the nursing care needed than the patient. The patient knows more about what he or she wants to be or become than the nurse. The nurse knows more about how the patient's present illness probably will affect the desired way of being. In addition, the nurse knows better what the patient is *likely* to experience due to the illness and the nature of the care. However, during the actual nursing care, only the patient is an expert concerning what he or she actually does experience. Thus, dialogue is required to give and to receive excellent nursing care which fosters the well–being of the patient.

If a nurse–patient relationship is a covenant one, then, in addition to requiring trust, it would require the patient as well as the nurse to agree to foster the patient's well–being. In nursing practice, however, patients often neither trust the nurse nor work cooperatively to foster their own well–being. In our study of fulfillment in nursing (Bishop & Scudder, 1987), we found that most nurses felt least fulfilled from relationships with uncooperative and unappreciative patients. In addition, Heron's (1987) autobiographical description of her nursing experience abounds with such patients. Yet she, like any competent nurse, continued to give those patients excellent nursing care in the absence of any covenant agreement from their side. In so doing, she fulfilled the moral imperative inherent in nursing practice even when the relationship between nurse and patient was one–sided. Can a relationship be called a covenant one when only one of the parties has agreed to foster the end which is supposed to be the basis for the covenant?

Even when a covenant is based on agreement by both parties, it can be morally questionable. For example, consider a patient who is a heavy user of drugs and is cared for by a nurse who also uses drugs. They both agree that the patient's stay in the hospital would be more pleasant if the patient were well–supplied with drugs. Since both are hedonists and therefore believe that pleasure is the highest good, their covenant is a moral one from their perspective. What would be morally wrong with this covenant? It obviously neglects the fact that the content of what the nurse agrees to offer a patient in any relationship, covenant or other, is directed and regulated, in the main, by the practice of nursing. Further, a nurse agrees to work within the responsibilities and control of the practice upon entering the profession of nursing when he or she professes to be a nurse. This profession to care applies to patients who will not cooperate in fostering their well–being, as well as to those who will. Thus, the nature of nursing practice indicates that a covenant relationship cannot adequately encompass all nurse–patient relationships.

The fact that the idea of covenant cannot encompass all nurse–patient relationships does not mean, however, that it cannot be productively used to articulate this relationship. Zaner shows us how it can be so used. He reports the following response of a patient suffering from a heart attack. "We were like a team and this was a campaign. I was a member of the team. I was the cause of all the trouble but I was also a member of the team. We were holding hands" (Zaner, 1985, p. 88). When the cardiac patient said "I was a member of the team," Zaner contends that "patient and nurse and physician had recovered themselves in their communality" (p. 88). He further maintains that in "this respect, it seems most appropriate and accurate to understand the patient-physician and patient-nurse relationship as a *covenant* and not as a contract" (pp. 101–102). Note that this covenant is based on *all* working together to foster the well–being of the one designated as a patient. Further, note that the basis for this covenant is participation in a community of nurse, physician, and patient—not merely the nurse–patient relationship in isolation from the health care team. Although Zaner does not mention it, this team relationship also implies a covenant relationship between physician and nurse, Thus, it seems to us that if covenant is used to articulate the nurse–patient relationship, it also should include the relationship of physician to patient and nurse to physician and not exclude them as Cooper seems to do in her criticism of our team approach. It is also significant that Zaner in his latest book (1988) treats health care ethics as clinical ethics, implying that although the nurse–patient relationship can be productively articulated as a covenant, nursing ethics should be rooted in nursing practice.

In Zaner's example, the covenant relationship requires that the patient share in the covenant to foster his or her well–being. Unlike a covenant relationship, a dialogical relationship does not assume a common purpose between both parties. Each person meets the other as they are present to each other as persons. They mutually respond to each other's presence in a relationship which recognizes the legitimate right of the other to be. This relationship has been described by Buber (1923/1970) as an I–Thou relationship, in contrast to an I–It relationship in which the person is treated as a thing to be categorized and used. I–Thou relationships are cultivated and developed through dialogue. When a nurse encounters an uncooperative patient in dialogue, he or she meets the patient as he or she is—an uncooperative patient. The nurse does not wait until the patient is cooperative enough to form a covenant relationship with the nurse to give nursing care. Of course, an uncooperative patient can learn to cooperate with the nurse through dialogue so that it is possible to form a covenant relationship—but then isn't this covenant agreement made possible by and incorporated in a dialogical relationship?

In addition to the problem of uncooperative patients, the very nature of the nurse–patient relationship itself poses problems for a covenant relationship. First, the nurse–patient relationship is fluid. Relations are always changing due to the fluctuation in the patient's well–being and to the encounters between patient and nurse. Thanks to Hildegard Peplau, we are well aware that nurse–patient relationships always have a period of introduction or orientation where the trust relationship is built between nurse and patient. This seems to us to be better described as a dialogical relationship in which trust grows out of the relationship rather than out of a covenant. Second, not only is the relationship between a particular nurse and patient fluctuating, the patient's care (in the hospital at least) usually is given by several nurses who are assigned to the patient. How could there be continuity in nursing care if each nurse made a particular covenant with the patient? However, in actual practice, when a particular nurse resumes her relationship with a particular patient, their dialogue and development of trust continues within a common nursing practice shared with other nurses who are also caring for the patient.

The dialogue they continue is primarily concerned with how to foster the patient's well–being. This does not, however, imply that their dialogue is confined to this subject. All good nurses joke with, chat with, and seriously discuss non–nursing matters of interest to the patient when it is appropriate. Neither the nurse nor the patient, however, have chosen each other as friends with whom to engage in personal conversation. The nurse–patient relationship is established by the patient's need for care and the nurse's special competency as a giver of that care. Thus, whether this relationship is called a dialogical one or a covenant one, it is a special one directed at a particular end, and that end is a moral one, fostering the well–being of the patient.

Cooper could rightly contend that a covenant relationship is more focused on achieving that moral end than a dialogical one. She could also justly request that we put dialogue to the same test we put covenant, namely, can it adequately articulate nursing as practiced? Actually we do not believe that Buber's conception of dialogue could pass such a test because, in his interpretation, dialogue has no end beyond itself.

DIALOGICAL CARE

Dialogical care is very different from Buber's dialogue in that it focuses on fostering the well–being of one of the partners. The relationship in dialogical care is not one that has no end beyond itself, as in Buber's treatment of dialogue, but is constituted, in part, by the end of fostering the well–being of one of the partners. For this reason, its structure can be better articulated as triadic dialogue (Scudder & Mickunas, 1985) in contrast to the dyadic dialogue of Buber. Dyadic dialogue cannot adequately articulate nursing practice because it has no end beyond itself; however, triadic dialogue can because it articulates a dialogue as constituted not only by the partners but by the end sought. Since we have treated triadic dialogue extensively elsewhere (Bishop & Scudder, 1990), we will focus our discussion on dialogical care, which is the central concern of this article. Care becomes dialogical when dialogue contributes to both nurse and patient an understanding of how the nursing care given this patient will foster his or her well–being. Therefore, this understanding could not come solely from personal dialogue between the partners but must be informed, ordered, and supported by a tradition of excellent nursing practice.

Dialogical care, sustained by excellent practice, is exemplified in the care given by Elizabeth Ashton to one of her patients (Ashton, 1988, p. 21). Ashton described a patient named Ben, who had a paralyzing spine injury at C3 and C4, as a very demanding patient who expected immediate attention. "His demanding ways made most of us want to avoid him, even if we felt guilty about it later" (p. 21). At the end of a particularly busy shift which was very understaffed, Ben's light was on once again. With many loose ends still to tie up before she could leave the hospital, Ashton went to answer Ben's light. He was somewhat frantic because of a mucus plug that needed to be suctioned. As Ashton suctioned Ben, wiped his eyes, and gave him a drink, she avoided his eyes in order that her impatience would not be obvious to him. Ashton proceeded to the nurses' station, but on her way down the hall, she could see Ben's light was on again, and she returned to his room. Ben motioned for his mouthpiece which he used to spell out words on an alphabet board. Usually Ben's use of the mouthpiece was frustrating to both Ben and the nurses because Ben was a poor speller and the process was time–consuming. Over Ashton's protests that she had to go, Ben insisted on spelling the words, "Thank you." Ashton relates, "I continued looking at him, surprised and delighted, but my eyes suddenly welled with tears. Personal contact—that was all he'd wanted" (p. 21).

In the above case, it is obvious that what the patient wanted was to communicate with his nurse in a way that well people take for granted. When someone does something for us, we normally respond by saying thank you. Due to his incapacity Ben was unable to do this without great effort. He appreciated the good care of his nurse and simply wanted to thank her. Note that her care was not exceptional, except that it was given on a busy night. One has the feeling that Ben tended to abuse the availability of his nurses who, knowing that patients like Ben could die from suffocation, feel compelled to answer the light. By responding to Ben, Ashton was doing the morally good work of any nurse who gives competent care to her patient. Although her return to his room was done begrudgingly, it certainly indicated that she was willing to give extra care to her patient in a difficult situation. However, perhaps her most significant moral activity was accepting his thanks by meeting his eyes and showing her gratitude for his appreciation.

THE MEANING OF CARE: PELLEGRINO

We can grasp the meaning of some aspects of caring in Ashton's case by using Pellegrino's interpretation of caring. Pellegrino describes four types of caring, all of which are integrally related in health care: (1) compassion for others, (2) doing for others what they can't do for themselves, (3) using professional understanding and skill for the patient's good, and (4) taking care in the sense of being diligent and skillful in actual practice (Pellegrino, 1985, pp. 11–12). Pellegrino's four senses of care can articulate the care given by Ashton. She cared for the patient by doing many things he could not adequately do for himself, such as wiping his tears and giving him a drink of water. She used her nursing skill in treatments, such as suctioning, and her understanding of the patient's condition to foster his well–being. She certainly was diligent in her care as shown by her availability, especially by responding to Ben's light at the end of a particularly busy, understaffed shift. Her compassion, while evident in many ways, was most evident in her meeting him face-to-face and accepting his gratitude appreciatively and graciously. In so doing, her dialogical care is not that of a caring physician but that of a nurse who engages in a practice of caring for an ill person, unable to care for himself, in a way that affirms both their common humanity and the worth of their personal way of being with each other.

In light of how Pellegrino's approach to care can articulate nursing in the above case, it may seem strange that Fry (1989) rejects Pellegrino's interpretation of care as inadequate for understanding the nurse–patient relationship. She contends that nurses should be wary of interpretations of caring that are based on a physician–patient relationship. Presumably, it was our previous use of Pellegrino's view of caring that led Fry to cite us, along with Cooper, as founding the nurse–patient relationship on a physician–patient model (Fry, 1989). Actually, Pellegrino claims that his treatment of caring in the work cited by Fry (Pellegrino, 1985) was intended for nursing as well as medicine. Perhaps Fry misinterpreted it as applying only to the physician–patient relationship, because it could be misconstrued to advocate a beneficent paternalistic care which occurs when compassion is not dialogical.

We will use Pellegrino's four senses of care in a way that we believe he never meant them to be used in order to show what happens when compassion is not dialogical. A nurse, out of compassion, diligently does for his or her patients what the patients cannot do for themselves, uses his or her nursing skill and knowledge for their good, and practices well the craft of nursing, but in his or her relation to them ignores the patients, their wishes, their values—in short their very being. In addition, the nurse's care for the patients is such that it fosters dependency rather than independence. In this case, care boils down to using skill and knowledge for the good of the other, in a way that fosters dependence, without being present to the other as a person.

In contrast to the above example of beneficent paternalistic care, in dialogical caring, compassion evokes *personal* availability when needed, as needed, and fosters self–direction. A patient is dependent on a nurse because the nurse has appropriated a practice that makes it possible for her or him to care in special ways. Fry is right in contending that Pellegrino's approach to caring is not adequate for the many forms of care involved in nursing. This is most evident in his treatment of the second aspect of caring which involves doing for others what they cannot do for themselves. This traditional function of nursing, as Pellegrino points out, has been turned over mainly to nursing assistants. If this aspect of concrete care is not being done by nurses, what remains for nurses other than to assist physicians in medical interventions? Nursing care has traditionally consisted of much more than doing for others that which they cannot do for themselves. First, and foremost, nurses have followed the primary direction set for them by Nightingale (1859/1946), who claimed that the primary purpose of nursing was to "put the patient in the best condition for nature to act upon him" (p. 75) to foster the healing process. This function of nursing has, in fact, become more important since World War II because of the injury done to the body by contemporary interventions, such as complex surgery and chemotherapy. Second, nurses have traditionally comforted patients by care which ranges from easing pain to fostering hope. Third, recently nurses have greatly expanded their traditional practice from taking care of patients to helping patients learn to care for themselves. Fourth, nursing primarily concerns a relationship between persons which is called a caring relationship. Any adequate treatment of nursing care must describe that relationship. Thus, we agree with Fry in her contention that an interpretation of care is needed that is specifically more appropriate to nursing care than Pellegrino's.

THE MEANING OF CARE: NODDINGS

We agree with Fry that Noddings' interpretation of caring is especially appropriate for articulating nursing care. In this brief article we do not have time to adequately show how appropriate Noddings' theory of care is for articulating nursing care. We have, however, demonstrated this in an extensive treatment of Noddings in a recently completed book–length manuscript. In this article we will merely indicate how Noddings can help us articulate nursing care. We will then show that for Noddings' theory to make its potential contribution to articulating nursing practice, it must be included in a context of caring practice.

Noddings' theory of caring is especially appropriate for this article on dialogical caring because Noddings draws heavily on Buber's conception of dialogue. Noddings' caring ethic stresses both mutuality and recognizing and fostering self–direction by the one cared for. Her caring ethic begins with natural caring which she defines as "that relationship in which we respond as one-caring out of love or natural inclination" (Noddings, 1984, p. 5). Caring appears when "we accept the natural impulse to act on behalf of the present other" (p. 83). The essential elements in the caring relationship are "*engrossment* and *motivational displacement* on the part of the one–caring and a form of *responsiveness* or *reciprocity* on the part of the cared–for" (p. 150).

Noddings articulates one–caring as first engrossment with another and then as motivational shift toward the other. When I am engrossed she says, "I receive the other into myself, and I see and feel with the other" (p. 30). I receive what the other shares without evaluation or assessment. When I care for others, my caring includes their experience of the world in Buber's sense of inclusion. How we care grows out of the "constellation of conditions that is viewed through both the eyes of the one–caring and the eyes of the cared–for" (p. 13).

Caring involves more than sharing in the patient's experience, however. Noddings contends that there also must be an actual motivational shift in which there is "displacement of interest from my own reality to the reality of the other." Then "we see the other's reality as a possibility for us" and "must act to eliminate the intolerable, to reduce the pain, to fulfill the need, to actualize the dream" (Noddings, 1984, p. 14). Eliminating the intolerable, lessening the pain, meeting the need, and actualizing the dream requires us "to act as one–caring . . . with special regard for the particular person in a concrete situation. . . . The one–caring desires the well–being of the cared–for and acts to promote that well–being" (p. 24).

A caring relationship not only involves the one–caring but also the response of the one cared–for. This response has been succinctly stated by Noddings. "The cared–for contributes to the caring relation . . . by receiving the efforts of one–caring, and this receiving may be accomplished by a disclosure of his own subjective experience in direct response to the one–caring or by a happy and vigorous pursuit of his own projects" (pp. 150–151).

Noddings interprets caring as a mutual relationship between the one cared–for and the one–caring initiated by the sentiment of natural caring. What if that sentiment is not present in the one–caring? If natural caring is not possible, then, Noddings contends, one should care out of the desire to be virtuous. She maintains that morality is an "active virtue" which requires two feelings. The first "is the sentiment of natural caring." The second sentiment is a feeling of imperative which grows out of a kind of remembrance of natural caring which "sweeps over us as a feeling—as an 'I must'—in response to the plight of the other and our conflicting desire to serve our own interests" (Noddings, 1984, pp. 79–80). When faced with such an inner conflict, "I have a picture of those moments in which I was cared for and in which I have cared, and I may reach toward this memory and guide my conduct by it if I wish to do so." Thus, an ethic of caring "strives to maintain the caring attitude and is dependent upon, and not superior to, natural caring" (p. 80). The sentiments of natural caring and of concern with being our best self are both sources of moral behavior. In the first case I act because I want to, in the latter because I ought to.

We can test the appropriateness of Noddings' theory of caring for articulating nursing by using it to interpret the case of Ashton and Ben. Ashton initially cared for Ben out of the ethical sense of "ought to." When Noddings' ethic of virtue is translated into nursing practice it means, "I care for my patient because I want to be a good nurse." Obviously the care Ashton initially gives to Ben is motivated by the desire to be a good nurse. Her conscientiousness as a nurse is emphasized by the difficult conditions under which she gives care. Her engrossment is the engrossment appropriate for ethical caring. She remembers the difficulties other patients have had when they were not suctioned promptly and knows first hand the danger involved. The remembrance of this past experience reminds her that she ought to give Ben prompt and excellent care. Ben responds to this excellent care "by disclosure of his own subjective experience" in writing with great difficulty, "Thank you."

The relationship between Ben and Ashton is transformed from ethical caring into one of natural caring by his appreciative thank you. Most people thank those who care for them, but Ben's difficulty in saying thank you accents his deep appreciation and may well indicate his recognition that his nurse needed appreciation at this particular time. By meeting his eyes, Ashton accepts his gratitude in a way that conveys to him that he is a person for whom she cares. This personal response is one of natural caring and it holds the promise of natural caring in the future. Significantly, Ben's appreciative response changed Ashton's caring from "ought to" to "want to," or from ethical caring to natural caring. Through dialogical caring, Ben became a person for whom Ashton cared in the way that, according to Zaner, all patients want, namely, that "those who care for them really care" (Zaner, 1985, p. 98).

THE PRACTICE OF CARING

Since Noddings' theory of caring brings into focus aspects of nursing care obscured by Pellegrino's approach to caring, it would appear that Fry is right in contending that Noddings' approach to caring is more appropriate for nursing than Pellegrino's. However, Pellegrino's interpretation of the relationship of caring to ethics is the same as Noddings' which, according to Fry, asserts that caring is "not an outcome of ethical behavior . . . but itself constitutes ethics" (Fry, 1989, p. 16). For Pellegrino, unlike Noddings, an ethic of practice, such as health care ethics, is not the outcome of general caring but itself constitutes caring. In contrast, Noddings' view of caring obscures the relationship of caring to practice that Pellegrino brings into clear focus.

Noddings' failure to recognize that practice can disclose the meaning of caring is evident in her treatment of caring in her own field of education. She regards education as a function rather than a practice. To her, students learn caring by practicing, thus practice for her becomes a form of learning by doing. In contrast, Pellegrino's conception of caring includes the essential aspects of medical practice. He recognizes that the knowledge, skill, and craftsmanship of medicine were developed to care for patients' well–being. Although the way in which he treats that knowledge, skill, and craftsmanship is more appropriate for articulating medicine than nursing, nursing scholars would do well to emulate his treatment of medical care by treating nursing caring in a way that discloses the essential ingredients of nursing practice as ways of caring. Noddings can make a significant contribution to this endeavor through her dialogical interpretation of caring, but it needs to be incorporated into a context of caring in nursing practice. Interpreting nursing in this way requires more extensive treatment than a brief article. We have, in fact, attempted to interpret nursing as the practice of care in a recently completed book–length manuscript.

CONCLUSION

We have examined the meaning of practice, care, and the nurse–patient relationshp through dialogical interpretation of the thought of Cooper, Fry, and Pellegrino. In treating nursing as a covenant relationship, Cooper rightly focuses nursing on the nurse–patient relationship in a way that does justice to the end of the relationship, namely fostering the well–being of the patient. However, a covenant relationship fails to adequately articulate nursing as it is practiced. A dialogical relationship can articulate the nurse–patient relationship in practice if it includes the patient's well–being as the focus of the dialogue. Dialogical care focuses the nurse–patient relationship on fostering the well–being of the patient. Dialogical care does, however, require an interpretation of caring appropriate for nursing care. We, like Fry, find Noddings' theory of care to be an appropriate one. However, we contend that for Noddings' theory to make its potential contribution to articulating nursing, it must include interpretation of nursing practice as ways of caring, as Pellegrino has done in his treatment of medical care. After interpretive response to Cooper, Fry, and Pellegrino, we are now prepared to answer the question raised in the opening paragraph: "Is the nurse–patient relationship to be defined by traditional nursing practice or a general interpretation of personal relationships?" We contend that it needs to be articulated in both ways, but that this articulation must make evident the integral relationship between nursing practice and dialogical care.

REFERENCES

Ashton, E. (1988). A simple message. *Nursing Life, 8*(2), 21.

Benner, P. (1984). *From novice to expert: Excellence and power in clinical nursing practice.* Menlo Park, CA: Addison-Wesley.

Bishop, A. H., & Scudder, J. R., Jr. (1987). Nursing ethics in an age of controversy. *Advances in Nursing Science, 9*(3), 34–43.

Bishop, A. H., & Scudder, J. R., Jr. (1990). *The practical, moral and personal sense of nursing: A phenomenological philosophy of practice.* Albany, NY: State University of New York Press.

Buber, M. (1970). *I and thou* (W. Kaufmann, Trans.). New York, Charles Scribner's Sons. (Original work published in 1923).

Cooper, C. C. (1988). Covenant relationships: Grounding for the nursing ethic. *Advances in Nursing Science, 10*(4), 48–59.

Fry, S. (1989). Toward a theory of nursing ethics. *Advances in Nursing Science, 11*(4), 9–22.

Gilligan, C. (1982). *In a different voice.* Cambridge, MA: Harvard University Press.

Heron, E. (1987). *Intensive care: The story of a nurse.* New York: Ivy Books.

Nightingale, F. (1946). *Notes on nursing.* Philadelphia: Edward Stern. (Original work published in 1859).

Noddings, N. (1984). *Caring: A femine approach to ethics and moral education.* Berkeley: University of California Press.

Pellegrino, E. D. (1985). The caring ethic: The relation of physician to patient. In A. H. Bishop & J. R. Scudder, Jr. (Eds.), *Caring, curing, coping: Nurse, physician, patient relationships* (pp. 8–30). University, AL: University of Alabama Press.

Peplau, H. (1952). *Interpersonal relations in nursing.* New York: G. P. Putnam's.

Scudder, J. R., Jr., & Mickunas, A. (1985). *Meaning, dialogue, and encultura-tion: Phenomenological philosophy of education*. Washington, DC: Center for Advanced Research in Phenomenology and University Press of America.

Zaner, R. M. (1985). "How the hell did I get here?" Reflections on being a patient. In A. H. Bishop & J. R. Scudder, Jr. (Eds.), *Caring, curing, coping: Nurse, physician, patient relationships* (pp. 80–105). University, AL: University of Alabama Press.

Zaner, R. M. (1988). *Ethics and the clinical encounter*. Englewood Cliffs, NJ: Prentice-Hall.

3

The Moral Foundation of Nursing: Yarling and McElmurry and Their Critics

Gary J. Foulk and M. Jan Keffer

"The Moral Foundation of Nursing," by Yarling and McElmurry (1986) has become well–known and much discussed since it appeared in *Advances in Nursing Science*. Unfortunately, given the valuable theses and proposals of this article, the discussion of it has to some extent been characterized by misunderstanding, conceptual confusion, and unjustified criticism. The purpose of this article is to contribute to and promote this discussion, using the method of philosophical analysis enlightened and guided by professional nursing knowledge, with a view to a critical clarification and examination of distinctions and points in accordance with the rules of logic and correct thinking. Since a goal of this method is to discover inconsistency, lack of precision or clarity, falsehood, and weak arguments, its employment and results may appear harsh or even pugnacious to those unfamiliar with or not fond of traditional philosophical argumentation and debate. However, we (the authors) feel that it is important for work in nursing ethics to take advantage of philosophical methods and skills for doing ethical analysis and construction, just as it is important for such work to be informed by knowledge and experience in nursing. The philosopher's critical and candid style does not reflect disrespect for those criticized, but rather the belief that truth is most likely to be found by means of vivacious, direct, and even warm discussion and debate among those who are, regardless of position or approach, equally dedicated to its discovery. While it is false that Yarling and McElmurry *never*, and their critics *always*, err, the attention here will be primarily on the weaknesses of the latter, with a view toward the clarification and elaboration of distinctions and points which should enhance the quality and usefulness of the ongoing discussion.

An error on the part of Yarling and McElmurry (1986) themselves, one so basic that one suspects that it was only a slip of their fingers, not of their thinking, must first be noted, since it involves the concept of freedom, which is at the foundation of their views. They say that, "...the concept of freedom, as in 'not free to be moral,' is not a reference to transcendental freedom of the *will*, for freedom in this sense is a necessary condition of even being a moral agent and having moral problems. The reference is rather to freedom of *action* in the sense that acts are free from *unforced* choice" (1986, pp. 63–64).

It is clear from this that Yarling and McElmurry accept the famous rule that "I ought" implies "I can" in the sense that, if it is impossible for one to do or impossible for one to refrain from X, then it cannot be the case that one ought to do or refrain from X, or that one faces a moral problem with respect to doing or refraining from X. There are, of course, different senses of possibility, such as technical, empirical, and logical, and various positions in the debate between determinism and libertarianism and about the concept of a free will. However, surely Yarling and McElmurry are right that, in some basic sense, freedom to choose and act must be possessed by one who is a proper subject of moral evaluation because of those choices and actions, and in thinking that nurses who practice in hospitals *do* have this freedom.

Rather, they are concerned with the concept of freedom upon which a famous comedy routine by Jack Benny depended for its humor. Having been confronted by a robber who demanded, "Your money or your life," Benny remained silent for a considerable amount of time while he tried to decide which alternative to choose. Part of the reason the joke was so effective was that we do not think of ourselves as having a choice in such a situation. To be sure, we think we have, in this case, what Yarling and McElmurry (1986, pp. 63–64) call "transcendental freedom of the will": we think that it is possible, that we could choose to die rather than comply, but there is such strong compulsion or *force* behind the latter that, with respect to what Yarling and McElmurry call "freedom of action" we do *not* think we have a free choice, and we would describe our giving our money to the robber as something we were forced to do, not something we freely chose to do.

But if the two different senses of freedom indicated by Yarling and McElmurry have been correctly described, then they should not have characterized the freedom of choice as that in which acts are free from *unforced* choice, but rather that in which acts are free from *forced* choice. It is interesting here to recall the position of soft determinism about the nature of free actions, namely that they are not *uncaused*, but rather *un-*

forced; not the result of external or internal coercion or force. Again, and especially since they later speak of nurses not being free from *forced* choice (Yarling & McElmurry, 1986) and themselves use the example of "Your money or your life" to illustrate a forced choice (1986, p. 70), this was surely just a mechanical slip by Yarling and McElmurry.

Criticisms By Bishop and Scudder

Turning now to the criticism of Yarling and McElmurry by others, Bishop and Scudder (1987) offer a distinction between health care in the sense of aiming at *cure*, and health care in the sense or aiming at *care*, and suggest that the nursing autonomy advocated by Yarling and McElmurry is more at home within the former model while the latter generates a contrasting, "traditional" view of nursing (Bishop & Scudder, 1987, pp. 34–35). However, in addition to possible problems in distinguishing between caring and curing, the thesis of Yarling and McElmurry seems applicable to both, as their case studies and clinical examples show. Where cure *or* care is the goal, and the nurse is aware of improper procedures or medications which are not only unlikely to promote cure or care but are likely to cause positive harm, their call is for the autonomy that will enable the nurse to take the moral action without fear of punishment. Further, in the case where the physician ordered the nurse not to grant the wish of her terminal patient to know her prognosis (Bishop & Scudder, 1987), presumably the goal is clearly *care*, not *cure*, and yet this case is a fine illustration of the need seen by Yarling and McElmurry for nurses to be free to do what morality demands. There is thus no good reason for thinking that their thesis is more compatible with the curing than the caring model, or contrasts or is in opposition to the latter. Bishop and Scudder are mistaken in thinking it is unfortunate that they did not specify which model they had in mind.

One is further at a loss to see the justification of the claim by Bishop and Scudder (1987) that

> The position taken by Yarling and McElmurry tends to denigrate the moral contributions made by nurses in their everyday work and blinds them to moral actions and reforms that can be made within the legitimate authority that nurses now possess or can acquire without the drastic reform of health care needed to give them full autonomy. [p. 36]

Nowhere do Yarling and McElmurry (1986) even suggest anything which tends toward the denigration of the morality manifested in everyday nursing practice. Indeed, they are prepared to describe the action of nurses who have the courage to act on principle in the face of the danger of the sacrifice of their prudential interests, as illustrated in some of their case studies, as heroic. To call the action of nurses heroic is hardly to denigrate them, and to call for the reform needed to reduce the unacceptable conflict between the prudential and the moral interests of nurses is neither to denigrate those who have risen to moral heroism in such conflict, or to blind oneself to other possible reforms or other morally praiseworthy actions by nurses. As for remaining within the legitimate authority that nurses now possess, it is possible to distinguish between *authority* and *power* in such a way that one could well claim that nurses already have autonomy by legitimate authority, and thus are remaining within the area of their legitimate authority in insisting on its recognition. What they lack, according to this perspective, is the power to exercise their legitimate authority. In this context it is interesting to note the use by Yarling and McElmurry (1986) of this word when they claim that

> [e]ither nursing must acquire sufficient *power* within the hospital, relative to medicine and administration, to create a balance of *power* in the control of the practice, or it must terminate its employee status with the hospital, move outside the hospital [p. 72, emphasis added].

They also speak of the goal as "liberation" (Yarling & McElmurry, 1986, p. 72), a word which suggests being freed from oppressive *power*.

The claim that Yarling and McElmurry stress "conceptual moral issues to the neglect of the moral issues in everyday practice" (Bishop & Scudder, p. 36) suggests confusion on the part of Yarling and McElmurry's critics about their thesis and what issues are logically relevant to it. True, they do not discuss the praiseworthy actions of the night nurses, referred to by Bishop and Scudder, who do their best under adverse conditions, but they in no way imply by what they *do* or do *not* say that these nurses do not deserve moral praise. To neglect something is not just to not discuss it, but to be obligated by one's research and thesis to discuss it adequately, and fail to do so. Yarling and McElmurry do not claim that the *only* area in which moral principles make a demand on, and are obeyed by, nurses is that where there is a conflict between prudential and moral interests. The focus of their discussion on this area of conflict is appropriate and suggests no lack of respect for the morality of the night nurse. Further, they do not say that nurses are never free to be moral, only that nurses often lack this freedom. They do not say that nurses often lack this freedom in all situations and settings, but that they lack it in those situations where

> [t]hey are forced to choose between patient interest and their

own self–interest, between their commitment to the autonomy and well–being of the patient and the autonomy and well–being of their careers, between moral integrity and professional survival [Yarling & McElmurry, 1986, p. 65].

It should be noted, however, that these situations *do* occur in everyday practice, so in discussing them Yarling and McElmurry have not neglected the moral issues in everyday practice.

With respect to the criticism that conceptual moral issues have been overemphasized, it must be remembered that such issues are crucial. It is true that nursing practice as experienced by nurses, is what nursing ethics is about, but one can hardly begin to think responsibly about this practice without facing and resolving philosophical, ethical, and conceptual issues. For example, Bishop and Scudder say that "[s]ince nursing practice aims at the well–being of the patient, the first moral responsibility of any nurse is excellent practice" (Bishop & Scudder, 1987, p. 36). However, the concept of the "*well*–being" of the patient is an evaluative concept which requires conceptual analysis, and the same is true of the concepts of "moral responsibility" and "excellent practice." Thus, one cannot even understand this statement, let alone experience its everyday application, without subjecting it to the conceptual analysis of evaluative concepts. In contrast to the claim that Yarling and McElmurry have overemphasized conceptual issues, a criticism discussed later is that they have underemphasized conceptual issues.

Points similar to those already made reveal the weakness of the criticisms that Yarling and McElmurry have neglected the autonomy inherent in the nature of the nursing profession and that they have misdirected the major moral thrust of nursing (Bishop & Scudder, 1987). Bishop and Scudder believe that being a professional nurse involves knowledge, skill, and commitment to and compassion for the patient, and that therefore "most professional, moral autonomy grows from within rather than from reform of bureaucratic structure and rules that regulate professions" (1987, p. 37). However, their premise provides no support for their conclusion, since whether or not a nurse has the professional characteristics listed, and whether or not a nurse has the power or freedom to exercise these characteristics autonomously are two separate issues. While the characteristics may be said to grow from within, the restrictions on their autonomous exercise seem to come from without, from the very direction in which Yarling and McElmurry have pointed. Further, just as they have not neglected the night nurse, they have not neglected whatever autonomy nurses have in advocating their thesis that in certain situations autonomy is lacking and is surely needed.

The fact that Yarling and McElmurry attribute to nurses as a primary responsibility patient advocacy hardly poses a dilemma for them in the face of abusive and unreasonable patients, as Bishop and Scudder (1987) suggest. Being a patient advocate does not require doing for or taking from the patient just anything, and again, the truth of Yarling and McElmurry's thesis is perfectly compatible with there being problems in the nurse-patient relationship. This criticism shares with several already discussed the confusion of thinking that issues or points about other aspects of, or situations in, nursing have been neglected by Yarling and McElmurry since they addressed *their* topic, not some other, and that truths about these other topics are incompatible with, or threats to, the independent points they make.

Of more general, and perhaps deeper, concern are the comments by Bishop and Scudder (1987), which suggest an insufficient grasp of the basic distinction between description and evaluation, between describing things as they are and prescribing things as they ought to be. They point out that the price one often has to pay to institutions for their rewards is a loss of moral freedom and autonomy, which is irrelevant to whether the price is too high and begs the question of its justice and whether it is a manifestation of legitimate authority or improper power. They further state that it is dangerous to be moral in many other fields, not just nursing, which is irrelevant to whether and to what extent being moral should be dangerous, and whether and to what extent, in particular, it is morally permissible for it to be dangerous in nursing. Again, they say that hospital bureaucrats do have some legitimate authority, which is irrelevant to the pressing question of what the proper limits of their bureaucratic authority are, and the distinction between their proper authority and their improper power. As another example, they say that there are other ways to produce change than those advocated by Yarling and McElmurry and that policy should be changed in desirable ways. This begs the question of which possible way of producing change is best, given the lack of moral freedom by nurses. One certainly doesn't gain such knowledge by the empty truisms that the best way is the desirable way or that the desirable way is the way that should be chosen.

The last example also calls for a reminder about what Yarling and McElmurry (1986) actually said or advocated about the methods for change, as opposed to the desirable goals to be reached by those methods.

> Precisely what policies and what structure are to be preferred in order to effect this liberation is not clear. It is a matter that will require extensive and ongoing deliberations in the councils of the profession.... The concern here is not so much the instruments and technologies of this liberation as the credibility

of this general analysis of nursing's moral situation. . . . [pp. 71–72]

It thus seems clear that the criticism of the methods for change advocated by them is unfair and uninformed by an accurate reading of their work.

Perhaps a more accurate reading would also have prevented some of the false dichotomies posed by Bishop and Scudder. They say that "exercising legitimate authority to foster the patient's well–being seems to us to make more sense than talking about autonomy" (Bishop & Scudder, 1987, p. 40). This statement overlooks the point that not only talking about but doing something about the latter is a means to promoting the former, an error of which they are also guilty in saying that "the primary concern of health care professionals ought to be the well–being of the patient and not the practitioner's autonomy" (Bishop & Scudder, 1987, p. 40). They further apparently think that there is a dichotomy between being autonomous, and working together with other health care professionals as part of a team (Bishop & Scudder, 1987), whereas in fact the two are quite compatible. Indeed, Benjamin and Curtis (1986) state that collaboration assumes that nurses are autonomous. It is interesting that Bishop and Scudder cite with approval the view of Habermas that teamwork is fostered by dialogue without domination (1987), since Yarling and McElmurry have shown that it is improper domination of nurses by *others* which can hinder their playing their legitimate role on the team.

Bishop and Scudder (1987) offer the perspective of the nurse as being "in between" in health care as being of value, and indeed claim this "in between" position is unique to nurses and thus not shared by the physician, hospital, or patient (pp. 40–41), although they are not clearly consistent about this. However, this perspective is inconsistent with the very view of health care as a team, cooperative enterprise which they advocate. If the physician, administrator, and nurse are each part of the team, cooperating with one another, then the nurse is no more "in between" the other members of the team than are the physician or the administrator. If the nurse has such a position, it is not unique but shared by the others. Here, in fact, is revealed in an interesting way the problem Yarling and McElmurry have posed and the need for its solution. In reading that the nurse is "in between," but not the doctor or administrator, one is reminded of the line from *Animal Farm* by George Orwell (1946) that "All the animals are equal, but some are more equal than others" (p. 148). On the one hand, teamwork by professionals with authority and power in different areas is offered as desirable, while on the other hand the offer is withdrawn by the claim that the nurse faces a certain limitation, namely being "in between," which is not faced by the other team members. It is to be suspected that this "in between" perspective is just another version of the threat to moral freedom and autonomy of which Yarling and McElmurry have warned.

CRITICISMS BY COOPER

Further criticism of Yarling and McElmurry (1986) is to be found in Cooper's "Covenantal Relationships: Grounding for the Nursing Ethic" (1988), where it is claimed that they have failed to provide a convincing account of the nature of the nurse–patient relationship and have overlooked the experience of and capacity for moral agency on the part of the nurse *within* that relationship. It is important in evaluating such a claim to again distinguish between *not* doing something, on the one hand, and neglecting or failing to do something or overlooking something, on the other. Something one does not do is only something one overlooked or failed to do if it is something one *should* have done, or that it was reasonable to expect one to do. Thus, whether or not Yarling and McElmurry (1986) failed to provide a convincing account of the nature of the nurse–patient relationship and overlooked the experience of a capacity for moral agency on the part of the nurse within that relationship depends on whether or not Yarling and McElmurry's thesis and the rules of relevance and logic obligated them to do so. Recalling the fact that their thesis was that nurses are often not free to be moral (Yarling & McElmurry, 1986), not that they never are, and that their topic was the threat to moral freedom posed by medical and administrative power, not areas or relationships where such power does *not* pose a significant threat, they do not seem to have been under such an obligation. To claim that nurses *do* have moral freedom in some areas is consistent with, and does not constitute a proper criticism of, the claim that often, and in other areas or ways, they do *not* have it. Further, an exposition and defense of the latter is not guilty of overlooking or failing to discuss the former, even if it is silent about it, since there is no rational requirement to do so. It should be noted in passing, that, if one's goal were to provide an account of the nurse–patient relationship, the standard of success should not be whether the account is convincing, but whether it is rational and true. It is important that one not confuse convincing or persuading, on the one hand, which may be accomplished by nonrational means, with proving or showing to be reasonable to believe, on the other hand. It is the latter that is the goal of rational inquiry. Finally, it should be noted that Yarling and McElmurry are not silent about the nurse–patient relationship. For example, they cite the views of medical students which suggest a negation and denial of the moral status of this relationship (Yarling & McElmurry, 1986), and some of their case studies reveal serious threats to it.

Although Cooper's (1988) extensive discussion of and citation of the views of others about the covenantal relationship between the nurse and patient is of interest in its own right, most of it has little bearing on and relevance to the evaluation of Yarling and McElmurry's views. What are very relevant, however, are such characteristics Cooper (1988) indicates to be involved in that relationship as safeguarding the patient, making promises, trust, and fidelity. Yarling and McElmurry make the point again and again, both by their case studies and in their general discussion, that fidelity to the patient, safeguarding the patient, respect for the patient's dignity and autonomy, earning and deserving the patient's trust, making and keeping promises, and honoring fidelity are all threatened by the nurse's lack of moral freedom. Thus, the covenantal relationship, as described by Cooper, is not some alternative to Yarling and McElmurry's views, but is that which they have shown to be threatened by the lack of moral freedom in nursing, and anyone who favors the former should be grateful to them for exposing the threat and directing efforts toward its elimination. Given Cooper's own characterization of the covenantal nurse–patient relationship, and given the threats to basic aspects of it shown by Yarling and McElmurry, Cooper (1988) is surely mistaken in saying that the capacity for moral agency within the nurse–patient relationship is "unimpeded by institutional restraints or demands of the health care team" (p. 49).

Given the points and clarifications that have been provided, the contrasts with which Cooper concludes are unjustified. She says that, unlike Yarling and McElmurry, her model "promises enrichment and benefit for the patient and nurse alike, but also undergirds the strong moral component of the prima facie duty of fidelity that helps guide the nurse in decision making" (Cooper, 1988, p. 59). However, this is precisely what Yarling and McElmurry want to do by promoting the moral autonomy and moral freedom for nurses which these things require. Again, Cooper says that "rather than focusing efforts on the enhancement of nursing autonomy in the work setting, the covenantal relationships model sets up the conditions for the individual autonomy of the nurse in relation to the patient" (Cooper, 1988, p. 59). Not only is this a curious contrast in virtue of the fact that a part of the enhancement of nursing autonomy in the work setting just *is* setting up the conditions for the individual autonomy of the nurse in relation to the patient, rather than the latter being in contrast with the former, but it is also an improper contrast with Yarling and McElmurry since they themselves are vitally concerned with the latter kind of moral autonomy.

CRITICISMS BY PACKARD AND FERRARA

In Packard and Ferrara's "In Search of the Moral Foundation of Nursing" (1988), one immediately encounters misunderstanding and unjustified criticism. They state that

> Yarling and McElmurry did not elucidate ways of knowing the moral foundation of nursing; illuminate the moral foundation of nursing; or reveal the political nature of nursing. Rather, they erred by equating the ideology of some nurses with moral reasoning; thinking that what nurses do is nursing; and assuming that professionalization is or leads to moral authenticity. [Packard & Ferrara, 1988, p. 60].

They go on to divide their discussion into parts corresponding to each of these criticisms, and the order they establish will be followed in evaluating them.

First, it was neither the goal nor an obligation of Yarling and McElmurry to engage in moral epistemology. To be sure, issues in the theory of knowledge, as well as issues in other areas of philosophy, such as metaphysics, are logically related to their views, but the development and defense of a thesis does not require, and is not defective because it lacks the development and defense of a position about every issue, question, or field of study to which it is logically related. Surely it was appropriate for them to just take for granted, in the context of their study, that we *do* know that the autonomy and well–being and interests and freedom from harm of a patient are at least prima facie goods which the nurse ought to promote, without making an excursion into the intricacies of metaethical theory to show how we know these things. Indeed, an examination of what Packard and Ferrara (1988) seem to offer as a more epistemologically superior alternative does nothing more, and sometimes less. They offer the empty truism that "one ought to desire the good" (Packard & Ferrara, 1988, p. 62) and judgments such as: life lived well is preferable to life lived poorly, one should live well, health contributes to living well, and nursing is related to health and is therefore good (Packard & Ferrara, 1988, pp. 61–62). These judgments are as much or as little in need, in the present context, of an elucidation of *how* we know them as those of Yarling and McElmurry, and tend to have the disadvantage of truisms; namely, that they lack the content and concreteness of the moral judgments of the latter authors.

Second, Packard and Ferrara (1988) provide no good evidence in support of their denial that Yarling and McElmurry (1986) illuminated the moral foundation of nursing, and this denial may grow out of the same error discussed above. It is true that they did not offer a complete moral epistemology and metaethical and normative ethical theory of nursing, but doing so was not a necessary condition for the illumination of a crucial issue at the very foundation of morality in nursing; namely, the issue of the freedom to do what moral principles in nursing demand, and they have illuminated this issue with admirable and needed light. Again, an examination of what Packard and Ferrara seem to offer as better illumination reveals mainly truisms such as: eliminating disease and healing injury are good, helping one to live well is right, and nursing requires right actions, knowledge, talent, and good will (Packard & Ferrara, 1988). These things may be obviously true, but they are of no help in illuminating and in solving the problem of the nurse's lack of freedom to act on this knowledge, use this talent, exercise this good will, and do the right actions.

Third, given the emphasis that Yarling and McElmurry (1986) placed on the political and social nature of the barriers and threats to moral freedom, and their call for political and social reform to promote and protect it, the claim that they did not reveal the political nature of nursing certainly seems implausible, and one would expect very good evidence in its support, which Packard and Ferrara (1988) nevertheless fail to provide. Indeed, in that part of their discussion where they elaborate on this criticism, they virtually withdraw it and agree that Yarling and McElmurry have revealed important aspects of the political nature and demands of nursing. This apparent contradiction is only excused by their suggestion that it is not clear that Yarling and McElmurry meant to reveal these aspects (Packard & Ferrara, 1988). Their suspicion of lack of clarity, however, seems based on a failure to pay close attention to what was said. They attribute to Yarling and McElmurry the claim that nursing is apolitical, and reply that nursing is by nature political and that "it would be incorrect to assume that both rank–and–file and influential nurses have not shaped public policy or social structures. In fact, they have exerted considerable influence in major and minor ways" (Packard & Ferrara, 1988, p. 65). However, Yarling and McElmurry make no such assumption. They say that rank–and–file nursing has been more personal than political, and predominantly apolitical—not that rank–and–file nurses have not shaped public policy or social structures. They recognize increasing political activity in this group. Further, they speak clearly of a distinct thread of social reform in nursing and name influential nurses who have been a part of it. Rather than denying or failing to be aware of this tradition and these reformers, they call for a stronger memory of, and greater recognition and honor for, it and them (Yarling & McElmurry, 1986).

Fourth, the supposed error of equating the ideology of some nurses with moral reasoning simply dissolves when subjected to careful thinking and conceptual analysis. A standard dictionary entry for "ideology" includes both "a systematic body of concepts" and "the integrated assertions, theories, and aims that constitute a sociopolitical program" within its meaning. It is both clear and appropriate that Yarling and McElmurry mean by "present–day ideology in nursing" and "the ideological revolution" in nursing education the moral principles and rules that should guide nurses and which, while having recently been embodied in nursing education, have not been sufficiently actualized and followed in practice because of sociopolitical forces (Yarling & McElmurry, 1986, p. 67). The recognition that some nurses accept these principles and rules no more equates moral reasoning with the ideology of some nurses than does the recognition that some professors accept moral principles about commitment to students and autonomy in the exercise of that commitment equates moral reasoning with the ideology of some professors.

Packard and Ferrara's (1988) confusion is revealed by their question "how can something be called an ideology and also be moral," and their concern about the fact that a racist ideology is of questionable morality (p. 66). This question and this concern are immediately resolved by seeing that whether something is an ethical theory, moral principle, ideology, or moral rule is logically independent of whether it is true or false, rational or irrational, or a good or bad theory, principle, ideology, or rule. Certainly some such things, such as the theory that the rightness of an act consists in the approval of it by society or the principle that might makes right, are incorrect, and other such things, such as the ideology that commitment to patients and the autonomy to exercise that commitment are good or the rule *primum non nocere* (first do no harm), are correct. With respect to the incorrect ones, they are not good guides to morality and adopting them may lead to immorality, while with respect to the correct ones, they *are* good guides to morality and following them may well, other things being equal, lead to morality. Thus an ideology, such as racism, may clearly be immoral, and an ideology, such as indicated and supported by Yarling and McElmurry, may clearly be moral. The cure for any discomfort felt in calling a moral principle immoral consists in recognizing the ambiguity of "moral." In one sense, a moral principle is a principle about morality, but a principle about morality may be unacceptable and thus in a second sense be immoral or lead, if accepted, to immorality. This is analogous to the case in biology where a principle may be biological in the sense of being about biology, but in another sense be said to be unbiological, or be, or lead to, bad biology because it is unacceptable in light of current knowledge.

Also in the context of their elaboration of their fouth criticism, Packard and Ferrara (1988) suggest that Yarling and McElmurry (1986) failed to show that patient advocacy, commitment to patients, and autonomy are morally defensible, that they did not draw the limits to the commitment to the patient which might rule out actions such as stealing and harming the patient, and that the idea of commitment to the patient is "inherently suspect" because it involves commitment only to the patient to the exclusion of other duties such as helping to prevent disease (Packard & Ferrara, 1988, p. 66). Again, one senses in these criticisms a failure to read carefully and think clearly. Yarling and McElmurry (1986) explicitly state at the beginning that their attention is, for the purposes of their discussion and thesis, confined to hospital practice, wherein the majority of nurses are found. Naturally, it is patients with which nurses are primarily concerned in this setting, but to focus on this setting and relationship in no way affirms or suggests that nurses, in or out of hospitals, are committed only to patients and have no other professional duties or goals or commitments. Further, even if one were only committed to patients, it is totally unjustified for Packard and Ferrara to say that this would be "almost totally self–serving" (1988, p. 66). As for not drawing limits to commitment which would rule out patient harm, Yarling and McElmurry (1986) explicitly speak of commitment to the well–being of the patient and protection of the patient from harm. One is reminded here of J.S. Mill's (1957) famous statement that "there is no difficulty in proving any ethical standard whatever to work ill if we suppose universal idiocy to be conjoined with it" (pp. 30–31). Surely, for the purposes of their discussion, it was permissible for Yarling and McElmurry (1986) to assume the absence of universal idiocy and not explicitly rule out all the possible misapplications of commitment to the patient, even if there are some interesting questions here that might be addressed at another time. Finally, the charge that they have not given an adequate defense of their moral acceptance of the patient advocacy and commitment, which they have shown to be realizable only by greater autonomy, has already been met in pointing out that, in a discussion aimed at revealing the importance of the latter, a sophisticated moral epistemology and ethical theory in support of the former was not required. If doing even some things required doing everything, then nothing would ever be done.

Fifth, one looks in vain in Yarling and McElmurry for any error about the relation between what nurses do and nursing. On the one hand, what nurses do when acting professionally in accordance with the proper standards and principles of nursing, both is and logically must be, nursing. On the other hand, not everything done by someone who is a nurse, regardless of its relation to that person's profession and its proper standards and principles, is nursing. Nowhere are Yarling and McElmurry guilty of confusion or error about these two obvious facts about the relationship between nursing and what nurses do.

Sixth, Yarling and McElmurry (1986) did not say or assume, and thus did not err in assuming, that professionalization is or leads to moral authenticity. What they said was that a strong sense of professional autonomy was a necessary, but not a sufficient, condition for the moral freedom of nurses. They thus made perfectly clear, by means of a standard logical distinction, that their view was that moral freedom, and the moral authenticity it permits, would not come about unless professional autonomy was strengthened, not that the latter just consisted in or would lead, with nothing else required, to the former.

As a final word about Packard and Ferrara (1988), it should be mentioned that their concern that professionalization among nurses fails as an element in the moral foundation of nursing, because it is seen as in conflict with commitment to people, is as odd as their suggestion that to be committed only to patients is self–serving. Yarling and McElmurry have shown that the need for greater professional autonomy grows out of the commitment to people and patients, which is frustrated by the lack of professional freedom and autonomy, rather than the latter being in conflict with this commitment.

CRITICISMS BY BRODY AND GREENFIELD

Misunderstandings of Yarling and McElmurry and errors about their subject matter have not been confined to substantive articles. In a letter to the editor Brody and Greenfield (1986, p. vii) say that "being forced to choose between limited or difficult options cannot be equated with lack of freedom or choice," apparently unaware of the clear distinction that was made between the complete lack of free choice and the lack of freedom from the necessity for self–sacrifice and moral heroism as the improperly imposed price for doing what is right.

An additional and very important shortcoming on their part is revealed by their statement "the choice between the well–being of the patient and the well–being of the nurse is not an ethical dilemma. Nurses know where their responsibilities lie" (Brody & Greenfield, 1986, p. vii). To be sure, where the choice is between moral obligations to the patient and nonmoral, prudential interests of the nurse, there is no ethical dilemma, since the latter require a conflict between duties or moral principles. However, conflicts between prudence and duty are those which Yarling and McElmurry emphasize as giving rise to the improper restrictions on the moral freedom of nurses, and there is no need for these to be ethical dilemmas in order for their thesis to be reasonable and true. It is crucial, however, especially given current concerns about AIDS, to recognize that one can have moral obligations to preserve and promote one's own well–being. All too many nurses feel embarrassed about their concern for self–protection because they feel that it is only a private, selfish, prudential concern, in contrast with their principled, moral concern for their patients. It is vitally important to eliminate this error by recognizing that nurses can have both indirect and direct *moral* obligations to themselves. Their indirect obligations to themselves arise out of their direct obligations to their patients. Illness or injury which they suffer tends to detract from their capacity to help their patients, so their obligation to do the latter generates an obligation to avoid the former. Further, nurses are themselves persons who have intrinsic worth and rights and to whom principles such as autonomy, beneficence, nonmaleficence, and justice apply. In virtue of these principles and this intrinsic worth as persons nurses have direct duties to themselves, so a conflict between the well–being of the nurse and the well–being of the patient *can* be a *moral* conflict and an ethical dilemma.

Brody and Greenfield (1986) also suggest that Yarling and McElmurry (1986) promote to some extent the nurse hiding from personal responsibility by giving the excuse "that they are not moral agents but victims of the system" (Brody & Greenfield, 1986, p. vii). However, anyone who finds support for such an attitude in their article is seeing something that isn't there, and had better look again and more carefully. Yarling and McElmurry make dramatically lucid that it is the strong and clear sense of *being* a moral agent and having personal moral responsibilities which gives rise to the conflict and frustration produced by the unacceptable suppression of the freedom to act morally and fulfill moral responsibilities. Rather than offering a hiding place, they call for nurses to come into full public and social and political view as advocates of a reform which is needed precisely because they are moral agents with moral responsibilities.

CONCLUSION

While it was admitted in the beginning, and illustrated with an example, that Yarling and McElmurry are not immune to criticism, it has been shown that much of the criticism directed at them is guilty of confusion, misunderstanding, lack of conceptual clarity, and the failure to pay careful and close attention to what they said and proposed. It is hoped that the above exposure of these defects will contribute to a more rational and just examination of and debate about their important thesis and call for reform. In closing, it is interesting to ask whether Yarling and McElmurry were guilty of anything, by way of commission or omission, which might account for, or have contributed to, their critics straying so far from the rational mark. One possibility is their citing as their topic, both in their title and throughout their article, the moral foundation of nursing, and their occasional talk of elaborating a nursing ethic. As said in their defense earlier, they *did* speak about and shed light on and elaborate these topics, and they had no obligation to say everything or answer every question about them. However, to accomplish, if possible, the latter, formidable, task and provide a comprehensive and complete moral foundation for an ethical theory of nursing *would* require the sophisticated moral epistemology, and metaethical and normative ethical theory which some of their critics found missing. As shown earlier, it was not a defect that it was missing or a failure on their part that it wasn't there, since their actual topic and thesis did not require it, but perhaps they could have avoided unfulfilled expectations and unjustified criticisms if they had described their topic in more limited and specific terms.

REFERENCES

Benjamin, M., & Curtis, J. (1986). *Ethics in nursing.* New York: Oxford.

Bishop, A. H., & Scudder, J. R., Jr. (1987). Nursing ethics in an age of controversy. *Advances in Nursing Science, 9*(3), 34–43.

Brody, J., & Greenfield, S. A. (1986). To the editor. *Advances in Nursing Science, 9*(1), vii.

Cooper, M. C. (1988). Covenantal relationships: Grounding for the nursing ethic. *Advances in Nursing Science, 10*(4), 48–59.

Mill, J. S. (1957). *Utilitarianism.* Indianapolis, IN: Bobbs-Merrill.

Orwell, G. (1946). *Animal farm.* New York: Harcourt, Brace & World.

Packard, J. S., & Ferrara, M. In search of the moral foundation of nursing. *Advances in Nursing Science, 10*(4), 60–71.

Yarling, R. R., & McElmurry, B. J. (1986). The moral foundation of nursing. *Advances in Nursing Science, 8*(2), 63–73.

4

Health Promotion, Caring, and Nursing: Why Social Activism is Necessary

Doris M. Williams

The notion that caring is the essence of nursing fits well with nurses' sense of professional identity. As Moccia (1988) and MacPherson (1989) point out, however, the social context of nursing practice has much to do with the operationalization of caring by nurses in their work. Whether nurses realize their potential for caring in interpersonal nursing practices may depend on social activism to shape a context that supports caring. The point that will be argued here is that when the concern of nursing is health promotion, social activism is the substance of caring itself. Some implications of this point of view for nursing practice and theory are discussed.

CARING AND HEALTH PROMOTION

Health, however defined, can be conceptualized as a continuum of states ranging from positive to negative. A positive state of health, as the term is used here, signifies an individual condition of integrity that provides the basic instrumentality for confronting the tasks, demands, pleasures, and joys of life.

As a basic instrumentality of humans, health status is a major factor in determining what Daniels (1982) calls the "opportunity range" of individuals, " . . . the array of life plans that it is reasonable to pursue within the conditions obtaining in a given society" (p. 72). Positive health, then, is an important enabling condition for the realization of human potential.

47

Negative health, on the other hand, by narrowing the opportunity range of individuals, creates inequalities in access and in freedom of choice and action that impede self–realization within a specific social setting. Wright (1982) argues that because health activates the human potential for freedom, equality, and justice, the health levels of a society can be used to judge its "goodness," by which he means its moral and political success.

A democratic society has a moral responsibility to undertake the actions that are necessary to maximize the occurrence of health among its citizens (Beauchamp, 1976; Milio, 1981; Wright, 1982). This moral responsibility arises from consideration of both individual and collective benefits to be derived from such actions. Positive health is a necessary, though not sufficient, condition for individual freedom and equality, and it is instrumental to both civic participation and economic productivity, both of which contribute to the common good.

Positive health is widely valued because, in addition to its instrumental value, it has intrinsic worth in meeting security needs in relation to comfort and survival. As Frankenberg (1974), Kelman (1975), and Milio (1983), among others, have noted, most people find the preservation of positive health preferable to the prospect, however likely, of its restoration. "Health promotion" is the term used most frequently to designate activities and arrangements that are aimed at increasing the probability of preserving positive health (Leavell & Clark, 1965; Terris, 1986; U.S. Department of Health, Education, and Welfare, 1979).

While the project of health promotion in this country is characterized by focusing nearly exclusively on individual behavior (Williams, 1987, 1989), some people conceive of health promotion as a much broader undertaking. For instance, the statement issued by the International Conference on Health Promotion in Ottawa, Canada, in November 1986, presents a comprehensive view of health promotion, one that is based on caring. This group proposed actions to promote health based on the following assumptions:

> Health is created and lived by people within the settings of their everyday life; where they learn, work, play and love. Health is created by caring for oneself and others, by being able to make decisions and have control over one's life circumstances, and by ensuring that the society that one lives in creates conditions that allow the attainment of health by all its members. [p. 2] The fundamental conditions and resources for health are peace, shelter, education, food, income, a stable eco–system, sustainable resources, social justice and equity. . . . Political, economic, social, cultural, environmental, behaviourial and biological factors can all favour health or be harmful to it. Health promotion

action aims at making these conditions favourable through *advocacy* for health. Health promotion action aims at reducing differences in current health status and ensuring equal opportunities and resources to *enable* all people to achieve their fullest health potential. . . . This must apply equally to women and men. [p. 1, emphasis in original.]

From the perspective of this statement, the promotion of health must be viewed as a collective undertaking with responsibility for caring about health distributed among many levels, from the individual to the whole social system. Further, the Ottawa statement clearly implies that the requirements for health impose structural imperatives on societies that care about the health of all their members; i.e., such societies must assume responsibility for seeing that people have the resources they need to give them an equal chance to be born healthy and to stay healthy. The project of health promotion, therefore, can be viewed as one of creating a health–making society. This view suggests the following definition: health promotion is the social construction of environments that interact with and respond to human needs and behaviors in such a way as to maximize the probability of preserving positive health and equalizing its distribution.

In a health–making society, all persons would have equal access to the resources needed for health, and individuals would not be exposed to health hazards beyond their personal control such as pollution, harmful biologic agents, intoxications of food and water, trauma, inducements for health–destructive personal behaviors, socioeconomic deprivations, and other health–assaulting conditions. Moreover, in a health–making society, individuals would be conditioned and motivated to care for and about their health and the health of others. Given that positive health is a precondition for realization of the democratic ideals of freedom and equality, a society committed to democratic values must regard a health–making environment as a basic human right.

One means for societies to exercise their responsibilities for health–making is to use the policy process to promote health. Health promotion

puts health on the agenda of policy makers in all sectors and at all levels, directing them to be aware of the health consequences of their decisions and to accept their responsibility for health. . . . It is coordinated action that leads to health, income and social policies that foster greater equity. Joint action contributes to ensuring safer and healthier goods and services, healthier public services, and cleaner, more enjoyable environments [Ottawa charter . . . , 1986, p. 1].

The promotion of health, then, is an explicitly political activity. Even health education programs, which some might think are apolitical, can be seen to be highly susceptible to the values and preferences of those who control the resources for such programs. This point is illustrated well by the example of AIDS where efforts to educate about risky behaviors related to sexual activity and illicit intravenous drug use have been obstructed by policymakers who openly admit that such educational programs effront their personal sense of morality (Stryker, 1989).

NURSING AND HEALTH PROMOTION

The promotion of health requires caring about the effects of social, political, and economic aspects of the environment on people's health. Caring at this level requires social activism. It demands a commitment to creating the environmental conditions and relations that enhance the possibilities for health. These ideas about caring and health promotion have implications for nursing education, research, and practice and for theories of caring. Some implications for nursing education and research have been discussed elsewhere (Williams, 1989). Here, the discussion will focus on nursing practice and theories of caring.

Social Activism as Nursing Practice

Because nursing has laid claim to a major role in health promotion, it must accept social activism as a *mode* of nursing practice, not merely as a background to it. While caring at an interpersonal level is a major and necessary nursing activity, it may not be sufficient nor even appropriate to accomplish health promotion. Individualistic health promotion, which concentrates on changing individual risky behaviors, fails to attend to contextual influences on either behavior or health, which may explain why it has had limited success and produced inequitable results (Milio, 1983; Williams, 1989). Though a preoccupation with individualistic health promotion has been evident in nursing (Williams, 1987), there are indications that a reconceptualization of health promotion by nurses is underway (Chopoorian, 1986; Milio, 1983, 1989; Williams, 1989).

Individually, nurses can advocate for health by engaging in a range of political activities, e.g., writing letters, making telephone calls, broadcasting opinions, lobbying, negotiating, testifying, picketing, boycotting, demonstrating, and engaging in civil disobedience. Such activities should be directed toward the appropriate policymakers, whether governmental or nongovernmental, and are often more effective when coordinated with similar activities by others. For this latter reason, individual nurses can amplify the effects of their political actions by belonging to or subscribing to the publications of organizations whose goals are the protection and promotion of health. Affiliation with organizations provides not only the basis for collective action, but also a means of keeping informed about issues and the status of any policy being developed or implemented.

Professional nursing organizations are necessary for the caring social activism of nurses. These organizations can supply not only the information and coordination needed to support individual efforts, but also the leadership and structure required to develop goals and plans of action for the profession's role in health promotion (e.g., the American Nurses' Association's Health Policy Agenda [Nursing's agenda . . . , 1989]) and the social critique necessary to make visible the forces arrayed against health (e.g., the mission statement of Nurses for Progressive Social Change [1986]). Because political strength is related to numbers, nursing organizations should continue to promote the professional unity essential to social activism. Consciousness–raising and consensus–building activities among nurses for major health promotion policy issues are critical pursuits for nursing organizations.

Organizations with interests related to health promotion include not just professional nursing organizations, but also broad–based health organizations, e.g., the American Public Health Association and the National Association for Public Health Policy; health–interested consumer and citizens' groups, e.g., Public Citizen, National Women's Health Network, Women's International League for Peace and Freedom, Citizen's Clearinghouse for Hazardous Wastes, Greenpeace, Action on Smoking and Health, and Center for Science in the Public Interest; labor unions; and political groups, e.g., the Health Commission of the National Rainbow Coalition. Individual membership in such groups is a valuable resource for social activism. Moreover, for both health and the profession, it is important that organized nursing be actively involved in the various coalitions that form around health promotion issues. The building of coalitions as the profession unites with other health advocates from all levels of society will create the broad base of caring that can support the social action needed for health promotion.

To promote health, nurses must advocate for health in social, economic, and political arenas. The focus of nurses' activism must be the conditions and resources fundamental to health as outlined in the Ottawa statement (1986). This necessarily results in a broad agenda for action. Some suggestions for this agenda are offered here with attention to activism that not only addresses current policy issues but also focuses on principles for social transformation.

Working to establish the principle of universal entitlement to an equal chance for health should be an important goal for nurses' political activity.

A step in this direction would be to support a national plan that assures universal access to health care. While personal health services are limited in what they can offer for health promotion (Milio, 1983), nevertheless, if it is established that health care is a right, then this idea can be generalized to the argument that keeping people healthy requires equal access to the resources that determine health. Moreover, among the efficacious preventive health care services are ones that are very important to promoting the health of pregnant women and children—prenatal and birthing care, immunizations, and physical and developmental examinations for children (Milio, 1983).

Nurses should support current efforts to produce federal legislation that would ban the advertising of all tobacco products (ASH proposal . . . , 1989). Not only would a ban on advertising tobacco protect people from persuasion meant to induce health–damaging behavior—aimed especially at youth, women, and blacks (Bailey, 1986; Blacks in debate . . . , 1987)— but it would also advance the principle that government should subordinate the interests of commercial actors to the public's health. The moral basis for this principle derives from the responsibility of a democratic government to promote health as a means of promoting individual freedom and equality. To further advance this principle, efforts should be directed at strengthening and extending existing laws and regulations that aim to control the health–affecting behaviors of commercial actors, e.g., tighter enforcement of toxic waste handling laws, revision of food labeling laws and regulations.

A policy strategy with the potential for a significant impact on health promotion is that of requiring health impact statements (similar to environmental impact statements) for all major policies developed by organizational policymakers, whether governmental or nongovernmental. Both Milio (1981) and Miller and Miller (1981) have made this proposal. Its merit lies in the explicit attention such statements would focus on the costs and benefits to health that major policy initiatives generate, for instance, the health effects of the unemployment and environmental degradation that result from present policies of military spending (Midgeley, 1989). Such information, widely disseminated among the public whose health would be affected, could create an activated constituency for health with which nurses, as well as other health advocates, could ally.

In addition to social activism in policy matters, nurses can promote health by acting as change agents in communities and work settings. In communities, nurses should establish their credibility as advocates for health by being visible and vocal participants in any community undertaking that affects health. Organizing citizen groups to become involved in political advocacy for health may be an important expression of nurses' caring about health.

To create the collective critical consciousness needed to support community organizing, nurses might need to rethink the purposes and content of health education. Health education might do more to promote health if, rather than focusing on individual behavior, it was geared to empower people for social action by giving them the information they need to understand the connections between their health states and their social situations. Ratcliffe, Wallack, Fagnani, and Rodwin (1984) emphasize the need for people to know about the risk–imposing behavior of others:

> Exhorting the worker to exercise personal safety in the midst of hazardous working conditions, asking adolescents to exercise mature judgment in the face of sophisticated advertising and social pressures to use (or at least try) government subsidized drugs, imploring poverty stricken mothers to feed their malnourished children a more varied and nutritious diet, and encouraging those who live near toxic waste dumps or nuclear plants to jog, quit smoking, and reduce cholesterol intake have not been demonstrated to be associated with positive health outcomes. . . . In whose life–styles are we going to intervene? Those who may be adversely affected by the risk–imposing behavior of others? Or those who, through enticing others to use harmful drugs or through the dumping of toxins in the environment, willfully expose others to health hazards? [pp. 69, 71]

Teach–ins, consciousness–raising groups, and community access television channels, in addition to individual/family teaching, are some methods useful for health education meant to empower.

Because nurses practice in all the settings important to health promotion, they are in advantageous positions to try to redirect existing programs of health promotion away from a singular focus on individual behaviors. Freudenberg's (1986) examination of the women's health movement suggests that the search for alternative health promotion programs should be concentrated on women's health services organized on feminist principles. He says that these services have resolved, in practice, what some have taken to be a philosophical dilemma of whether to change individual behavior or social conditions. The women's health movement, says Freudenberg, does both. He comments,

> In the final analysis, the totality of the feminist contribution to public health practice is greater than the sums of its individual parts. Consciousness raising, health education as a right, alternative institutions and a critique of the system are more than

separate elements of the women's health movement. Together they combine to offer a vision of a different social order—where women and men are equal, where health care and health education are rights, and where making health is a collaborative effort involving the individual, society and health care workers. [p. 30]

Nurses can coordinate comprehensive, community–wide programs of health promotion. As part of this effort, nurses and the agencies they are associated with need to take the initiative in developing linkages with minority, low–income, and women's groups to provide opportunities for these people to participate in the design of health promotion programs.

The resources needed to undertake the preceding strategies for social activism, admittedly a partial list of the possibilities for gains in health promotion, require that health advocates come together. For some issues, nursing might take the lead in organizing coalitions, while for others, it might support the efforts of others. In either case, for nurses to perceive the primary importance of this level of advocacy for health promotion, a broader view of what constitutes nursing practice is required and the development of theories of caring needs to be anchored in this broader view.

Theories of Caring

Benner and Wrubel (1989) maintain that nursing "theory is derived from practice" (p. 19). From this perspective, the definition of what constitutes nursing practice is critical to what a theory developed from practice will explain, describe, and interpret. Activity that falls outside definitional limits for practice will not be interesting to theorists as a source of knowledge for theory development. An assumption that nursing practice is completely constituted by focusing on interpersonal relations and transactions appears to be widely held by practitioners and theorists. Given what is known about the effects of physical, social, political, and economic environments on people's health and given nursing's aspirations to a leadership role in health promotion, it is necessary to challenge this assumption.

In the promotion of health, both nurse–patient and nurse/nursing–environment relationships are important. A theory of nursing derived from a view of nursing practice as exclusively interpersonal caring, however, would not be likely to capture the experiences and knowledge of nurses who engage in social activism to advocate for health. A theory thus derived would not provide analytic or prescriptive frameworks for nurses to promote health at the social level of caring. Such a theoretical deficiency might explain Benner and Wrubel's exclusive focus on individual level strategies to promote health in their recent book, *The Primacy of Caring* (1989).

An interpretation of practice as interpersonal caring likewise has implications for ethical theories of nursing. Fry (1989) argues that a theory of nursing ethics ought to be grounded on the idea of caring and that such theory "will become an essential part of a yet–to–be–formulated philosophy of nursing" (p. 10). If ideas of caring do not encompass concerns about health beyond the level of the individual, then ethical theories in nursing will not provide a basis for nurses to inquire about or to know what constitutes ethical decisions and behavior in social activism.

Because of the nature of the project of health promotion, a nursing theory of caring that would serve nursing's commitment in this area must be based on a definition of nursing practice that encompasses both interpersonal and social caring. While the content of such a theory remains to be developed, there are three features that such a theory must have. First, given the requirements of health promotion—the building of a health–making society—the theory must be grounded in a broad conceptualization of environment, one such as suggested by Chooporian (1986) or Stevens (1989). Second, the theory must be developed from a critical stance; i.e., those who would generate this theory must be committed to identifying and changing the oppressive social, economic, and political conditions that affect both health and behavior. This means that nursing practice must also be subjected to critique to determine both its relationship to health and the effects of social context on the realization of the potentials for caring in practice.

Finally, the embeddedness of caring in social context must be explicitly addressed at a theoretical level. Caring, like health, is a human potential; it is neither a necessary nor an inherent feature of a universal "human nature." The possibilities for caring are shaped, like those for health, by social, economic, and political aspects of the environment. Tronto (1987) contends that the social context for a theory of care must be specified.

> Among the questions a convincing theory of care needs to address are the myriad questions crucial to any social and political theory. Where does caring come from? Is it learned in the family? If so, does an ethic of care mandate something about the need for, or the nature of, families? Who determines who can be a member of the caring society? What should be the role of the market in a caring society? Who should bear the responsibility for education? How much inequality is acceptable before individuals become indifferent to those who are too different in

status? How well do current institutions and theories support the ethic of care? [p. 661]

Caring is conditioned by and realized within historically specific social, political, and economic circumstances. We learn to care—or not—and we are enabled or constrained in our caring by social situations that may be beyond our control, like social hierarchies and divisions of labor based on gender, race, and class. Moreover, in a social context where caring work is culturally undervalued, those who do it, which in most cases is women, will likewise be undervalued. From her historical study of nursing, Reverby (1987) made explicit the oppressive potential inherent in caring in such a context when she concluded that the central dilemma for American nursing is "the order to care in a society that refuses to value caring" (p. 5).

The idea of caring is ascendant in nursing. As theories of care develop, it will be necessary to base them on broad definitions of nursing in order to include all nursing activities that promote health. Such theories must attend to the primary role of social context in shaping both health and the possibilities for nurses to realize caring in their practices.

REFERENCES

ASH [Action on Smoking and Health] proposal adopted by tobacco ad foes in Congress. (1989, May–June). *ASH Smoking and Health Review*, p. 3.

Bailey, B. (1986). Tobaccoism is the disease—Cancer is the sequela. (Editorial) *Journal of the American Medical Association, 255*, 1923.

Beauchamp, D. (1976). Public health as social justice. *Inquiry, 3*(3), 3–14.

Benner, P., & Wrubel, J. (1989). *The primacy of caring.* Menlo Park, CA: Addison-Wesley.

Blacks in debate on tobacco industry influences. (1987, January 17). *New York Times*, pp. 1,9.

Chopoorian, T. (1986). Reconceptualizing the environment. In P. Moccia (Ed.), *New approaches to theory development* (pp. 39–54). New York: National League for Nursing.

Daniels, N. (1982). Equity of access to health care: Some conceptual and ethical issues. *Milbank Memorial Fund Quarterly/Health and Society, 60*, 51–81.

Frankenberg, R. (1974). Functionalism and after? Theory and developments in social science applied to the health field. *International Journal of Health Services, 4*, 411–427.

Freudenberg, N. (1986). The women's health movement—Lessons for health educators. *Health/PAC Bulletin, 16*(6), 30.

Fry, S. (1989). Toward a theory of nursing ethics. *Advances in Nursing Science, 11*(4), 9–22.

Kelman, S. (1975). The social nature of the definition problem in health. *International Journal of Health Services, 5,* 133–144.

Leavell, H., & Clark, E. (1965). *Preventive medicine for the doctor in his community.* New York: McGraw-Hill.

MacPherson, K. (1989). A new perspective on nursing and caring in a corporate context. *Advances in Nursing Science, 11*(4), 32–39.

Midgeley, J. (1989). *The women's budget.* Philadelphia: Women's International League for Peace and Freedom.

Milio, N. (1989). Developing nursing leadership in health policy. *Journal of Professional Nursing, 5,* 315–321.

Milio, N. (1983). *Primary care and the public's health.* Lexington, MA: LexingtonBooks.

Milio, N. (1981). *Promoting health through public policy.* Philadelphia: F. A. Davis.

Miller, A., & Miller, M. (1981). *Options for health and health care: The coming of post-clinical medicine.* New York: John Wiley & Sons.

Moccia, P. (1988). At the faultline: Social activism and caring. *Nursing Outlook, 36,* 30–33.

Nurses for Progressive Social Change. (1986). Statement of purpose. Breckenridge, ME: Author.

Nursing's agenda calls for accessible care (1989, January). *American Nurse,* 19.

Ottawa charter for health promotion. (1986). Drafted by participants in the First International Conference on Health Promotion, November 17–21, 1986, Ottawa, Ontario, Canada.

Ratcliffe, J., Wallack, L., Fagnani, F., & Rodwin, V. (1984). Perspectives on prevention: Health promotion vs. health protection. In J. Kervasdoue, J. Kimberly, & V. Rodwin (Eds.), *The end of an illusion: The future of health policy in western industrialized nations* (pp. 56–84). Berkeley: University of California Press.

Reverby, S. (1987). A caring dilemma: Womanhood and nursing in historical perspective. *Nursing Research, 36,* 5–11.

Stevens, P. (1989). A critical social reconceptualization of environment in nursing: Implications for methodology. *Advances in Nursing Science, 11*(4), 56–68.

Stryker, J. (1989). IV drug use and AIDS: Public policy and dirty needles. *Journal of Health Politics, Policy, and Law, 14,* 719–740.

Terris, M. (1986). What is health promotion? (Editorial) *Journal of Public Health Policy, 7,* 147–149.

Tronto, J. (1987) Beyond gender difference to a theory of care. *Signs: Journal of Women, Culture, and Society, 12,* 644–663.

United States Department of Health, Education, and Welfare. (1979). *Healthy people: The Surgeon General's report on health promotion and disease prevention.* Publication No. (PHS) 79–55071, Government Printing Office.

Williams, D. (1987). *Nursing and health promotion: Contradictions between the goals of the profession and its model of health promotion* (Dissertation). College of Urban Affairs and Public Policy, University of Delaware.

Williams, D. (1989). Political theory and individualistic health promotion. *Advances in Nursing Science, 12*(1), 14–25.

Wright, W. (1982). *The social logic of health.* New Brunswick, NJ: Rutgers University Press.

5

Caring for the Environment: The Ecology of Health

Martha N. Smith and Gail M. Whitney

If in 1965 Rene Dubos could say confidently, "the search for environmental determinants of disease is not a fashionable topic and carries little scientific prestige" (Dubos, 1965, p. 357), he could no longer do so today. The intervening 25 years have not made the search any more glamorous, but time has indeed made it much more immediate and urgent—"fashionable," if necessity can be considered a matter of fashion. Since Dubos' writing, enough scientists have in fact pursued the unfashionable to stake out the undeniable: Massive evidence supporting the relationship between today's illnesses and diseases and predominant characteristics of modern life; specifically, environmental changes of all types, small– and large–scale (Last, 1987). The tables have turned: The emphasis on medical technology and drugs is "out," their glories and value recognized, but recognized, too, as finite (Dever, Sciegaj, Wade, & Lofton, 1988) or simply non–applicable. The relationship between the state of the world—its undeniable environmental problems—and the state of human health, on the other hand, is "in." Everybody is talking about it.

Of course, the environment and environmental determinants of disease are not quite the same thing. One is context—situational, the conditions in which a person lives. The other is cause and effect—relational, the interactions that occur between or among elements of the context. To learn anything about either, one must observe both. In nursing care, practice, and discourse, emphasis has been placed on the client's personal or immediate environment and the cause and effect relationships between various factors and the client's state of health. In its most basic sense, this personal environment may be deemed "healthy" or "unhealthy" for the individual client, just as some coping behaviors are determined "healthy" or "unhealthy." High–risk factors may be fixed, so to speak, as with hereditary risk factors or long–term occupational exposure to toxins. Or, high–risk factors may be changeable, increasing and decreasing in proportion to the quality of a client's self–care habits or in proportion to the degree the client sets out to change factors within his or her immediate environment. A thorough health assessment and intervention plan will treat not only the client, but also the client's personal environment, with the client acting as the agent of change, and the health professional as helper and advocate.

The aim of this article is to redefine the client's environmental determinants or personal environment by detailing *as personal* the client's relationship with what remains beyond the bounds of most current client health assessments and nursing care plans: the biosphere itself, that part of the earth and its atmosphere in which living things exist. A grand idea, surely. Then again, consider that few nurses or doctors working in a metropolitan area these days can feel truly confident advising the client to "get a bit of fresh air." Where will the client have to go to get it? To the moon? How far away? According to the March–April 1990 issue of *International Wildlife*, "the World Health Organization estimates that fully 70 percent of the globe's urban population breathes air made unhealthy by high levels of smog, sulfur dioxide, nitrogen oxides and other pollutants" (Moore, 1990, p. 14). The 1990 *World Almanac and Book of Facts* states that "the long, hot summer of 1988 saw the worst air pollution in decades. Smog . . . appeared in record proportions far from its usual city haunts" (Hoffman, 1989, p. 214).

As all sectors of modern society and all peoples everywhere face the task of curbing (or abandoning altogether) those practices which contribute to or exacerbate environmental problems and, in their place, adopting new methods, techniques, behaviors, habits, and life-styles, nurses are well–suited to provide leadership. As educators, counselors, advocates, researchers, and clinicians, nurses are already addressing core issues defining health: individual, occupational, family, community, and public health; physical, mental, emotional, and spiritual health. Perhaps more than any other health professionals, nurses have direct, frequent interaction with clients. Perhaps they will promote a new kind of informed consent. So much depends upon information.

What if, silly as it sounds, the nurse or doctor prescribed "for starters, a good drought of fresh air if you can get to Nevada, taking the bus to work or carpooling three days a week, and a letter from you and ten of your friends addressed to City Hall—and to the Governor, while you're at it"? The client might laugh out loud, find another medical center, dismiss the ideas, and find a new doctor or nurse who will mind her or his own business—or maybe the client will do it. What if, in the waiting room, magazines about the environment, wildlife, conservation, socially conscious companies, and alternative, environmentally kind products were available? Patients who may be subscribers could donate their old copies for others to read. What if brochures published by the city or state listing companies that will accept aluminum, glass, or paper for recycling were available at a health center? If the state's list is out of date, perhaps a local high school student club might be recruited to create a list. Can a health center facilitate a community's efforts to create quality jobs that promote, rather than relinquish, the health of the environment and hence the community's long–term economic health and the health of its residents? Is the highly political, economic nature of environmental issues a conflict of interest on behalf of the health care provider? If so, how? According to whom, and whose logic? City Hall's? The Licensing Board's? The electric company's?

The question, really, is whether and why nursing care should incorporate caring for the environment at large. Certainly it is difficult to imagine measuring the pulse of a tree or discussing its health habits; certainly other professions are more specifically dedicated to the care of tall pines and grasses and to monitoring the population of spotted owls or the "unexplained losses of amphibians around the world" (Cowen, 1990, p. 142). Nursing, on the other hand, is dedicated to health. Defined by Virginia Henderson, nursing is

> the practice in which a nurse assists the individual, sick or well, in the performance of those activities contributing to health or its recovery (or to a peaceful death) that he [or she] would perform unaided if he [or she] had the necessary strength, will, or knowledge. And to do this in such a way as to help him [or her] gain independence as rapidly as possible [cited in Urdang, 1983, p. 752].

If this is so, and if nursing, according to the American Nurses' Association, is defined as "the diagnosis and treatment of human responses to actual or potential health problems," two things call for further consideration: (a) the "activities contributing to health or its recovery" that the client "would perform if" and (b) "actual or potential health problems." Who can say what these are, the activities or the problems? Who can say what someone else would do, had she or he the strength, will, or knowledge, or what, precisely, he or she would consider to be a health problem, actual or potential? No one has the authority to say, not anybody. The nurse's professional authority rests with what the nurse has learned, with experience, skill, knowledge, observation, and personal and professional judgment. The facts are in: The environment is suffering; people are suffering; animals and fish are suffering and dying; economic booms promised to small communities by new, large industries are offset by the costs of the health hazards of working for those industries; the antibiotics fed to mass–produced chickens decrease the drugs' effectiveness in humans who eat those chickens and agribusiness puts small, family farmers out of work; the unemployed become the indigent. No one can argue infallibly that environmental issues are none of nursing's business.

Treating the client requires assessing environmental factors affecting the client, but interventions and outcomes of treatment depend also on factoring in the client's effect on environmental factors affecting the client. The outrageous prescription, then, of trying to find some fresh air is analogous to advising that a non–smoking spouse of a smoker address the issue of whether the spouse will smoke in the house. Or, to consider another example, when people changing their eating habits are advised to place foods not included in the menu behind cupboard doors, the same principle is at work. The client is advised to affect his or her personal environment because the personal environment in turn affects the client and the client's health. But this is no chicken and egg riddle at work, it is the riddle of relationships. It is called ecology.

ECOLOGICAL PRINCIPLES: PRINCIPLES OF HEALTH

Ecology is the science of the relationships between organisms and their environments, and an invaluable resource for health professionals. Within the study of ecology can be found the most complex interactions, where no one element is entirely exempt from the influence of another. In 1870 German biologist Ernst Haeckel, to whom the term is largely credited, described ecology as

> the body of knowledge concerning the economy of nature—the investigation of the total relations of the animal both to its inorganic and to its organic environment; including above all, its friendly and inimical relation with those animals and plants with which it comes directly or indirectly into contact—in a word, ecology is the study of all the complex interrelations referred to by Darwin as the conditions of the struggle for existence [Kormondy, 1969, p. pviii].

Since then, Charles Elton, a British ecologist, has described ecology as "scientific natural history" and the "sociology and economics of animals." Frederick Clements, an American plant ecologist, described ecology as "the science of the community."

"Sociology," "economics," "relationships," "community": in their more usual contexts, these words do not immediately call up visions of the animal or plant kingdoms—lions on Wall Street or grassland communities electing local, reedy officials. Rather, they are more often encountered as descriptors of society, a human phenomena. As Bookchin says, "ethics presupposes the presence of volition, the intellectual ability to conceptualize and the social ability to *institutionalize* communities, not merely to *collect* into a community. These capacities are uniquely human and deserve emphasis as such" (Bookchin, 1986, p. 10). And yet, notwithstanding the obvious differences in the application of meanings and hence the role of terminology, nor the inherent pitfalls of wholesale applications of paradigms (dangers of distortion, oversimplification, generalization, and plain inaccuracy) it is informative still that ecologists should say:

> just about everyone knows that, ultimately, *survival of the human species* depends upon all of us *understanding and obeying* the basic principles of ecology. You can learn these principles by studying a stream, a pond, a forest, or a meadow.... The importance of that dark quiet world under our feet is *indisputable* [emphases added] [Davies, Stoker, Windsor, Ashcroft, Coburn, & Andrews, 1973, p. v, 2].

The "struggle for existence" and "survival of the human species" are hefty topics, but that they should depend upon "that dark quiet world under our feet" and requires obedience, of any sort, seems ludicrous, an infringement of the rights of our species, a denial of human power and influence. But, in fact, to say such things is a recognition of such influence, an influence so fantastic as to alter genetic material, the pH of rain in most regions of the world, and the shapes of mountains. Indeed, human influence is so fantastic as to induce or discourage illness merely by changing the surrounding environment, if the environmental conditions affecting health are altered sufficiently. Florence Nightingale recognized health as a condition reflecting obedience to certain laws of cause and effect of certain conditions; the principles of ecology can be considered similarly.

Mostly, the principles of ecology involve one basic principle, interaction. Consider the world ecosystem and its most basic interactive factors, climate, soil, plants, animals, and humans:

> *Interaction* is the key word in understanding what is happening in an ecosystem. No factor is independent of the others. Therefore a change in any one factor results in changes in all the other factors that are directly or indirectly related to it. [Davies et al., 1973, p. 3]

The interactions themselves may be extremely complex, but the same kinds of interactions occur on the large and small scales. In Ray Bradbury's short story, "A Sound of Thunder," a man traveling through a time machine to a prehistoric past steps on a butterfly and with the untimely death of the butterfly changes history. The world the time travelers return to is not the world they left. Travis, the time machine travel guide, had warned the travelers not to touch so much as a blade of grass and that, should someone kill a thing so small as a mouse, parent to ten (now) unborn mice:

> For want of ten mice, a fox dies. For want of ten foxes, a lion starves. For want of a lion, all manner of insects, vultures, infinite billions of life forms are thrown into chaos and destruction. . . . Fifty–nine million years later, a caveman, one of a dozen on the entire world, goes hunting wild boar or saber–toothed tiger for food. But you, friend, have stepped on all the tigers in that region. By stepping on one single mouse. So the caveman starves. . . . He is an entire future nation. . . . With the death of that one caveman. . . . Perhaps Rome never rises on its seven hills. . . . Step on a mouse and you crush the Pyramids. . . . Who knows? Who really can say he knows? We don't know. We're guessing. But until we do know for certain whether our messing around in Time can make a big roar or a little rustle in history, we're being careful. [Bradbury, 1962, p. 60-61]

Now consider this, remembering that it was published in 1973 and that by now, 17 years later, "be able to cause" must be rephrased to "have caused":

> The human species has accumulated enough technological skill to be able to cause serious changes in the world ecosystem. One of the most important tasks now facing [hu]mankind is to learn how to predict the ultimate effect of a change in one factor in the system before an irreversible step is taken. [Davies et al., 1973, p. 6-7]

Travis, finding the butterfly in the mud on the bottom of his shoes, "glistening green and gold and black . . . very beautiful and very dead," says, "Not a little thing like that! Not a butterfly!" (Bradbury, 1962, p. 68). Meanwhile, in 1990, the protective layer of global ozone in the stratosphere "all but disappears each spring" at certain altitudes over parts of Antarctica, and "the increase in ultraviolet light is already at levels high enough to harm planktonic life in southern oceans" (Moore, 1990, p. 15). Here is the butterfly, Bradbury's (then futuristic) mouse.

In just such a manner, through such complex interactions, does illness occur, by "accumulation" of toxins, say, or "the ultimate effect of a change in one factor in the system," the failure of a kidney or liver or the unstemmed growth of a massive tumor, resulting in an "irreversible step"— chronic illness, death. It does not necessarily occur all at once, but rather is a matter of crossing that terribly significant threshold. Likewise, "the eighties in general, with 1988 in particular, could be considered as the decade when the planet struck back" (Hoffman, 1989, p. 214).

The principles of ecology are in many ways natural models of cooperation rather than competition, diversity and participation rather than an aggressive, necessity–ruled survival of the fittest. Unimpeded, nature is abundant and diversified, a rich genetic bank (Morell, 1990); impeded, promoted, altered, it responds in proportion to the degree and kind of human intervention. Twenty years ago (and surely before that), commentators were using the word "crisis" and applying cause to "the outlook of western man, in particular" which considers land and nature, the oceans and air, as

> his adversary to be conquered, as his servant to be exploited for his own ends, as a possession of rightful and eminent domain, and, most importantly, [as a] land [or sea or sky] of unlimited capacity. These concepts must give ground to an ecological conscience, to a love, respect, admiration, and understanding for the total ecosystem of which we are part; our course, otherwise, is one of collision, an inexorable Armageddon [Kormondy, 1969, p. 196].

That word, inexorable, is absolutely appropriate: "Incapable of being persuaded by treaty; unyielding," just like so many diseases contracted, progressed beyond that threshold, just like the absence that answers a rare bird's mating song.

LAWS OF ENERGY: LAWS OF HEALTH

While humans have discovered that species can be destroyed all too easily, humans have also discovered "energy" cannot be, according to the laws of thermodynamics. Whether the natural world is blossoming or dying, the manner in which "energy is changed from one form to another" is at work. The First Law of Thermodynamics states that "energy can neither be created nor destroyed, even though it may be changed from one form into another" (Nadakavukaren, 1986, p. 21). The Second Law of Thermodynamics states:

with every energy transformation there is a loss of *usable* energy (that is, energy that can be used to do work) . . . The Second Law introduces the concept of *entropy*, the idea that all energy is moving toward an ever less available and more dispersed state" [Nadakavukaren, 1986, p. 22].

Published in 1980, Jeremy Rifkin's *Entropy: A New World View* dispels the beliefs associated with the present, crumbling, mechanical world view, summarized basically as a logic concluding that "the more material well–being we amass, the more ordered the world must be getting" (Rifkin, 1980, p. 28). Rifkin explains further:

Progress, then, is the amassing of greater and greater material abundance, which is assumed to result in an ever more ordered world. Science and technology are the tools for getting the job done.

But can we call such "progress" orderly? What of the "smog" evident at the Arctic Circle as early as the 1950s? The Environmental Protection Agency indicated last year that "half the streams in the mid–Atlantic and southeastern states—areas not previously considered in the acid rain zone—were either acidic or on the verge of becoming acidic" (Hoffman, 1989, p. 214). In Madagascar, "where 80 percent of the flowering plants are species found nowhere else in the world, more than half the original forest cover has been lost or seriously degraded. . . . the rosy periwinkle [native to Madagascar] provides some of our most important anti–cancer drugs" (Morell, 1990, p. 7). Human–set fires to clear forests are so massive they can be seen from space. Why are the poor only getting poorer, and the hungry, hungrier? What, according to the Second Law, is happening?

In nature, whenever one element of an ecosystem multiplies or grows out of proportion to its proper functioning relationship with the rest of the elements in the system, it robs other life forms of the negative entropy (available energy) they need to survive. By doing so, it threatens the continued existence of the entire system. [Rifkin, 1980, p. 195]

Again, the interactions within an ecosystem could as well describe the balances of health or the debilitating effects of long–term or chronic illness on the body as an ecosystem. Temporary or minor illnesses seldom, in themselves, go so far as to alter the entire functioning relationship of organs or cells. But continue the illness over time and something else may go wrong, too, something more serious, with the body having been weakened by continued stress.

DEFINING THE PERSONAL: WHOSE HEALTH?

Rifkin applies the Law of Entropy to society as a whole:

When certain individuals or institutions capture an inordinate amount of the society's energy for themselves, their gross accumulation of wealth and power robs the rest of the members of society of the available energy they need to survive. [Rifkin, 1980, p. 195]

In a February 1990 *Close-Up Report* delineating the cruelty and waste of intensive confinement farming, "the corporate takeover of America's farms," the Human Society of the United States puts the basic idea another way: "What's good for animals is good for people" (The Humane Society of the United States, 1990). Intensively confined farm animal flesh, the report states, supporting its contention with numerous facts and examples, is neither good for animals nor for people. Peter Singer, author of *Animal Liberation*, points out

the raising of animals for food by the methods used in the industrial nations does not contribute to the solution of the hunger problem. On the contrary, it aggravates it enormously.... The food wasted by animal production in the affluent nations would be sufficient, if properly distributed, to end both hunger and malnutrition throughout the world [Singer, 1975, p. 171].

Of course, the world population of humans was somewhat less in 1975—roughly 4,103,000,000 compared with today's figure of 5,320,000,000.

Nevertheless, "saving the environment does not pit people against nature but goes hand–in–hand with improving the lot of the world's poor and downtrodden" (Carey, 1990, p. 5). There are a great many solutions to the troubles that afflict the world, many of these troubles directly attributable to the manner in which people live: As if there were no law of entropy, as if there were no ecosystem, as if there were no marginal peoples, as if the plankton will always thrive, no matter what is or is not done.

To the World Health Organization, "health is the state of complete physical, mental, and social well–being, not merely the absence of disease or infirmity" (Turshen, 1989, p. 18). To Florence Nightingale, it was an additive process, the result of a physical, environmental, and psychological process. To Rogers, both health and sickness are "expressions of the process of life" (Rogers, 1970, p. 85). And to Dubos, "health can be regarded as an expression of fitness to the environment" (Dubos, 1965, p. 350). Last, writing in *Public Health and Human Ecology*, suggests "health is a state of equilibrium between humans and the physical, biologic, and social environment, compatible with full functional activity. This definition recognizes the ecologic foundations upon which health must rest" (Last, 1987, p. 6).

Nursing care can be described by four principal characteristics:

> The phenomena that concern nurses; the use of theories to observe the need for nursing interventions and to plan nursing action; the nursing action taken; and an evaluation of the effects of the action relative to the phenomena. [Urdang, 1983, p. 752]

Environmental health is the phenomenon discussed here; the theories needed for observation and planning may be derived from ecological principles or from current practices that incorporate more commonly accepted environmental factors, and it is likely, too, that current and past nurse theorists have had much to say which is applicable. The nursing action taken can begin with the nurse and be suited to the client's or community's health concerns and interests; evaluation of effects, for example, could consider measuring the well–being of people who have something to take care of, something that depends on them.

Twenty–five years ago discourse regarding environmental problems was, as often as not, considered alarmist, but the old tale of the shepherd boy who cries "wolf" now has a new twist. Today, while the wolf ravages not only the sheep but the village itself, the water supply, the fish, the air and the land, much of the governmental, commercial, and industrial sectors continue to call for further study or, more popularly, for "balancing" industrial and environmental concerns (and the balance remains tipped far in the favor of industry and the status quo). Even so, private citizens, professionals, and organizations are helping each other to change their living and buying habits and have either continued or joined the fight against the wolf—not the mysterious and wildly legendary canine beauty, for it has receded with the wilderness, but a sad invention of our own mechanical world–making, a kind of Robo–Cop gone mad.

REFERENCES

Bookchin, M. (1986). *The modern crisis*. Philadelphia: New Society Publishers.

Bradbury, R. (1962). A sound of thunder. In *R is for rocket* (pp. 57–68). New York: Bantam.

Carey, A. (1990, March–April). Fighting to save a fragile earth. *International Wildlife*, 5.

Cowen, R. (1990). Brooding over Australian frogs. *Science News, 137*(9), 142.

Davies, N. D., Stoker, D. G., Windsor, D. E., Ashcroft, M. T., Coburn, M. C., & Andrews, W. A. (Eds.). (1973). *Contours: Studies of the environment (series). A guide to the study of soil ecology.* Englewood Cliffs, NJ: Prentice-Hall, Inc.

Dever, G. E. A., Sciegaj, M., Wade, T. E., & Lofton, T. C. (1988). Creation of a social vulnerability index for justice in health planning. *Family and Community Health, 10*(4), 23–32.

Dubos, R. (1965). *Man adapting.* New Haven: Yale University Press.

Hoffman, M. S. (Ed.). (1989). *The world almanac and book of facts 1990.* New York: Scripps Howard.

Kormondy, E. J. (1969). *Concepts of modern biology series. Concepts of ecology.* Englewood Cliffs, NJ: Prentice-Hall.

Last, J. A. (1987). *Public health and human ecology.* East Norwalk, CT: Appleton & Lange.

Moore, C. A. (1990, March–April). Fighting to save a fragile world: Atmosphere. *International Wildlife*, 14–15.

Morell, V. (1990, March–April). Fighting to save a fragile world: Rain forests. *International Wildlife*, 6–7.

Nadakavukaren, A. (1986). *Man and environment: A health perspective* (2nd ed.). Prospect Heights, IL: Waveland Press.

Rifkin, J. (1980). *Entropy: A new world view.* New York: Bantam.

Rogers, M. (1970). *Introduction to the theoretical basis of nursing.* Philadelphia: F. A. Davis.

Singer, P. (1975). *Animal liberation.* New York: Avon.

The Humane Society of the United States. (1990, February). Intensive confinement: Cruel to animals, destroyer of the environment. *Close-Up Report.*

Turshen, M. (1989). *The politics of public health.* New Brunswick, NJ: Rutgers University Press.

Urdang, L. (Ed.). (1983). *Mosby's medical and nursing dictionary.* St. Louis: C. V. Mosby.

6

Caring and Not Caring: the Question of Context

Nancy P. Greenleaf

A caring act, carried out by one person to benefit another person,. both influences and is influenced by the social context in which the act occurs. The act influences the context by validating it as a context in which caring can and does occur and thus enhancing the moral definition of the context. This in turn benefits others, connected to the context but not directly involved in the caring act itself, by giving them reason to take pride in their family, their school, their workplace or whatever defines their social context. Taking pride in the particular context occurs whether or not the caring act itself is witnessed as long as it is presumed to have happened. We may simply take it for granted that caring acts will occur and only occasionally give recognition to them. Still, we benefit in our associations with places where caring happens. Our world is made a better place.

Caring itself is influenced by the social context in two ways. First, by the expectation that caring acts will occur within that context and second, by the resources brought to support such acts. If, for instance, we establish an AIDS hospice to provide a humane place for people with AIDS who are dying, the intention is for caring acts to occur there. In fact, the expectation

Portions of this paper were presented at the Politics of Caring conference co-sponsored by the Women's Studies Department and the School of Nursing at Emory University and the Emory University Hospital Division of Nursing, in Atlanta, GA on October 12, 1990.

is so strong, so unequivocal, that it seems to be stating the obvious to even mention it. The notion of caring acts is so deeply embedded in the meaning, the intent, of *hospice*, that it usually remains unstated. The taking for granted of such caring acts, this notion that they are inherent in certain social contexts renders the acts themselves, and the people who perform them, invisible. An important characteristic of caring acts is that they are most noteworthy in their absence, when neglect, indifference or even abuse, alert us that something is missing.

Contextual resources brought to support caring acts are, on the other hand, easier to see, to count. If we establish an AIDS hospice but lack the money to pay the rent, buy the medicine, coordinate the volunteers and otherwise fail to bring moral and material support for the caring activities we expect to occur, then the enterprise will fail and the intention will be subverted. Intent is not enough. Simply stated, caring acts require material support if they are to be sustained.

Caring and not caring characterize relationships between individuals where caring is central, and poses caring acts as the principle activity of the relationship. In such relationships, not caring cannot be benign. If the expectation is to care, to take care of, to engage in caring acts, then failure to care, failure to take care of, omission of necessary caring acts constitutes indifference or neglect. When caring is embedded as an unspoken but clearly present expectation of gender role, as in, men make—women take care, the potential for not caring is vast, and women may be automatically indicted. No wonder the fantasy to go out on strike is so pervasive among feminists. No wonder the dynamics of caring and the politics of caring are of such vital interest to women.

For this analysis, it is important to distinguish between a single caring act, and sustaining caring acts and attitudes throughout relationships over time. The single caring act, or even a caring attitude, may be considered and analyzed in isolation, but I will argue that such an analysis has limited value for understanding sustained caring. Sustained caring cannot be adequately understood apart from the social context.

The politics of caring, then, are best understood when the relation between caring acts, and the contexts in which they occur is clear. Caring acts have an influence on their social context and are influenced by them. Furthermore, the relation is not an equal one. Caring acts can enhance, or by their absence diminish the moral definition of the context. They can make the context, and thus the world, a better place or a meaner place. The social context on the other hand, must provide the necessary supports if caring acts are to be sustained. If the social context establishes an intent for caring acts to occur but fails to provide the necessary resources to sustain them, caring will fail in spite of the most heroic efforts of individuals to sustain it alone. It is easy to imagine how individuals may then be held responsible for the failure of caring even when the breakdown is in the supportive system or context. The potential for, and some would say actual, scapegoating of women—who perform most of the caring acts—for system failure is great.

Failure to recognize the relation between caring acts and their social context keeps hidden from view the civilizing contributions of caring. It keeps hidden the power that caring has for altering not just the reality for individuals within the caring act itself, "the caring one" and "the cared for" in Noddings' (1984) terms, but also to alter the meaning of the context, and the world beyond it by making them more humane.

Tronto addresses the need for a contextual theory of care, stating that "[a]s a fully developed moral theory, the ethic of care will take the form of a contextual moral theory" (1987, p. 658). Contextual moral theories move the central questions away from a centrality of universal moral principle and rather ask "How will individuals best be equipped to act morally" (1987, p. 657). She argues convincingly that the ethic of care is dependent on the adequacy of the social and political theory in which it is embedded.

The purpose of this paper is to analyze the relationship between caring acts and the contexts in which they occur. The analysis will be limited to employment situations where carework is the socialized expression of caring. The term carework is used here to emphasize that caring acts, performed in the context of a job, require physical, mental, and emotional labor that takes up time. Carework carries with it a contract that calls up standards of care and holds the worker accountable for maintaining these standards.

CARING AND CAREWORK–DEFINITIONAL AMBIGUITIES

Inherent in the idea of caring is an inclination toward other. What is important is that the other matters and holds one's attention whether the inclination is perceived as a burden, a care, love or joy. The opposite of a caring attitude is one of indifference, the opposite of a caring act is neglect. Graham notes that the definition of caring carries with it distinct, though overlapping, dualities of psychological and material; of identity and activity; of love and labor (1983). Pulling apart these dualities or meaning clusters helps locate and clarify ambiguities that confound the work of caring, including its temporal qualities and its attitudinal expectations, with a person's more private or intimate experiences. Caring is different at home than at work. Caring relations in families are ongoing, in the work setting they are limited, more proscribed. This does not mean that the demands of caring in employment do not impinge on the private realm. Hochschild (1983) describes the estrangement from self that results when jobs demand emotional labor; acting *as if* one cares deeply for clients or customers as one would care for family or friends. This type of job expectation that requires deep acting, and conflates the private and public realms of caring is particularly exploitive. It asks the worker to care for the stranger as if the stranger were his or her own.

Carework refers to the work entailed in caring as it has been socialized and brought into the realm of paid labor. Although meant as a generic construct to refer to human service work, examples will be drawn from the field of nursing work. Although variation in skill is recognized in nursing work, no distinction of skill level is made here. What is important for this discussion is the work entailed in caring, carework performed for compensation and in the context of a job.

Socialized caring capitalizes on an impulse to care for others that arises out of family experiences. It relies on this impulse to carry out the social intent of corporations established to provide care. That carework has become socialized (Caplan 1989)—is bought and sold in the marketplace along with other commodities—is readily apparent in such terms as health care provider, medical care, custodial care, nursing care, intensive care, long-term care, skilled care, and even in the bald, market substitutes of self–care and family–care. From the affective realm we meet with feelings and concerns, attitudes toward, compassion for, causes for anxiety, suffering of mind, regard and esteem, solicitude and worry. All imply responsibility toward another. Carework does not dismiss the affective aspects, rather it incorporates them, counts on them. To provide effective nursing care for instance, the nurse must attend to the needs and responses of the other, while at the same time helping the other, doing for him or her those things he or she would do if able.

Carework in nursing combines doing, which takes time, as in feeding a patient who cannot otherwise eat, moving a person who is immobile, washing a patient who cannot otherwise be cleansed, while at the same time attending to the responses of each person both to these activities as well as his or her responses to the actions of medications, medical and nursing treatments, disease processes within his or her body, and all other internal and external impositions on the person. In addition, the careworker needs time to listen, to focus, and to reflect on the assessment of the situation and effectiveness of his or her activities—to teach.

The magnitude and complexity of expert carework, or caring practice as described by Benner & Wrubel (1989) on the one hand, is countered by the invisibility of the work and the workers on the other (Fagin, 1987). Carework is most noticed when it is absent. We are more apt to see the results of neglect than the results of carework. Carework, unnoticed, is taken for granted. It's what the careworker is paid for—even if that pay in no way reflects the expertise or effort.

Nowhere does the specification, the measurement of carework get more attention than in the organization that manages, that buys and sells it. It is in the act of measuring and quantifying carework that the definitional ambiguities become most apparent. The flaw in the quantification effort that focuses on behavioral tasks, measuring them by the level of skill required to perform them and the duration of effort required for each task, is two–fold. First is the impossibility in capturing the essence of *attention–toward* in a time dimension, and its consequent dismissal. If it can't be timed, it doesn't count and thus cannot be counted. Secondly, tasks by themselves fail to take into account the planning and evaluating that require assessment and reflection and that also take time and focus. When employers fail to account for a particular essential aspect of carework, the worker is placed in a position of needing to compensate for the omission by grabbing or stealing time from here or there to stop and listen, to focus, to attend to, to teach. Nurses in a study done by Foshay (1988) noted that patient classification systems used by their hospitals to measure their work, failed to include what they themselves considered *caring*. Foshay characterizes the stealing or grabbing of time from here and there as the hospital's means of extracting surplus value from the nurses. When the stealing of time is impossible, then carework fails altogether—for both the caring one and the cared for. The result is, in Noddings' words, a diminished "ethical ideal of the one caring" (1984, p. 81) and disappointment, neglect, or even abandonment for the cared for. Such partial accounting for carework erodes the caring ideal of the worker, cheats the cared for, and subverts the intent of the social context.

SOCIAL VALUE OF CARING—THE CONTEXT

If we think of caring and caring acts as attitudes and activities of individuals, then the notion of a caring society or a caring context—community, school, hospital—is at best, a metaphor. The question is not how does society care? but, as Tronto (1987) suggests, how can society best equip individuals to act morally? What conditions are necessary to support caring acts? What resources must be brought to create a context where caring may occur? Caring, for society, is not just a matter of value in its immaterial sense. Rather, it is a matter of actual material valuing that is called for to *equip* individuals to do carework. To provide carework, workers need access to a potential cared–for and also space, beds, blankets, medicines, bandages, food, crutches, soap, water, and any number of specialized items as well as time. When Reverby says nurses are "order[ed] to care in a society that does not value caring," (1987, p. 5) she doesn't mean people think caring isn't, in itself, important, or that it isn't noticed in its absence as neglect. Rather, she indicts a society that fails to *equip* careworkers, to allocate them the necessary resources to do carework.

For the purpose of this analysis, the context is defined as the social enterprise in which carework is provided. The simple distinction is made between the supportive context, that is, the context that does provide the resources necessary for the provision of carework and the non-supportive context, where necessary resources for the provision of carework are lacking or insufficient. Present in both contexts is the expectation that carework will take place. This distinction is, admittedly, artificial. It is most likely the case that a particular context may in fact provide the necessary resources at one moment and fail to provide them at another. Also, the assumption that the immediate social context, that is, the organization or employer, is in and of itself responsible for provision of resources, is used to simplify analysis. It is recognized that the context, in this sense, may also be dependent on a larger context. These realities complicate indictment, but must not be dismissed or allowed to obscure the relationship between caring acts and their contexts.

The caring and not caring of individual careworkers is next examined in terms of supportive and non-supportive contexts. The emphasis is on the relationship between the social context and the individuals engaged in caring acts.

CARING AND NOT CARING IN SUPPORTIVE AND NON-SUPPORTIVE CONTEXTS

The following matrix has been developed to aid the analysis.

CONTEXT	CARING	NOT CARING
SUPPORTIVE	A	B
NON-SUPPORTIVE	C	D

In cell A, carework is provided to those in need of care in a context that furnishes the necessary resources. Carework here succeeds as expected. If an accident occurs and a patient is inadvertently harmed, we assume that the cause was not due to the actions or inactions of the careworker. The main issue here is that when things work the way they are intended, the whole business is enhanced: we think, "that's a good hospital" or "a high quality facility." Credit for such quality or goodness is most often given to physicians or administrators, the actual carework entailed remains invisible.

In cell B, the context is supportive of caring, but caring fails because the careworker does not provide care as expected. A classic example of this is the night nurse who falls asleep on the job. Harm may or may not befall a neglected patient, depending on the situation, but if it does, it is a clear case of breach of duty by the careworker.

The liability of careworkers becomes an issue in our legal system which may ignore the need for a supportive context. The danger is that careworkers may in fact be scapegoated for system failures. Having said that, it is also true that careworkers may be negligent or show deliberate indifference to needs of those in their care. In Mitler vs. Beorn (1990) an inmate of the Virginia Correctional Center for Women with a known history of angina was repeatedly sent back to her dormitory room by the clinic nurse when she presented herself with complaints of chest pain, dizzyness, weakness, and headaches. Finally the inmate was admitted to the clinic and the doctor notified. He ordered a tranquilizer and observation. Six hours later she was found dead on the floor by her bed. The finding against the nurse was "deliberate indifference." This case turned on the nurse's failure to take the inmate's complaints seriously, to diagnose the implications of the presenting symptoms, and to communicate the same to the physician.

In Phillips vs. Eastern Maine Medical Center (1990), a case with similar implications, a recovery room nurse failed to respond immediately to symptoms of wheezing and pain experienced by a postoperative patient who had had esophageal surgery. The nurse's failure to understand the symptoms as indicative of an esophageal tear and to immediately notify the surgeon delayed treatment. The patient suffered massive infection and subsequently died.

These two cases, used here to illustrate careworker negligence are also interesting in their demonstration of the relationship of carework to medical work; of nurses to physicians. They contradict the conventional notion that physicians diagnose and tell nurses what to do. Here, nurses are held accountable for failure to diagnose the seriousness of presenting symptoms, and to communicate their urgency to the physician.

In cell C we have a situation where the careworker attempts to care but the context is non-supportive to caring. In such a case the worker may be overwhelmed by too many demands, too many patients, have insufficient or faulty equipment, or lack support staff to do housekeeping work. Harm to those dependent on care, the cared–for, may well occur. In cases that fall into this cell, careworkers may be held accountable for negligence by the courts, in spite of how we might judge them here.

To care, or attempt to provide carework in a non–supportive context invites despair. The caring ideal of the one caring is diminished and the well–being of the cared–for is endangered. The legal system, reflecting ideologies of the dominate culture, has placed careworkers—who are mostly women—into incredible binds. Nor have the courts managed to sort out issues of accountability between careworkers and their employers. Holding careworkers accountable for failures to provide adequate support for carework—whether such holding occurs in the courtroom or simply in the minds of employers and employees themselves—makes the world a meaner place.

The binds are real. For instance, a nurse is told she must not leave her duty post until the relief nurse arrives. If the relief nurse fails to arrive, she must stay, must not abandon the patients. This same nurse is, by being held past her time on duty, forced to abandon her own children for whom she had provided care until the end of her shift but no longer. This is not a choice—this is a bind. Records of an arbitration finding in a case brought against a hospital by a union (Massachusetts Nurses Assoc. vs. St. Elizabeths, 1980) describe a bind that nurses often face. In this case, an intensive care nurse reported on duty to find she was the only person there to take care of patients when there should have been five. Her repeated attempts to get hospital administration to send help failed. All patients on the unit were critically ill, and there was no possible way that she alone could provide adequate care for them. During the course of her shift, one patient died and another had to be resuscitated twice. For this nurse to leave the situation would have been abandonment and clear disaster for the patients, to stay in the situation she must witness neglect. Here she must choose between the lesser of two bad situations. Her choice was to stay and later file a grievance with the union against the hospital. The arbitrator's finding sustained the grievance and ordered the hospital to develop special procedures for staffing intensive care units. The recurrence of short staffing in hospitals and nursing homes where a great deal of carework is provided makes one wonder if such findings have much effect on assuring the resources to sustain caring activities in institutions whose intent is to provide care.

Cell D, the situation of a non–caring worker in a non–supportive context, so distorts the notion of caring, of civilization, that we are compelled to look away. We picture Romanian orphans neglected and abused by a corrupt regime and apparently attended by non–caring workers. But what's wrong with this picture? Is it even possible to think that workers could care in such a context?

Consider for instance Timerman's (1981) description of the corruption of caring language used by the physician who attends him during torture. "I'm your friend," says the physician, "the one who takes care of you when they apply the machine" (p. 54).

Who among the careworkers should we indict? The Romanian attendants in the orphanage or the physician colleague of torturers?

More importantly, the danger in using non–caring extremes such as those above allows us to remain blind to more subtle extremes in our own culture that we participate in, however unconsciously. For instance, our high–tech tertiary care health system is governed in no small way by a right to life ideology. This emphasis on rights inhibits true caring. It replaces caring about the quality of life with the imperative to save life. This imperative casts careworkers, however reluctantly or unintentionally into roles and behaviors not unlike torturers.

So the old woman who has lost most of her memory, her home, her freedom to take laxatives when she wants to, or have a small glass of sherry in the evening before she retires; who has lost her friends and lifetime companions, her sense of usefulness to herself and others, is forced to see a psychiatrist when she expresses a wish to die. She is rushed in an ambulance to the emergency where she must sit in a straight chair for three hours before she is seen because she refuses to eat; has gone on a hunger strike. She is chided for feeling depressed, cajoled into false cheerfulness. Here the missing resource is our will to focus away from the "right to life" and toward a more humane and caring attitude toward life as it ebbs. It is not hyperbole to liken the consequence of this lack of will to torture.

SUMMARY

The intent of this analysis, this placing of caring and not caring side by side to supportive and non–supportive contexts is to make more visible the policy implications for the social value of caring and to suggest a grounding for feminist social philosophy in the practical activities of carework. It is critical that we make more visible the expectations and indictments of women in their socially constructed roles of menders and tenders.

INTELLECTUAL AND POLITICAL WORK
ON NURSING AND CARING

Increasing attention to caring in the nursing literature shows its description and analysis to be a major intellectual project within the field. Although there has been attention to the care concept for some time, especially by the work of Leininger (1980) and the transcultural movement in nursing, the last decade has shown a remarkable increase in attention. The works of Watson (1985, 1988), Benner (1984), Benner & Wrubel (1989), Bevis & Watson (1989), Wheeler & Chinn (1989), Moccia (1988), MacPherson (1988), and others have developed and criticized the concept of caring with an enormous impact on nursing and nursing education.

There also has been attention paid to the politics of caring from within nursing. "Nursing: The Politics of Caring," is the title of a film (Ilex Films, 1978) exploring nursing work, nursing image, medical dominance, collective bargaining, and other political actions of nurses. An entire issue of the topical journal, *Advances in Nursing Science* (1980) was devoted to the "Politics of Care." The collective bargaining movement within nursing has consistently addressed political issues in caring. Recently, a group calling themselves Nurses for Progressive Social Change claimed, as part of their statement of purpose, " . . . that society is at a faultline where trends and forces that have shaped contemporary life can neither sustain or nurture individuals or civilization." Further, this faultline may be seen " . . . in nursing, where the intensified exploitation of a female labor force renders caring impossible" (Nurses for Progressive Social Change, 1987). Moccia (1988) gives an excellent analysis of this crisis in caring and challenges nurses to include social activism in their definition of caring.

CONCLUSION

The central themes emerging from this analysis are the civilizing characteristic of caring acts, their ability to make the world a more decent place, and the invisibility of caring and carework. Noticed only in its absence, caring is not recognized for its contribution to civilization.

Work, as defined by Arendt (1958), refers to the production of material artifacts and excludes carework—the production of service for people. According to Arendt, carework is seen as labor, distinct from work or political activity. Labor is tending to the body or life's necessities, and was seen by the ancient Greeks as embarrassing, something citizens should be freed from. Labor was for beasts of burden, slaves, and women. Freed from such necessity, men could make real artifacts, do real work, create a civilization.

In the 1844 manuscripts, Marx focused on the production of material goods in analyzing work or the labor process. For Marx, such material production creates community, mediates between people, and, significantly, creates civilization (McClellan, 1975) He doesn't say much about caring, or the work involved therein except as it is relegated to the domestic sphere and ignored rather than analyzed.

Scarry (1985) vividly describes how torture deconstructs civilization by creating pain which takes away artifacts such as language and ideas and turns material artifacts into weapons. Still, when Scarry turns her attention toward constructing civilization, she, like Marx, focuses on the production of artifact, the creation by human effort of something else— something that stands outside of persons.

Human effort that provides comfort for another person, that brings another out of pain or helps bear the burden of that pain, that heals—is invisible and unrecognized in Scarry's discussion about making the world. In a modern university of the late 20th century, I found myself, as dean of a nursing school, wondering why it seemed that the school's accomplishments were ignored; why our struggle for recognition and resources seemed so constant, so demeaning; why I so often felt like nursing was an embarrassment to others in the university. It certainly was not because of our academic record. Our students were among those with the highest grade point averages in the university, often captured the top academic awards at graduation, were among the outstanding leaders on campus. The answer is very connected, I'm sure, to the fact that the school is seen as a woman's place and represents carework.

It seems that in 20th century America carework is as despised as it was for the ancient Greeks. What is it that makes the work entailed with tending to the biological needs of others so embarrassing; so overlooked as work even as it is praised and sentimentalized? Why is Mother Teresa so beloved while millions of other women who daily care for others amidst squalor are ignored? Why is it that social theories are predicated on a definition of work as the creation of material artifact? Why is a description of the work of tending and mending so completely absent from the construct civilization?

The feminist project called for here requires that we act as if carework counts, as if caring matters—for if it really matters, it must be supported. We need a feminist theory of civilization that counts, and accounts for, caring and the work it entails.

REFERENCES

Arendt, H. (1958). *The human condition.* Chicago: University of Chicago Press.

Benner, P. (1984). *From novice to expert: Excellence and power in clinical nursing practice.* Menlo Park, CA: Addison-Wesley.

Benner, P., & Wrubel, J. (1989). *The primacy of caring: Stress and coping in health and illness.* Menlo Park, CA: Addison-Wesley.

Bevis, E. O., & Watson, J. (1989). *Toward a caring curriculum: A new pedagogy for nursing.* New York: National League for Nursing.

Caplan, R. L. (1989). The commodification of American health care. *Social Science and Medicine, 28*(11), 1139–1148.

Chinn, P. L. (Ed.). (1980). Politics of care. Advances in Nursing Science, 2(3), entire edition.

Fagin, C. M. (1987). The visible problem of an "invisible" profession: The crisis and challenge for nursing. *Inquiry, 24,* 119–126.

Foshay, M. (1988). Professional nurses' perception of their caring activities and their perspectives of the ability of patient classification systems to measure their caring activities. (Master's Thesis, University of Southern Maine School of Nursing).

Graham, H. (1983). Caring: A labour of love. In J. Finch & D. Groves (Eds.). *A labour of love: Women work and caring.* London: Routledge & Kegan Paul.

Hochschild, A. R. (1983). *The managed heart: Commercialization of human feeling.* Berkeley, CA: University of California Press.

Ilex Films. (1978). *Nursing: The politics of caring.* Cambridge, MA.

Leininger, M. (1980). Caring: A central focus for nursing and health care services. *Nursing and Health care, 1*(3), 135–143, 176.

Massachusetts Nurses Association vs. St. Elizabeths. (1980). Brief on behalf of MA Nurses Association on case no. 1130–2066–79, Wm. J. Fallon, Arbitrator.

MacPherson, K. I. (1988). Looking at caring and nursing through a feminist lens. Address presented at the University of Colorado Science Center, School of Nursing, Center for Caring.

McClellan, D. (1975). *Karl Marx.* New York: Viking.

Mitler vs. Beorn. (1990). Deliberate indifference: Civil rights issue. *The Regan Report on Nursing Law, 30*(2), 1.

Moccia, P. (1988). At the faultline: Social activism and caring. *Nursing Outlook, 36*(1), 30–33.

Noddings, N. (1984). *Caring: A feminine approach to ethics and moral development.* St. Louis, MO: Mosby.

Nurses for Progressive Social Change. (1987). Statement of purpose. Breckinridge Conference Center, York, ME.

Phillips vs. Eastern Maine Medical Center. (1990). Delay in detecting esophageal tear: Death. *The Regan Report on Nursing Law, 30*(9), 4.

Reverby, S. (1987). A caring dilemma: Womenhood and nursing in historical perspective. *Nursing Research, 36*(1), 5–11.

Scarry, E. (1985). *The body in pain: The making and unmaking of the world.* New York: Oxford University Press.

Timerman, J. (1981). *Prisoner without a name, cell without a number.* New York: Knopf.

Tronto, J. (1987). Beyond gender difference to a theory of care. *Signs, 12*(4), 644–663.

Watson, J. (1985). *Nursing: Human science and human care.* New York: Appleton-Century-Crofts.

Watson, J. (1988). Of nurses, women and the devaluation of caring. *Medical Humanities Review,* 2(2), 60–62.

Wheeler, C. E., & Chinn, P. L. (1989). *Peace and power: A Handbook of feminist process* (2nd ed.). New York: National League for Nursing.

7

Caring Conceptualized for Community Nursing Practice: Beyond Caring for Individuals

M. Patrice McCarthy, Carol Craig,
Linda Bergstrom, Elizabeth M. Whitley,
Martha H. Stoner, and Joan K. Magilvy

Caring, as it is currently conceptualized, is inadequate for nursing in relation to the growing awareness of global interconnectedness. Caring has been conceptualized primarily as occurring between individuals. Strong support exists in the literature for caring to take on an individual focus in theory, practice, and research (Gaut, 1983; Noddings, 1984; Watson, 1985). Rich concept analysis and theoretical work on caring have informed nursing practice at the individual level; however, nursing practice extends to the community and global level. To accomplish this extension, further exploration of the paradigm concepts: person, environment, health, and nursing, is indicated. In this paper, the concept of person is expressed as community. Emphasis is placed on environment being integral to the health of a community. Further, environment is viewed by the authors as a client of nursing care as well as a physical, social, and political setting for practice. The authors propose that caring serves as the exemplar for nursing—the interactive mode that relates the other three concepts of the paradigm. The purpose of this paper is to explicate the concept of caring at the community level and to illustrate how this conceptualization may occur in and influence nursing practice. Selected paradigm concepts will be examined in turn, followed by examples of how knowledge gained in this examination could inform nursing practice.

CARING: THE COMMUNITY AS CLIENT

Historically, the idea of person in the paradigm has been translated to mean a single person or perhaps a small group such as a family. Schultz (1987) argues for extending the concept of person to include "pluralities of persons." She distinguishes between aggregates and pluralities based on the idea that aggregates lack the "person qualities of any collectivity of humans" (p. 78). A plurality of persons is more than those individuals with common characteristics, such as aggregates of young mothers or people with cancer. Pluralities of persons could be used to designate the clients of nursing practice in the community.

Interaction between people is a key concept that forms the foundation for the conceptualization of person (Schultz, 1987). Meleis (1985) also identifies interaction as an important defining concept in nursing. Schultz (1987) further emphasizes that while interaction is possible in communities, organizations, and groups, it is not necessarily present in all pluralities. Although both pluralities and communities could be viewed as clients of nursing, Schultz states that for the meaning of these groups to be "compatible with the meaning of person as defined in the nursing literature, the idea of a multidimensional, interactional whole must be present" (p. 78). A major premise of this paper, then, is that the basic paradigm concept of person be extended to mean groups of persons such as communities, and further, that this extension imply the naming of community as a client of nursing care. The naming of community as a client of nursing has been debated over the last several decades.

In the Division of Nursing sponsored Consensus Conference (1985), representatives from several major nursing and public health organizations grappled with the definition of the terms public health nursing and community health nursing. While some consensus was achieved, the definitions derived at the conference did little to advance nursing's understanding of community as client. The authors have elected to use the term public health nursing because it more closely approximates the position of the authors that community is the client. Research in community health has been limited by nursing's focus on community as the setting of practice rather than the community as client. This perception has limited nursing's ability to conduct theoretically based research that goes beyond population assessment or program planning (Sills & Goeppinger, 1985).

For the practice of public health nursing to progress, the paradigmatic concept of person must be extended to the community and even global perspective. Such a perspective could embrace a concept of client that includes a small town or rural community, a large urban center, nations, or even the world as a community. Interaction occurs in these geographically based communities through activities such as conduct of commerce, communication through mass media, and delivery of health care services. Interaction may not always be visible or voiced in these larger communities. Attitudes and practices that affect the lives and health of community members may represent interaction just as laws and policies might constrain or enhance community life and health.

Interaction can also serve as an essential component of non-geographically based communities; these communities might be underserved populations named as the client of nursing care. Non–place communities are recognized as the vulnerable populations that become the focus of community health nursing practice. Migrant workers and their families are communities in transit. Homeless persons, medically indigent individuals and families, young parents and their babies, and persons living with AIDS are examples of non–place communities that command attention and intervention strategies in public health nursing practice.

One of the earliest nursing theorists stressing interaction was Peplau (1952). However, interaction was then and remains today focused on the uniqueness of the particular people involved in a given situation. In the literature of public health nursing, interaction between nurses and families or small groups has received considerable attention. However, the notion of a nurse's interaction with an entire community is only beginning to be recognized (Williams, 1977; Goeppinger, 1984; Marchione, 1986). Interaction as a caring intervention with communities is even less well explored. More work in this area of community–nurse interaction is indicated; this paper represents a beginning exploration of these ideas.

When community is viewed in the traditional sense as the setting in which nursing care is delivered, nurses are primarily involved in providing care to individuals and small groups. The question to be addressed in this paper is "Can a nurse interact in a caring manner when the community itself is the client of care instead of the setting for care?" Interaction is generally considered a communication act that occurs between two individuals. However, in the case of community, the concept of interaction needs to be extended to a broader perspective. Although the nature of communication varies, communities do communicate. For example, spokespersons may be used to tell others about a town's history, customs, and resources. Newspapers contain information about government, recreation, housing, employment, and politics. Billboards communicate lifestyles. Town meetings promote interaction among residents and others with a vested interest in the community. All of these examples are observable communication and interaction patterns at the community level.

Patterns of communication can provide critical information about community interaction. If nurses are to intervene with a community as a client, we must recognize patterns of interaction and analyze their association with the health of the community. For example, in a community in which drug traffic and associated crime are prevalent, residents may be isolated as a result of fear. This isolation disrupts interaction among residents and thus further hinders community problem solving.

The public health nurse's awareness of these interaction patterns facilitates alternative approaches to interventions aimed at promoting health. Community meetings might be held at schools or churches, convened by a partnership of public health and school nurses and community residents. Strategies for making the community safe and healthy might be identified by those in attendance. Communication of these strategies might then take place through school newsletters, church bulletins, fliers, and the local media.

In summary, the paradigm concept of person should be extended beyond individuals and families to include pluralities of persons in interaction, such as communities. The notion of a broadly defined geographic or non–place community as client is compatible with this redefinition of person. Nursing intervention with the community level of client involves recognition of patterns of interaction that affect the health of the community.

CARING: THE ENVIRONMENT AND COMMUNITY

Currently, the paradigm concept of environment is considered to be merely the setting where nursing care happens and where people live. Chopoorian (1986) discusses the inadequacy of this conceptualization, especially when environment is viewed as if it were a static reality with a comparatively small impact on the health of the persons in the community. Through her analysis, she concludes that considering the environment as "setting" means that "the sphere for enactment of the nursing role is individualized, to a degree privatized, and situationally or institutionally oriented . . . as a result the social, political or economic world in which the person is an actor . . . has not been the focus of attention or conceptualized as a field, as a panorama for intervention and action by nurses" (p. 45). Persistent allegiance to the conceptualization of environment as static ignores current knowledge about the impact of the environment on health as well as the impact of communities on the environment. In this paper, the authors propose that the environment itself can also be identified as a client of public health nursing.

When the focus is on the environment as client, the public health nurse considers the environment as an entity that must be cared for in order to promote health. An example of this kind of caring can be found in cultural practices of some Native Americans. Decisions that affect the tribe are understood to affect the environment, and all decisions are made with a reverence for the gifts of the land so that the environment is given the same care as the tribe (Hobday, 1981). If the tribe were a community level client of nursing, interaction with tribal members would entail caring directed toward the environment, as well as the community, because of the regard for the environment as an integral part of the community.

A public health nurse might care for the environment by opposing the development of a strip mine because it is detrimental to the health of the environment., not just because the mine might be a potential source of ill health for community residents. This example illustrates a relevant point related to community caring. A definition of community as client should include the understanding that communities extend in time and include traditions and histories of persons who are no longer alive as well as those people yet to come. Caring for the environment of a community entails caring for the health of future generations by caring for the place where they will live and attending to the resources they will need.

The environment is not just the natural world but includes social, political, and economic realities. Attention to the social environment includes identification of caring actions which enable the development of political and economic health in community life. Caring for the social environment would require heeding the patterns of social interaction that reflect on the community as a whole.

An example related to the social and political environment is a public health nurse who works in a community known for its tourist-based economy. The nurse might work with community leaders and citizens to promote fundraising (or taxation) to improve the water treatment facilities and ensure water safety. This environmentally related caring action would not only affect the physical health of the community but also contribute to the economic well–being of the community by assuring continued tourist dollars. Another example of caring actions that facilitate political, economic, and social health in community life is the response of one state to the Institute of Medicine's (1988) report on the future of public health. The State of Colorado recently held a multidisciplinary conference to address critical issues about the future of public health in the state. Nurses from a variety of practice settings played a key role in developing health policy and planning strategies to improve the health of the state as a community. There may, however, be competing perceptions of what constitutes health across the political, social, and economic dimensions of a community.

CARING: COMMUNITY HEALTH

Health, another major paradigm concept, is conceptualized in this paper as the health of communities. Nurses cannot practice public health nursing without identifying what constitutes "health" for a particular community. Community health has been defined by Goeppinger & Schuster (1988) as product (quantitative measures of morbidity and mortality), as structure (services, resources, and utilization patterns) and, in the most modern definition, as process (functioning and problem solving). Process-based definitions have concentrated on the idea of community "competence." A competent, and therefore healthy, community is one that is self-aware, communicates effectively, has high participation from members, and manages conflict between members and the larger society (Spradley, 1985; Newman, 1986). Interaction and communication as described earlier are integral to the community competence approach to community health.

Caution needs to be exercised in relation to the definition of health, however, as the standards of healthy practice demonstrated by communities may be different across communities. For example, two communities may approach services for older adults in very different ways. One community may decide to use a senior center to house activities such as socialization, meal programs, and other recreation and health services. The center is well used and seen as an important asset by the older population. In another community, older adults are so well integrated into community life that they would object to the provision of a facility "just for seniors." In each community, the standards of health for the older population are determined by the values and norms of the community.

Community competence is remarkably similar to a definition of community health based on Newman's (1986) theory of health as expanding consciousness (Marchione, 1986). Newman defines consciousness as "the informational capacity of the system: the capacity of the system to interact with its environment" (p. 33). In Marchione's (1986) definition of community health, health is understood as a pattern of the whole. Expansion of Newman's theory to the community level implies that the health of the community is expressed as an explicate pattern of an implicate order. In other words, what is seen externally (explicit order) is a reflection of the underlying (implicate pattern) values and beliefs held by the community. A behavior pattern within a community, such as drug abuse with no efforts toward addressing the problem, would be an expression of an implicate pattern and would be reflective of its values about having a drug free community. This behavior pattern would serve as one of many possible indicators of the health of a community.

Conversely, a community in which relationships are reflective of expanding consciousness might be identified as a healthy community. The healthy community has an increased awareness of relatedness between members, effective communication, and adequate means for dealing with problems (Marchione, 1986). This community might approach the drug abuse problem with multiple interventions demonstrating networking from diverse elements of the community, such as: schools, judicial system, health agencies, churches, and businesses.

Community health as expanded consciousness enables exploration of patterns of community expression that are unique to that community. Discovery of rhythmic patterns of energy exchange, communication, relational style, and the manner in which knowledge is incorporated into the community provides a foundation for understanding the unique nature of a community (Newman, 1986). Through a connection with underlying patterns, a discovery of meaning, values, and relational processes can be articulated and used to expand the repertoire of responses available for, and necessary to, the dynamic evolution of community health.

Increasing consciousness, as an indicator of health, becomes the task of the nurse who practices with a community as the client. The challenge for nursing is to expand community consciousness (improve community health) through caring on a community level. Caring requires that nurses practice in a collegial, reciprocal manner. The identification of health problems, therefore, is accomplished by the nurse and community engaged in dialogue. The values expressed through the community's patterns may then be discovered and explored for their health implications.

In summary, the focus for practice will be the use of nursing expertise to: (1) study the explicate pattern of community health and bring it to the community's awareness; (2) assist in facilitating communication; (3) encourage participation in community processes; (4) promote effective interaction and change within the larger community environment; and (5) facilitate effective problem solving.

One example of a caring nursing intervention to improve the health of the community as client is a series of community analysis studies conducted by the University of Colorado Health Sciences Center School of Nursing graduate program in community health nursing. Each year, students and faculty conduct Project GENESIS, a combined ethnographic and epidemiological community analysis of a rural community or population group within a community (Magilvy, McMahon, Bachman, Roark, & Evenson, 1987; Magilvy, 1987; Schultz & Magilvy, 1988). Patterns of risk factors, strengths, needs, and values influencing community health are explored. The qualitative methodology facilitates assessment of multiple variables influencing health: environment, politics, socioeconomic, communication, health care resources, and other factors from the perspective of community members and nurses working collaboratively on the study. The resulting recommendations developed by the research team in interaction with the community provide a foundation on which to plan future health programs.

A second example of nursing intervention at the community level relates to a non–place community of persons living with AIDS. Nurses initiated a project to enhance the overall health of this community and meet some of the community–identified needs. The Denver Nursing Project for Human Caring is a cooperative effort of four institutions that provides a home–like setting for socialization, group support, and access to medical treatments without requiring hospitalization. Strong community involvement exists in the Nursing Project; all plans and activities are jointly determined by the nurses and the community members.

CONCLUSION

Recognition that the client of nursing care lies beyond the individual, family, and small group is essential as the world becomes a community. Similarly, the environment is identified as a client beyond the context within which nursing takes place. The effectiveness of caring, and the visibility of nursing in the community arena, is enhanced by nurses entering into a partnership with community members, thereby empowering the community to make changes in patterns that promote its overall health.

REFERENCES

Chopoorian, T. J. (1986). Reconceptualizing the environment. In P. Moccia (Ed.), *New approaches to theory development* (pp. 39–54). New York, National League for Nursing.

Committee for the Study of the Future of Public Health, Division of Health Care Services, Institute of Medicine. (1988). *The future of public health.* Washington, DC: National Academy Press.

U.S. Public Health Service, Department of Health and Human Services. (1985). *Consensus conference on the essentials of public health nursing practice and education.* Rockville, MD: Author.

Gaut, D. (1983). Development of a theoretically adequate description of caring. *Journal of Nursing Research, 5*(4), 313–324.

Goeppinger, J. (1984). Community as client: Using the nursing process to promote health. In M. Stanhope & J. Lancaster (Eds.), *Community health nursing: Process and practice for promoting health* (pp. 317–404). St. Louis: C. V. Mosby.

Geoppinger, J., & Schuster, G. (1988). Community as client: Using the nursing process to promote health. In M. Stanhope & J. Lancaster (Eds.), *Community Health Nursing.* St. Louis: C. V. Mosby.

Hobday, M. J. (1981). Seeking a moist heart: Native American ways for helping the spirit. In Matthew Fox (Ed.), *Western spirituality: Historical roots, ecumenical routes* (pp. 317–329). Santa Fe: Bear & Co.

Magilvy, J. K., McMahon, M., Bachman, M., Roark, S., & Evenson, C. (1987). The health of teenagers: A focused ethnographic study. *Public Health Nursing, 4*(1), 35–42.

Magilvy, J. K. (1987). Health of adolescents: Research in school health. *Issues in Comprehensive Pediatric Nursing, 10*(5–6), 291–302.

Marchione, J. M. (1986). Application of the new paradigm of health to individuals, families and communities. In M. A. Newman, *Health as expanded consciousness.* St. Louis: C. V. Mosby.

Meleis, A. I. (1985). *Theoretical nursing: Development and progress.* Philadelphia: J. B. Lippincott.

Newman, M. A. (1986). *Health as expanded consciousness.* St. Louis: C. V. Mosby.

Noddings, N. (1984). *Caring: A feminine approach to ethics and moral education.* Los Angeles: University of California Press.

Peplau, H. E. (1952). *Interpersonal relations in nursing.* New York: G. P. Putnam's Sons.

Rodgers, S. (1984, December). Community as client—a multivariate model for analysis of community and aggregate health risk. *Public Health Nursing,* 210–222.

Schultz, P. (1987). When the client is more than one: Extending the foundational concept of person. *Advances in Nursing Science, 10*(1), 71–86.

Schultz, P. R., & Magilvy, J. K. (1988). Assessing community health needs of elderly populations: A comparison of three strategies. *Journal of Advanced Nursing, 13,* 193–202.

Sills, G. M., & Goeppinger, J. (1985). The community as a field of inquiry in nursing. *Annual Review of Nursing Research, 3,* 3–24.

Spradley, B. W. (1985). *Community health nursing concepts and practice.* Boston: Little, Brown & Co.

Watson, J. (1985). *Nursing: Human science and human care: A theory of nursing.* Norwalk, CT: Appleton-Century-Crofts.

Williams, C. A. (1977). Community health nursing—what is it? *Nursing Outlook, 25,* 250–255.

8

The Role of Context in Culture-Specific Care

Anna Frances Z. Wenger

Culture context is a useful window through which to view the phenomenon of care. It is generally thought that the survival of a culture is related to the beliefs and practices of care among its members (Leininger, 1978). Leininger contends that "human caring is a universal phenomenon, but expressions, processes and patterns vary among cultures" (Leininger, 1981, p. 11). Given this assumption and the belief that caring is the central focus of nursing (Leininger, 1984; Watson, 1985; Benner, 1989; Joel, 1990), it seems imperative for nurses to give attention to the relationship between culture context and culture-specific care.

In some cultures, the contextual boundaries are maintained in such a way that the differences between insiders and outsiders are overtly recognizable. Cultures which emphasize kinship ties, intergenerational relationships, shared language styles, and deeply held religious values, create a cultural context that encourages bonds to develop among members of the culture. It seems likely that care patterns would be deeply embedded and

The major tenets of this article were first presented at the annual conference of the Transcultural Nursing Society, October 8, 1986, Chicago, IL.

This research was partially funded by Sigma Theta Tau Lambda Chapter, by Miller–Erb Nursing Fund, and by Goshen College Faculty Research Grants.

mutually shared among members of such cultures. If that is true, then care expressions and patterns would also be less well known to outsiders.

Nurses and other caregivers who are outsiders to a particular culture need research-based knowledge about care meanings and functions in a particular culture in order to provide professional nursing care that fits the beliefs and values of that culture. Identification of the meanings and functions of care in one culture can lead to comparative studies in other cultures, and subsequently to theoretical postulations concerning care and culture context.

This article focuses on the relationship between culture context and care, using a conceptual framework based on Leininger's Cultural Care theory (Leininger, 1988) and Hall's concept of high and low cultural context (Hall, 1976). Selected findings from an ethnographic and ethno-nursing study on the phenomenon of care in the high context culture of the Old Order Amish (Wenger, 1988) are used to illustrate the theoretical concern about context and care.

These theoretical definitions derived from Leininger (1988) and Hall (1976) will be used throughout the article:

Culture context refers to the environment or situation which is relevant to the care beliefs, values, and practices of the culture under study.

Culture-specific care refers to the assistive, supportive, and facilitative acts through which meaning is derived from the shared lifeways of a particular group. These lifeways are transmitted from one generation to the next and change over time.

CULTURE CARE

Since 1966, Leininger has postulated that care is the essence of nursing, and that nursing as a practice profession and as a scientific discipline should consider cultural diversity (Leininger, 1978, 1980). She recognizes the importance of both folk and professional health care systems and the need for nurses to base their nursing practice on the principles of culture care preservation, accommodation, and/or repatterning. In addition, transcultural nursing research and practice are influenced by sociocultural factors in language and environment contexts and worldview (Leininger, 1978, 1981, 1984, 1988).

"Leininger first made explicit the link between nursing, care, and cross-cultural variation" (Aamodt, 1984, p. 75). Aamodt (1984) suggests that Leininger's contribution of the concept of care to nursing theory is an example of Kuhn's (1962) description of the development of a new paradigm. This means that the concept of care now needs to be clarified and its theoretical relationships postulated.

Care has been postulated to be an essential human need for growth and development, health maintenance, and survival of human beings in all cultures (Leininger, 1978). Mayeroff (1971) describes caring as an essential means for self-growth through helping others. A major assumption of Watson's (1985) nursing theory is that effective caring promotes health and individual or family growth. Gaylin (1976) uses a psychoanalytical, biological, and cultural explanation to describe the loving and caring capacity, which is developed in infancy and almost inevitably is carried into adult life. The capacity to care may be nurtured or thwarted by one's culture, but it is believed to be universally observable in the daily behavior of human beings, as well as in biology and literature (Gaylin, 1976).

Leininger's theory of Cultural Care Diversity and Universality is focused on culture care which integrates values, beliefs, and practices that make it possible for lifeway patterns within the culture to be nurtured, maintained, or improved (Leininger, 1988). The ultimate goal of the Cultural Care theory is to promote the provision of culturally congruent care. A meaningful and satisfactory fit of culture care beliefs, values, and practice between health care providers and care recipients is needed in order to preserve, maintain, or change care practices for the benefit and satisfaction of clients (Leininger, 1978, 1981, 1984, 1988).

Leininger (1988) predicts that the different dimensions of the social structure have an impact on care that influences health or well-being of clients. Social structure factors are interrelated and include economic, educational, political, kinship, religious/philosophical, technological, and cultural values. Although these factors are interrelated within a given culture, the theorist predicts that variability and diversity exist in the way that specific social structure factors influence care and health.

The social structure features are discovered within environmental and language contexts, according to Leininger's theory. The environment includes both structural and functional components such as geographical setting, family and social constellations, sociocultural boundaries of the culture, and the general milieu in which care is expressed. Since care values and beliefs are believed to be deeply embedded in the culture, it follows that language would be an essential element in discovering culture-specific care.

Care occurs within folk and professional health care systems. The folk health system reflects the use of indigenous care practices in a specific culture. These practices are influential in identifying care values, beliefs, and practices essential to professional nursing knowledge. The professional system has health care providers who have been prepared through formal education, often requiring licensure to practice. The folk and professional care systems may exist side by side within a culture and sometimes are in conflict with each other. Care phenomena can be discovered by examining the worldview, social structure, language, and folk and professional health care practices of a specific culture.

CULTURE CONTEXT

Spiro (1965) is one of the major anthropologists to focus on context and meaning. He cites as his mentor, Edward T. Hall, who studied the relationship of kinship to selected contextual factors, such as economic and political system factors, which influence the kinship pattern. Hall (1966, 1976, 1983) has increasingly elucidated his conceptual framework of high and low context. Although his major work focuses on cultural communication, he has also identified criteria for high and low context cultures.

Hall (1976) contends that only basic patterns can be sketched because more research is needed. His research has focused mainly on intercultural communication with French and German businessmen, and with Japanese and American businessmen (Hall, 1983). Hall (personal communication, April, 1983) stated that the French, German, and Japanese have been more receptive to his theory and research than have American researchers.

High and low context refers to the level of context–dependency in the human–environment interchange (Hall, 1976). For instance, a high context communication is one in which most of the meaning is explicit in the context. When people are acquainted over a long period of time and/or share many life activities they tend to use high context communication. Conversely, people who are mobile, know little about each other, or have few life experiences in common, use low context communication in which the meaning is explicit in the transmitted message.

Although all cultures have degrees of high and low context communication, specific cultures have general characteristics that tend to be lower or higher in context (Hall, 1976). These characteristics influence all lifeways of the people. Table 8-1 lists the major characteristics contrasting high and low cultures that help to focus attention on specific sociocultural factors. Persons in high context cultures are deeply involved with each other. This high level of involvement produces a greater degree of context. When people share many aspects of their lives such as work, leisure time, and knowledge of kinship, there is less variability in cultural lifeways. Hall (1976) states that high context people expect more of each other than low context people do because they share contextual knowledge and experience with many levels of meaning that are not made explicit. For instance, a person may seem to talk obscurely, often skirting an issue, expecting the

Table 8-1
Characteristics of High and Low Context Cultures

Characteristics	High Context	Low Context
Relationships	long-term	minimal acquaintance
Shared life activities	many	few
Meaning of message	implicit in context	explicit in transmission
Linguistic code	restricted	elaborated
Variability in cultural lifeways	more	less
Intergenerational kinship knowledge	more	less
Social control and support	high	low
Sociocultural boundaries	insider/outsider distinction marked	blurred
Integration of new situations	take more time	more quickly completed
Rate of change	slow	rapid

interlocutor to know what the personal nature of the problem is without specific data being given (Hall, 1976, p. 113). In sociolinguistics this form of communication is referred to as restricted code, in which words and sentences are collapsed because of shared contextual understanding (Bernstein, 1975; Trudgill, 1974).

In high context cultures, the bonds which tie people together are so strong, that when problems occur there is flexibility within the system to accommodate the situation, so that the cultural lifeways of the people are preserved in a manner that is often not understood by outsiders. This limited flexibility within the system is in part controlled by the authority vested in the designated leaders. Persons who are in leadership positions by virtue of position or kinship status are personally responsible for the actions of their subordinates (Hall, 1976). This level of social control and support tends to create greater distinctions between insiders and outsiders than in low context cultures.

Change tends to occur slowly in high context cultures. The high levels of context in social and cultural networks, often involving several generations, seem to require more time in dealing with new situations. New situations are accepted only if approached in great detail, because of the need to process and integrate the new concepts into a highly contexted matrix of sociocultural concepts, which are understood and accepted by the culture. "High context actions are by definition rooted in the past, slow to change, and highly stable" (Hall, 1976, p. 93).

Levels of technology should not be equated with high and low context cultures. For example, the Japanese culture tends to be high context, but also uses high technology similar to the Anglo-American culture, which is relatively low context. Similarly, French are high context and Germans are low context, a fact that becomes apparent in human interactions in transcultural settings. In German and American cultures people are more mobile, use more effort to articulate meaning overtly in transmitted messages, are more outcome–oriented, more monochronic in terms of time and energy, and incorporate change and technology at a faster rate than do French and Japanese. If Hall's statement that the Anglo-American culture is low context is accepted and it is known that much of the professional health care system is based on Anglo-American middle class values, then professional nurses should be especially concerned about the interface of professional health care with high context cultures.

RELATIONSHIP OF CARE AND HIGH CONTEXT

Knowledge about the context or "fit" within specific cultural systems adds to what is known about health care, including the care as well as the boundaries of the concept (Aamodt, 1984, p. 78). In a high context culture, where people share many aspects of their lives over extended periods of time, it seems logical that the nature of care responses to health and illness would be significant in the maintenance of that culture. In order for family and community life to be enhanced and to be durable, some effective forms of care are likely to develop and even become ritualized. These care expectations may vary among high context cultures depending on the influence of specific sociocultural factors, but a care system would need to be present in order for the ongoing relationships within the family and community to endure.

The care system within the high context culture affects how the cultural group members seek and respond to health care services. If people know each other well and have many intergenerational contacts, care expectations will probably be associated with other family and community role expectations. In high context cultures where the sociocultural boundaries make distinctive differences between insiders and outsiders, the availability, choice, and use of professional health care services is most likely determined by more than individual preference. The nature of professional nursing and other health care service is, in part, determined by the care beliefs and practices in the high context culture. Indeed, in order to provide culture-specific nursing care, professional nurses need to understand the cultural beliefs and practices about care which are related to cultural context.

OLD ORDER AMISH

A study of care patterns of the Old Order Amish illustrates the beginning of a body of research-based knowledge about culture care and culture context. The Old Order Amish constitute an ethnoreligious group who live in settlements in 20 states of the United States and in Ontario, Canada. From a small group of 5,000 in 1900 they have grown to more than 100,000 persons (Krabill, 1989). The settlements are not communal economically but rather are geographically intentional so that their farms are often contiguous, with some non-Amish homes and farms dispersed throughout the community.

Hostetler (1980) has suggested culture context as one of several models for understanding Amish society. He suggests that the Old Order Amish culture provides a highly selective screen between itself and the outside world. "What Amish pay attention to (contexting) and what they ignore are different from the choices made in low contexting cultures" (Hostetler, 1980, p. 19). It is interesting to note that contemporary Amish fit Hall's definition of a high context culture, even though ethnically they are of German origin and they still use a German dialect among themselves, speaking English only with outsiders and in school. According to Hall (1976, 1983), contemporary German culture is low context. The shift for the Old Order Amish toward becoming more high context and for Germans, in general, toward becoming more low context has taken place slowly over several hundred years.

CONTEXT AND OLD ORDER AMISH

The separation of the Old Order Amish from the dominant culture through the years since their migration from Europe to the New World in the 17th and 18th centuries has in effect increased the contextualization of their culture. Religious solidarity, the use of a common dialect, geographical proximity, and shared family and community values all contribute to frequent and sustained intergenerational contact and communal contextual understanding. The Anglo-American culture, with which the Amish interact selectively, has increasingly become more low context in that families are more mobile with less intergenerational knowledge. People share fewer life activities and there is a lower level of social control and support. Therefore, the highly contextualized culture of the Amish becomes ever more sharply contrasted with the surrounding dominant culture.

In a high context culture like that of the Old Order Amish, where people share many aspects of their lives over extended periods of time, it seems logical that the nature of care response to health and illness would be significant in the maintenance of that culture. In order for family and community life to be enhanced and to be durable, some effective forms of care are likely to develop and even to become ritualized.

Yet the Amish are dependent on the Anglo-American culture for professional health care services such as medical, nursing, dental, and mental health services because they have no professionally educated care providers among their own number (Krabill, 1989; Wenger & Wenger, 1988). Professionals often find it difficult, or choose not to learn, about indigenous care beliefs and practices and, thus, prescribe culturally incongruent and sometimes duplicative care and cure treatments.

RESEARCH DESIGN

An ethnographic/ethno-nursing study was conducted in an Old Order Amish settlement in Northcentral Indiana over a three-year period of time. Intensive ethnographic interviewing, participant observation, and life histories were done with 13 families whose children attended one of the 21 Amish schools. The key informants were the 13 mothers, and the general informants included ten fathers, 34 children, five grandmothers, two grandfathers, and two Amish healers.

Entry into the field was accomplished through carefully planned cultural–congruent activities by first meeting with the author of the local Amish directory, which lists names, households, and homes of all persons in the settlement. This led to meetings with selected persons such as the bishop of the church and the chairman of the school board. After being invited to attend a parent-teacher meeting to explain the project, ethnographic interviews were initiated with 13 of the 17 families represented in the school. Four families chose not to participate for personal reasons, and because of a concern that Amish might be misrepresented, as frequently happens in the news media. At least four interviews per family were held with 11 of the 13 participating families, in addition to interviews with five grandparents and two Amish healers.

Continuous confirmation, an earmark of qualitative research, was part of all interviews, life histories, observation, and participation. Field notes were recorded following each interview and observation. A computer program using Data Base III Plus was developed for the microcomputer to process the data. This computer program was adapted from an earlier version of the Leininger-Templin-Thompson software program (Leininger, 1990). Leininger's data analysis model was used throughout the study (Wenger, 1988). This model includes four phases as follows:

1. Collecting and documenting raw data through use of a field journal and computer.

2. Identifying and coding descriptors and components from raw data.

3. Analyzing patterns and categories.

4. Abstracting themes and theoretical formulations.

This continuous analysis process resulted in the discovery of patterns and themes about culture care and high culture context. A full description of the research study is available in other sources (Wenger, 1988; Wenger, 1991).

Many characteristics of high culture context related to culture care became evident throughout the study. These Amish characteristics were compared with Hall's characteristics of high context culture. High context features of Amish culture were identified in relation to culture care. Long-term relationships, shared cultural lifeways, and boundary maintenance will be discussed as evidence of high context in informant interviews and participant observations.

HIGH CONTEXT THEMES

Long-Term Relationships

This study revealed that the Amish value long-term relationships which are constantly nurtured. Social events are planned which bring people together frequently. Time and energy are spent on these relationships. Friendship quilts were identified by five informants as important in their relationships. Young women design and sew together quilt blocks with their names embroidered on them for a friend. Then they get together to do the quilting. The recipient has a life-long visual remembrance of her friends' caring action. Young children are taught to be aware of the Amish network of relationships. Some children use the local Amish directory to learn the relationships of families to church districts and to schools. An 11-year-old child examined the directory for children with the same birth-date as hers. Relationships developed in childhood often continue throughout the adult years. These long-term relationships increase shared knowledge of care needs and lifeways.

Shared Cultural Lifeways

Intergenerational relationships were found to be encouraged consistently. For example, all elderly in this study were respected and included in the everyday life of the community. At the school Christmas party, the grandparents were given fruit baskets by the children, as they said, "Because the grandparents do so much for us." One granddaughter, age 23, gave her grandfather shoulder and back massages, and he in turn gave her foot treatments.

Many houses are constructed so as to include grandparents in the lives of the extended family. A great-grandfather living in the *daadi haus* (a house attached to the main house for the grandparents) was known to relate best to the two-year-old child living in the main house. The mother recognized the benefits of this care relationship to her, the child, and the great–grandfather. In another example, four young adult single women each chose an 8-to-10-year-old child and took them to a metropolitan science museum for a day. This required hiring a driver with a van. However, this was considered worthwhile because it nurtured intergenerational relationships (an indication of high context) and was discussed by an informant as a caring action. Care is expressed by sharing experiences, knowledge, and by being interested in and concerned for others.

Community awareness is part of the social structure of the Amish. People generally live in close proximity to each other. For those who live in other geographical areas, social contacts are maintained through frequent visits and letters. During one interview, out-of-state relatives of the informants stopped in unannounced. No one present reacted with surprise. It seemed as though they had so internalized their bonds with geographically distant kin that an unexpected visit could be dealt with quite matter-of-factly. Both practicality and intensely conscious social networking were evidenced as the researcher was asked before leaving to pass on information of the visit to another relative. Family members to whom the visit was reported wanted to know how long the visitors were staying, who was along, and when they had left their home. It was understood that contact could not be made with all eleven family members. Care is expressed by "keeping in touch," which is highly valued by the Amish and is a characteristic of high context. Outsiders need to remember that Old Order Amish have no telephones in their homes and own no cars, thus requiring considerable effort to maintain these highly valued, high context care expressions.

A constant awareness of people and their movements in the community was observed. Reports of social events usually included accounts of who was present. During interviews, the informants looked out the window to check who was passing by in a buggy. One informant had her sewing machine positioned so that she could view the road and the school, thus increasing her awareness of community activity. People regularly read the Amish newsletters which report church services, funerals, weddings, accidents, illnesses, and card and gift showers. This intense interrelated community awareness promotes opportunities for culture care and shared knowledge in the culture, evidence again of high context.

Boundary Maintenance

Huntington (1987), Hostetler (1980), Krabill (1989), and other researchers have discussed various aspects of boundary maintenance as a key to understanding Amish culture. There is general agreement that differences between insiders and outsiders are pronounced in the Amish community. *Deitsch*, a German dialect, is used as the language with insiders and English is used with outsiders. Distinctive Amish dress and use of non-motorized transportation are constant reminders of the boundary between Amish and non-Amish. When Amish work outside the community, often there will be several Amish working in the same industry, thereby increasing their support of each other. One informant family had six men from the same *friendschaft* (extended three-generation family) working in the same trailer factory. Although Amish have regular contact with outsiders, they are sometimes wary of persons who want to relate to them through providing services. On five separate occasions, informants questioned whether such persons were wanting to spy, steal, or influence the Amish with "worldly ways."

Group cohesiveness and internal consistency are important in high context cultures. Amish want to "fit in," thus promoting community similarity rather than individual distinctiveness. The "Amish way" is reinforced daily. One informant said, "You see things and you do it. You do not want anyone to say, 'she doesn't go along with things.'" The value of "fitting in" encourages persons constantly to be aware of group expectations which create shared lifeways and caring interactions. Persons who do not "fit into the culture" experience withdrawal of group sanction, which may be perceived as non-care. However, if culture care is viewed within the framework of the Amish world view, then protection of group norms is essential. To care is to help people who want to fit into the culture.

Upholding tradition is a part of boundary maintenance. Amish are often not aware of their historical roots, but they are keenly aware of tradition. The *ordnung* (set of unwritten rules) of each church district helps people to maintain traditional and accepted behaviors in each community. One informant discussed her interest in becoming a nurse, but that did not fit with being Amish. "No one says you can't, but people who study, usually change. There are things that just don't fit. If you could just take care of people, but it's not that simple," she explained.

There is flexibility within the culture which allows for infractions of expected behavior. Young adults sometimes drive cars, use radios, dress in non-Amish clothes and still live at home. The value of family unity and community cohesiveness is so great that infractions are tolerated for a period of time in the hope that these persons will eventually embrace "the Amish way." If pregnancy occurs before marriage and the couple wants to get married, their church districts may alter their church calendars to allow for baptism to these persons so that marriage rites and the wedding can take place as soon as possible. Such examples of flexibility in social sanctions and cultural expectations are evidence of culture care and high culture context with a pragmatic bent toward cultural maintenance and survival. Hall (1976) states that high context cultures exhibit internal flexibility that allows for considerable bending of the system because the bonds between people are so strong. This high context feature accounts for the expressions of care identified when cultural infraction had occurred.

CULTURE CARE THEMES

Centrality of Care

Four major themes of culture care were identified that were related to high culture context. The first theme focused on the idea that care was at the core of the Amish worldview and social structure. This care set was found to be representative of this theme: (1) giving care involves both obligation and privilege, and (2) receiving care involves both expectation and humility. Young people grow up knowing their obligation to care for parents. Parents fulfill their obligations by teaching their children how to work and consequently how to care, thus socializing them for this present life, while spiritually preparing them for eternal life hereafter. The duty to care is a privilege. Amish informants discussed the benefits of caring, including feeling good. Good health, good crops, obedient children, and financial solvency are considered gifts of God. Therefore, to help others puts one in a privileged position not to be taken lightly.

The counterpart to an obligation to give care is the security of the expectation to receive care when needed. Amish who remain in the culture can expect to receive care throughout their lifetime. This assurance of care does not permit persons to be lax in caring for their own needs. Rather, to be Amish also means that they will be responsible for their families, and do everything to be productive members of the group. The lifelong expectation of care is, therefore, coupled with humility. For the Amish, humility, which is a highly valued virtue, means a personal submission and obedience to God and a consideration of others before oneself. This requires persons constantly to be aware of others who may need care more than they do.

Anticipatory Care

The second theme is anticipatory care, which refers to care whereby persons develop care patterns that allow them to maintain high context relationships and knowledge about other persons' needs, thus developing the ability to sense people's care needs. A complex network of social events functions to help people anticipate and predict each other's needs. These may be role-related, intergenerational, familial, or communal. These actions are undergirded by their religious and cultural beliefs that they are a separate people ordained by God to be "not conformed to this world" (Romans, 12:2). The deeply held belief that the Amish belong together is a principle that guides them to care for each other in every way they can, thus fulfilling God's will for them. The value of sensing when care is needed (preferably without being told) links up with this belief about Amish belonging together to promote anticipatory care.

Active Participation

The third theme is active participation. Amish actively participate in care actions and options. Health is highly valued, and treating one's body as the temple of God (I. Cor. 6: 19–20) is taken seriously. Amish informants considered and selected from an array of health care options which included folk, professional, and alternative care. They did not relegate care decisions to outsiders unless extreme trust was invested in the health professional. Rather, the Amish were actively involved in care decisions throughout the illness episode and often used folk and professional health care services simultaneously. Professional health care providers may prescribe care and cure treatments, but Amish clients want to understand and enter into the care process by choosing from among options that fit their worldview.

Principled Pragmatism

The fourth and last theme is principled pragmatism, which means that care attitudes and actions are influenced by practical day-to-day consequences. This pragmatic approach was based on moral and ethical principles as well as on expediency. The prevailing general principle seemed to be "if it helps, it's good, and if it does not help, it will not hurt" Pragmatism was also noted in caring in times of cultural infractions. There was flexibility in care actions, so that deeply held care beliefs and values could be upheld in situations where there was infraction of selected cultural norms. These actions resulted in flexibility and cultural resilience that helped promote togetherness and family/community well-being, which have a higher priority for all concerned. This finding is consistent with Huntington's (1987) analysis of pragmatism and flexibility in boundary maintenance during times of health care crisis. Hall's (1976) high context concept includes the dimension of intracultural flexibility, which promotes substantial bending of rules within the system precisely because the bonds between people are so strong. "To do all we can to help in the Amish way" was the guiding principle in such pragmatic situations.

High Context and Amish Care Patterns

The high context features of the Old Order Amish culture promote cultural care patterns that help them maintain their identity and encourage cultural survival. The highly contexted matrix of intergenerational relationships helps Amish to sense each other's care needs, whereby they respond with obligation, privilege, expectation, and humility.

Care becomes culturally ritualized as "the Amish way." Non-Amish professional (medical, nursing) and alternative (chiropractic, reflexology) health care services are used simultaneously with traditional care. The selective choice of non-Amish health care services is highly influenced by the opinions of Amish family and friends. The high context features of the culture aid in the selective use of non-Amish care services, always reminding the people that they are promoting "the Amish way."

CONCLUSION

Theoretical and empirical support has been discussed regarding the relationship between culture care and culture context. The Old Order Amish culture is only one of many high context cultures with which professional nurses interact. Transcultural communication is especially difficult in the interface between low context and high context cultures, such as when care providers from the Anglo-American health care system, which is low context, relate to clients from a high context culture. Only when nurses understand the indigenous care patterns and cultural context, can they provide culture–specific professional care. The care patterns manifested in the culture, which are beneficial, need to be promoted. Professional caring should always supplement, and not substitute for, culturally beneficial indigenous care. This kind of caring interaction then will be economically, ethically, and culturally responsible.

Eventually, with an adequate research base, it should be possible to identify some universal high context and low context cultural themes with related care themes specific to several similar cultures. For example, are the care themes identified in this ethno-nursing study of Old Order Amish found in other Amish groups? What are the differences in care themes and contextual features among other high context cultures? What are differences in care values, beliefs, and practices between similar high context and low context cultural groups such as rural Anglo-American and Old Order Amish? These and other questions will guide further research studies.

REFERENCES

Aamodt, A. (1984). Themes and issues in conceptualizing care. In M. M. Leininger (Ed.), *Care: The essence of nursing and health.* Detroit: Wayne State University Press.

Benner, P. E. (1989). *Primacy of caring: Stress and coping in health and illness.* Menlo Park, CA: Addison-Wesley.

Bernstein, B. (1975). *Class, codes and control.* New York: Schocken Books.

Gaylin, W. (1976). *Caring.* New York: Avon Books.

Hall, E. T. (1966). *Hidden language.* Garden City, NY: Anchor Press/Doubleday.

Hall, E. T. (1976). *Beyond culture.* Garden City, NY: Anchor Press/Doubleday.

Hall, E. T. (1983). *The dance of life: The other dimension of time.* Garden City, NY: Anchor Press/Doubleday.

Hostetler, J. A. (1980). *Amish society* (3rd ed.). Baltimore: Johns Hopkins University Press.

Huntington, G. E. (1987, November). *Cultural interaction during times of crises: Permeable boundaries and Amish cultural success.* Paper presented at annual meeting of the American Anthropological Association, Chicago.

Joel, L. (1990, February). NCNIP/Advertising council campaign challenges resistant stereotypes: President's message. *American Nurse, 13.*

Krabill, D. B. (1989). *The riddle of Amish culture.* Baltimore: Johns Hopkins University Press.

Kuhn, T. (1962). *The structure of scientific revolutions.* Chicago: The University of Chicago Press.

Leininger, M. M. (1978). *Transcultural nursing: Concepts, theory and practices.* New York: John Wiley and Sons.

Leininger, M. M. (1980). Caring: A central focus for nursing and health care services. *Nursing and Health Care, 1*(3):135–143.

Leininger, M. M. (Ed.). (1981). *Caring: An essential human need.* Detroit: Wayne State University Press.

Leininger, M. M. (Ed.). (1984). *Care: The essence of nursing and health.* Detroit: Wayne State University Press.

Leininger, M. M. (1988). Leininger's theory of nursing. Cultural care diversity and universality. *Nursing Science Quarterly, 1*(4), 152–160.

Leininger, M. M. (1990). *Leininger-Templin-Thompson qualitative ethnoscript software: User handbook.* Detroit: Wayne State University Press.

Mayeroff, M. (1971). *On caring.* New York: Harper & Row.

Spiro, M. (1965). *Context and meaning in cultural anthropology.* New York: The Free Press.

Tridgill, P. (1974). *Sociolinguistics: An introduction.* New York: Penguin Books.

Watson, J. (1985). *Nursing: Human science and human care.* Norwalk, CT: Appleton-Century-Crofts.

Wenger, A. F. Z. (1988). The phenomenon of care in a high context culture: The Old Order Amish. *Dissertation Abstracts International, 50/02B.*

Wenger, A. F. Z. (1991). The cultural care theory and the Old Order Amish. In M. M. Leininger (Ed.), *Cultural care diversity and universality: A theory of nursing.* New York: National League for Nursing.

Wenger, A. F., Wenger, M. R. (1988). Community and family care patterns of the Old Order Amish. In M. M. Leininger (Ed.), *Care: Discovery and clinical community uses.* Detroit: Wayne State University Press.

9

A Phenomenological Investigation of Caring as a Lived Experience in Nurses

Carol Green-Hernandez

Caring—what is it? What does it mean to give caring? To receive caring? What does giving caring feel like to the giver and receiver? Over the last several years much nursing research has focused on caring as it is practiced by nurses, while some has also investigated how such caring affects patient-family recipients. Both Leininger (1977) and Watson (1979) assert that caring is nursing's essence, and yet one might ask how it is that caring is what defines the profession? Curiosity about the foregoing questions led to the current investigation of the concept of caring as a lived experience from human and, more specifically, nursing perspectives.

PURPOSE AND RESEARCH QUESTION

The above questions provided the impetus for the study's purpose, which was to discover whether the nurse's caring exists as a direct and intentional professional process, or as a spontaneous human response, or perhaps as a combination or integration of both of these.

The research question of this phenomenological inquiry was: What is the experience of caring in professional nursing, and of caring outside of nursing, as lived by the nurse? An additional subquestion was: Is the lived experience of professional caring a direct and intentional process or a spontaneous human response?

CONCEPTUAL ORIENTATION

The disciplines of theology, philosophy, psychology, medicine, and nursing each share a common tradition of caring. Theology's notion of caring originated in the *Old Testament's* biblical shepherding activity of God. The *New Testament's* message of *agape* is one of caring in its most basic, human expression of shared fellowship (Nygren, 1932). *Agape* provides both the basis and the forum for experiencing Divine healing. Such healing is integral to human connection with a God-centered universe (LeShan, 1966).

Philosophy's view of caring is perhaps more concrete; here caring provides meaning and orderliness to life. The caregiver helps another grow and actualize while inevitably changing and, sometimes, becoming self-actualized as a result (Mayeroff, 1971). Sharing is inherent in this experience of reciprocal change and actualization which Mayeroff asserts is the basis for a philosophy of caring. Noddings (1984) adds that the caring individual makes acts of commitment through caring acts. Although the recipient may perceive these caring acts, that individual may not acknowledge the commitment underlying them. Caring, then, can occur only when it is mutually seen as caring (Noddings, 1984).

In contrast to the theological and philosophical notions of caring, psychology's perspective of caring derives from empathy, which is unidirectional rather than bidirectional in its client focus. Empathy requires that the therapist accept the client, entering into the other's reality. Empathy is caring to only a very limited extent because the individual expressing empathy is not expected to change or grow as a result of therapeutic interaction with the other (Rogers, 1961). Empathy provides a foundation for helping the other heal when it occurs within the confines of a formal, therapeutic relationship (Ashbrook, 1985). Rogers (1961) tells us that this therapeutic relationship is built on nonjudgmental acceptance of the other. Such acceptance can promote the carer's social support of the other. Social support is the vehicle by which the caregiver helps the other (Dimond & Jones, 1983).

Traditionally, nursing's vision of caring shares psychology's approach in that nursing requires nonjudgmental acceptance of the patient–family (Henderson, 1978; Peplau, 1952). Nursing's view of caring moves beyond psychology's view, however, in that nursing's caring combines theology's and philosophy's notions of *agape* and self-actualization. Nurse caring interweaves the therapeutics of healing, helping, empathy, and social support in caring for the patient and family (Leininger, 1977, 1984, 1985; Watson, 1979, 1981, 1989).

REVIEW OF LITERATURE

The body of caring research in nursing does not clearly differentiate the related concepts of healing, helping, empathy, and social support from that of caring. Further, whether or not caring is different when professionally practiced has not been clearly considered in the nursing literature. However, scholars are now beginning to discover important elements of caring's meaning to nursing. Gaut (1979, 1983) believes that caring is indirect because it occurs by means of other activities. In other words, caring is "mediated action" (Kerr & Soltis, 1974, cited in Gaut, 1979). This notion of caring logically includes the concept of helping.

The helping aspect of caring is rooted in Nightingale's work (1969, first published in 1860). For Nightingale, the goal of nursing is to assist nature in helping the patient get well. This is a powerful assertion, for it implies that the nurse must work in concert with nature in order to achieve a desired outcome. Zderad (1969) sees such helping as arising from the nurse's empathy for the patient. The purpose of empathy is "understanding and neutral acceptance" of another (Zderad, 1969). No further action need occur.

Although helping has not previously been clearly differentiated from caring in the literature, its humanistic essence is well-described. Reflective of Nightingale's (1860) goal for nursing, Watson (1981) defines caring within a humanistic framework of ten carative factors, which provide the structure necessary to the caring process in nursing by which patient health and positive change are promoted. Leininger's (1977, 1981, 1985) view of caring similarly builds on Nightingale's goal for nursing and also validates Mayeroff's (1971) notion of caring. Leininger's examinations of the nature of nursing define care/caring as assisting, supporting, and facilitating those actions necessary to meeting another's need(s), which also logically provides social support.

The nurse's ability to help others derives sustenance from the ability to care for oneself (Mayeroff, 1971; Leininger, 1984, 1985). Hyde (1976) asserts that the nurse's conscious choice to care for oneself in turn facilitates one's caring for the patient. Similarly, Bevis (1978) sees the nurse–patient relationship as nurse–caring and holds that this relationship is unidirective, in that the main focus of the nurse's caring is the patient. The unidirectionality of this focus might imply that caring is intentional because of the therapeutic nature of the nurse–patient relationship. Despite the proposal that caring in nursing is intentional (Kerr & Soltis, 1974, cited in Gaut, 1979; Gaut, 1983), the nature of this intentionality has not yet been described.

Traditionally, the term intentional action refers to any action that is intended; implied is a connection between the action and the intention to act (Gustafson, 1981). One's intention to act may thus generate one's behavior (Thalberg, 1984). In order to be therapeutic there should be little disparity between what one intends to do and the action one takes as a result. Any meaning ascribed to the action itself derives from the intention rather than a mediating circumstance (Gustafson, 1981; Thalberg, 1984). That an action's meaning is derived directly from intentionality is thus in opposition to the view that meaning occurs via "mediated action" (Kerr & Soltis, 1974, cited in Gaut, 1979). Intentionality, then, engages with reality when an action occurs because it was intended. Intentional action, therefore, requires that one know that such action will occur (Gustafson, 1981).

An individual develops the capacity for intentional caring action through first learning a variety of specific natural human caring actions (Gustafson, 1981). An example of this learning can occur during the lived experience of parental nurturance while growing up. Because of this lived experience, an individual learns how to be a nurturing parent and so can, in turn, intentionally provide nurturance to one's own child. An individual learns how to intentionally give natural human caring because one has a lived experience of that caring. In contrast, the intentional actions of a profession are taught as a repertoire of intentional actions to those who are members of that profession (Gustafson, 1981). "In both human development and in human learning, intentional action that is deliberate, thoughtful, and performed for a purpose occurs only following . . . the development of natural capacities of voluntary movement and acquired modifications of such natural capacities" (p. 43).

This study postulated that intentional caring action(s) given by a non-nurse differ from that of a professional nurse possessing a developed skill and knowledge base in nursing. This postulate built on Gustafson's (1981) assertion that the capacity for intentional action does not extend to individuals who are untried or untrained. The premise was therefore made that an intention, as well as a desire for and belief in that which is intended, are requirements for intentional action's performance.

DESIGN, METHODOLOGY, AND JUSTIFICATION
FOR THE STUDY

This was a qualitative study which used the structural phenomenological method as described by Colaizzi (1978; Polkinghorne, 1989). This method seeks to uncover both what people know and how they organize their knowledge by approaching the research question(s) from the point of view of the person who has lived the experience (Harris, 1968; Norris, 1982). The researcher used this process to abstract the property description of professional caring in nursing (Hinshaw, 1979).

Sample

Colaizzi (1978; Polkinghorne, 1989) advises that subjects can participate in a phenomenological study provided they have experience of the phenomenon under investigation and are both willing and able to articulate that experience. The researcher used participant self-report of these Colaizzi requirements as a criterion for study participation. Data were collected over a period of three months from a purposive sample of 20 nurses who stated that they had experienced caring and agreed to participate in the study (Field & Morse, 1985; Bogdan & Biklen, 1982). The purposive sampling technique includes both yea and nay sayers who have experienced the research phenomenon. This study's purposive sample consisted of nurses who at time of sample selection were asked whether they primarily valued their caring (i.e., yea sayers) or their technical skill ability (i.e., nay sayers) in their nursing. Additional criteria for subject selection included: holding a baccalaureate degree in nursing; history of full-time employment as a staff registered nurse for a minimum of three years (validated by subject self–report); and willingness to discuss the experience of non-nurse versus nurse caring openly and freely (Kruger, 1981).

Redundancy of findings occurred from the seventh interview onward. That is, despite repeated probing using open-ended interview and cue questions, data which differed in thematic content were not elicited from respondents. Bogdan and Biklen (1982) believe that a minimum of two interviews should be conducted after such redundancy is reached. This researcher chose to interview five rather than two subjects beyond redundancy in keeping with Colaizzi's (1978) suggestion that sample size " . . . depends on various [unnamed] factors that must be tried out in each research project" (p. 58). In this study, these factors included investigator curiosity regarding whether thematic redundancy had indeed been reached and, ultimately, a belief that 12 subjects was a more salient sample size than nine.

Participants were female, caucasian, and ranged in age from 29 through 40 years. Ten were married and nine had one or more children, none of whom were younger than nine months of age. Two participants were unmarried and had no children. Two subjects held master's degrees in nursing; a third individual was enrolled but not matriculated in a graduate program in nursing. A fourth participant had completed course work but not her research project requirement for her master's degree in nursing. Eight subjects worked full-time, while four worked part-time in nursing three to four days per week. Each nurse's natural caring background was uniquely her own. Nine reported growing up in rural poverty. Nine subjects discussed their rich family lives experienced while growing up. Three nurses clearly experienced their early years in dysfunctional home environments. Eleven subjects expressed contentment in their adult personal lives. One individual denied feeling adult life contentment. She shared that she grew up in an urban dysfunctional family outside the study's geographic region. Participants' rights were protected.

Procedure for Data Collection and Validity and Reliability

The researcher used Goodwin and Goodwin's (1984) criteria for establishing validity and reliability in qualitative research. Prior to undertaking the investigation, the researcher posed the research question as well as the subquestion to herself in order to " . . . uncover [her] presuppositions about the investigated topic" (Colaizzi, 1978, p. 58). Called bracketing, this process supported the investigator's attempt to suspend or make inoperative her preconceptions, beliefs, and biases about the study's phenomenon (Colaizzi, 1978; Polkinghorne, 1989). The researcher addressed her assumptions head-on in order to facilitate "reflective awareness" through the process of "bracketing and rebracketing" (Valle & King, 1978). This attempt to reduce preconceptions about caring continued throughout the study in order to: (a) separate investigator from respondent beliefs and preconceptions, and (b) assist in the continued development of probing questions as new preconceptions emerged (Colaizzi, 1978; Polkinghorne, 1989).

Bracketing provided the foundation for exploring three different experiential areas of the lived experience of caring in nursing and outside of nursing in three subjects who formed a pilot group. These three experiential areas included recall of: a recent nurse-patient relationship; a nurse–patient relationship that developed during the first year of professional practice; and caring both prior to and since professional entry. The researcher used both tape recordings and field notes in an effort to remain true to subjects' exact words. Interviews lasted approximately one and one-half hours. Each interview was transcribed verbatim. The researcher also included field note observations of participant nonverbal behaviors and investigator impressions in each transcript.

The researcher then integrated her own as well as pilot subjects' bracketed presuppositions about the lived experience of caring, returning to the subjects to validate whether this integration was consistent with their lived experience of caring. This integration provided the substance for creating the study's research question and subquestion, to which the three pilot subjects were invited to respond fully in order to ascertain if they had anything to add to their stories. These individuals were subsequently integrated into the study as the first three respondents.

Each of the study's nine succeeding subjects was asked to describe her lived experience of the two nursing experiential areas as fully as possible until she felt they were fully described, probing whether this was for her a lived experience of caring. Memories of what was done, what it felt like, and what meaning each participant connected to what she had done were explored as fully as possible. Thoughts and actions associated with each scenario were also explored. This latter discussion was used as a springboard for the respondent's exploring what, if any, association existed between these and her nursing actions. The same process was followed for exploring each participant's lived experience of caring outside of nursing as fully as possible, comparing and contrasting that experience with the lived experience of caring in nursing.

The researcher asked questions at appropriate times throughout an interview if she needed to clarify content. Cue questions explored what feelings and meanings each participant associated with her experiences. Cue questions such as "what did this mean to you?" or "what did this feel like for you?" or "such as?" were meant to uncover data that might otherwise not appear. This technique was also useful in uncovering the real meaning perceived by subjects of their lived experience of caring, not just what they thought they should feel or say to the researcher (Colaizzi, 1978). Leading, suggestive, and close–ended questions were avoided. Finally, each respondent was invited to add any other thoughts or perceptions that had not occurred to her while telling her story about her experience of caring both in nursing and in life (Colaizzi, 1978).

DATA ANALYSIS

Data were analyzed using the Colaizzi (1978) method. Data analysis within this framework involves reducing the data while addressing emergent themes. These themes are then organized into categories, each of which is descriptive of those themes contained within its boundaries.

Analysis began with reading each subject's transcribed interview (termed a protocol) in the effort to make sense of the data. Each protocol contained descriptions of natural as well as professional nurse caring situations, actions, and feelings. Following several rereadings, and using respondents' own words, significant statements about these descriptions were extracted from each protocol. The researcher then constructed a general restatement of each significant statement, which she used to develop a formulated meaning statement. Each formulated meaning statement was examined in concert with continual referral back to the original significant statement. For example, one subject said that in growing up: "I always felt accepted and encouraged by my parents and brothers while growing up. Someone was always there. I got lots of hugs at home!" The researcher restated this as: Growing-up years were characterized by feelings of familial belongingness, encouragement, and love. These feelings were reinforced through touch. The formulated meaning statement that emerged from this data analysis stated: It was important to feel accepted and encouraged by family; touch via hugs was used to nonverbally express caring.

Concurrently, rereview of the related literature facilitated continued insights into data. Bracketing was used as an on-going process to help the investigator avoid imposition of her preconceptions into the formulated meaning statements, in order that each such statement would remain faithful to the original protocol data. These formulated meaning statements were then submitted to three experienced qualitative research judges for validation (Colaizzi, 1978; Goodwin & Goodwin, 1984).

Clusters of themes were derived from each protocol's formulated meaning statements (Colaizzi, 1978). The researcher referred back to each original protocol in order to validate their occurrence. The following example demonstrates one protocol's formulated meaning statement about caring's professional practice. As proscribed by Colaizzi (1978), this formulated meaning statement was used in substantiating the subsequent theme clusters which emerged from this statement.

Formulated Meaning Statement:

Caring was always valued, and both verbal and nonverbal behaviors used to transmit that caring were perceived as direct and intentional, as exemplified by deliberate use of verbal reassurance in order to calm a patient experiencing profound hypotension. As a new graduate, the goal of her nurse caring actions was perceived as both self- and patient-focused, because she was concerned that her patient like her, and that she met his physical needs safely. With development of feeling technically competent as she has become more professionally experienced, she now feels that her caring actions are patient–focused. She tries to consider all aspects of her patient, including psychological and spiritual needs. She tries to anticipate patient needs but also reassures each patient that she is there for him, and that he is safe. She backs this reassurance up by making both scheduled and unscheduled patient checks during her work shift. She tries to include the family in planning, giving, and evaluating her nursing care. She bases much of her care on giving health teaching and believes in her role of patient-family advocate.

Theme Clusters:

Professional caring as holistic.
Expression of caring through touch.
Technical competence must underpin the nurse's feeling of giving nurse caring.
Communication of caring can be verbal and/or nonverbal.
Therapeutic listening expresses nurse caring.
The nurse must be physically available to the patient.
Professional nursing experience enables the nurse to forget the self in order to focus caring energy on the patient.
Empathy for the patient–family derives from the nurse's own life and professional experience.
Support of the patient-family includes health teaching, being reassuring, providing for safety, security, and professional advocacy.

These theme clusters were then submitted along with all raw data, transcribed interviews, and formulated meaning statements to the aforementioned judges (Goodwin & Goodwin, 1984). This process of theme validation proved to require minimal judge–directed suggestions for language clarification. Following this process, the researcher collapsed the theme clusters into larger theme categories (Colaizzi, 1978; Polkinghorne, 1989). For example, the last theme cluster described in the protocol presented here was collapsed into the overall theme of social support (Dimond & Jones, 1983). All overall themes were then resubmitted to the research judges for final validation (Goodwin & Goodwin, 1984).

RESULTS

Table 9-1 lists the six themes that emerged as descriptive of the lived experience of natural caring. Table 9-2 lists the 14 themes of professional nurse caring.

The following discussion will highlight the significant differences as well as similarities between natural caring and professional nurse caring that emerged through analysis of the data. Instances in which professional nurse caring included an integration of natural caring's themes will also be presented.

Table 9-1
Themes of Natural Caring

Theme	Number of Protocols in Which Theme Emerged
Being There	12 out of 12
Touching	10 out of 12
Social Support	10 out of 12
Reciprocity	6 out of 12
Time/Extra Effort	3 out of 12
Empathy	2 out of 12

Holism

Unlike the lived experience of natural caring, professional nurse caring requires that the nurse address the patient-family as a whole. Subjects described the need to use their whole bio-psycho-spiritual self in order to feel successful in giving nursing that they perceived to be caring. As one nurse described this need:

> I have to consider what my patient needs from *his* perspective.... I think caring for the whole person—not just his "gallbladder" or whatever—I think that's nursing to me.... I care differently when I'm caring as a nurse, I think, because of this. When I'm not working, my caring may not be "holistic" because I'm not thinking about "total patient care" ... when I'm caring at home ... I might try to make my little boy's sore throat feel better, but I'm not thinking about anything but his throat and how much it hurts.

Being There

All participants stated that the lived experience of natural caring required significant others being there for them in order to feel physically and emotionally safe. Being there does not need to be verbally stated in order to be felt in natural caring relationships, perhaps because of the long–term nature of many such relationships. This contrasts with subjects' descriptions of being there as nurses for their patients. Out of 12 respondents, 11 felt that professional caring requires the nurse to both verbally state and nonverbally demonstrate being there for the patient-family. As one subject stated:

I always felt that someone was there for me while growing up. I don't need my husband to tell me he's there for me because what he *does* for me tells me that. . . . [as a nurse] I do whatever it takes to reassure my patient that I'm here for him, but I know I can't just say that—I have to actually do it, like wheeling him to a phone so he can call his wife, or just checking back on him [at the time] when I told him I would.

Touching

Touching enabled all participants' to both feel and communicate the experience of caring. Touching was not found to be a requirement for every participant's experience of feeling natural caring, but there was universal agreement that one's professional caring was frequently transmitted nonverbally through touching that was neither rushed nor rough. Although it was discovered that the capacity for touching may arise out of the lived experience of natural caring, touching can also be deliberately learned. This can occur through either formal or informal learning and/or professional experience. Nine subjects felt that their nursing education enabled them to touch more therapeutically than would have occurred through informal learning (e.g., role modeling) alone. Eleven nurses believed that

Table 9-2
Themes of Professional Nurse Caring

Theme	Number of Protocols in Which Emerged
Holism	12 out of 12
Touching	12 out of 12
Technical Competence	12 out of 12
Communication	12 out of 12
Listening	12 out of 12
Being There	11 out of 12
Professional Experience	11 out of 12
Empathy	10 out of 12
Social Support	10 out of 12
Reciprocity	10 out of 12
Involvement	10 out of 12
Time	9 out of 12
Formal and Informal Learning	9 out of 12
Helping	8 out of 12

their professional experience strengthened their skill in using touch effectively. As one individual shared:

> I'd get smiles at home, but not a lot of hugs or kisses. We weren't "touchy" ... I'm still not in my home life. But I do use touch with my patients a lot because I've seen how well patients respond ... they seem to get calmer.

Yet another subject declared:

> [As a nurse] I learned the value of touch from watching the [nurse] midwives use it. I've learned that touch works with labor patients but I have to work to be comfortable with it.

Technical Competence and Professional Experience

An important study finding links the themes of technical competence and professional experience to the capability for direct and intentional practice of professional nurse caring. At the time of its undertaking, this was the first documented study to elicit this finding from the professional nurse's perspective, although several studies had earlier indicated that patients valued receiving care from those nurses whom they perceived as technically competent (Henry, 1975; Larson, 1981; Gardner & Wheeler, 1981; Haase, 1985). The development of technical competence for providing professional nurse caring is attained through professional experience. This process is illustrated by the subject who observed:

> I try to incorporate my caring and my skills all into one to help my patient—that's total care that I certainly couldn't give if I weren't a nurse.... [But] as a new grad it was hard to coordinate my nursing skills with my ability to really help someone—I didn't have as much to give him. I was ... stressed at just trying to be competent.... It was at least a year before I really felt that I was reasonably competent in my skills, and able to start focusing on other things my patient might need besides my ability to give safe technical care.

Formal and Informal Learning, Communication, and Listening

Psychosocial theories learned in baccalaureate education provided the foundation for acquiring formal (e.g., didactic) and informal (e.g., role-modeled) learning. Therapeutic communication and listening skills were similarly obtained. A nurse, whose basic education was a diploma program, stated:

> Going back to school [for a BSN] really made a difference to how I view my patients. I don't just try to get the work done. . . . I use therapeutic communication, active listening . . . I really enjoy what I do.

All respondents discussed similar experiences that helped them in learning actions expressive of nurse caring. For example, all subjects related that they used touching, communication, and listening as expressions of natural caring when first practicing nursing. Formal and informal learning in nursing, as well as professional experience with therapeutic professional modalities, were described by respondents as the means for transforming natural caring into professional nurse caring. Similarly, participants reported that they believed that giving nursing care through nursing therapeutics such as active listening, therapeutic communication, and physical nursing modalities such as post-operative management directly and intentionally transmitted professional nurse caring which differed from natural caring. As one subject stated:

> When I was a new grad it was hard to coordinate giving caring the way I had personally experienced caring. . . . I was worried about my technical skills, so I didn't have as much reserve to give [caring] to my patient. My actions were technical . . . no way could I have used "therapeutic communication!" I wasn't secure enough in my skills to be other-centered. With experience, though, I can now put the technical skills together with my caring as a nurse . . . but I think my caring is different from what I do [i.e. caring] with my family and friends. My caring when I'm nursing is tied up in my nursing—you can't separate them. When I'm not at work, my caring is still caring but it's different, too. I'm not nursing when I'm home.

Empathy

Empathy was also integral to the practice of professional caring, discerning the modus of professional caring from natural caring. One subject asserted:

> As I've gotten older, I find I'm more tolerant and less impatient. But my patience in nursing is, I think, also due to the fact that doing technical things in here [ICU] doesn't throw me anymore.

I can be caring *and* technically expert at the same time because I'm an experienced nurse . . . and that's nursing to me.

In other words, life as well as professional experience can provide the nurse with opportunities for learning how to provide caring. Such experience is central to the empathy inherent in professional caring.

Social Support

The theme of social support was another factor integral to both natural and professional nurse caring, although it appeared to mean several things to the majority of subjects. Foremost among support components was nurse advocacy of the patient's worldview, regardless of whether one agreed with this view. Participants expressed that the nurse must accept the patient at that individual's developmental level in order to interact with the patient as an individual. Nurse–matriarchal intervention on behalf of the patient did not emerge as consistent with such support in this study. Conversely, the support of natural caring was found to be related to parental nuturance and advocacy from the perspective of what the parent views as best. As one nurse described this difference:

I'm a real patient advocate. I do my best to give my patient the nursing care he needs . . . health teaching, everything. I go to bat for my patients when it's needed . . . [but] I'm not going to tell my patient what to do. I try to help him or his family member come to a decision if that's what's needed, but I don't make his decisions for him, or tell him "you must do this" or, "you must do that." I think that's horrible . . . it's taking away a person's right to make his own decision.

Reciprocity

The theme of reciprocity emerged as important to both natural caring and professional nurse caring. As a requirement to professional caring's reciprocation, ten subjects agreed that one must first be caring toward the self. One individual shared that:

If I have problems at home, or if I'm feeling down or haven't been taking care of myself, I won't be able to be caring [at work], just technical, because I won't have the energy. If someone tries to be caring to me, I may just not even be able to feel it.

Ten participants shared the view that giving caring is facilitated when the patient–family respond favorably. Another nurse stated that:

> It takes a lot of energy to be a *caring* nurse, not just giving physical care. It helps when you know your patient appreciates what you're doing . . . like when one patient I just took care of told me [at discharge from ICU] that he thinks he made it through his stay because I was his primary nurse. That's what I mean by getting the energy back [to continue caring].

Three individuals stated that they needed to feel a reciprocation of caring when involved in close patient–family relationships; ten asserted that they believed that an important means for feeling that their caring is reciprocated should occur in two ways. First, they believed that a balance of personal with professional life was important to the lived experience of feeling the reciprocation of natural caring. Second, they believed that the capacity to practice professional caring required caring reciprocation from fellow professionals, which could occur through peer validation that subjects' nursing was either proficient or particularly effective. One subject for example believed that her patient had reciprocated her caring, but added that:

> . . . it's important that my peers know that I'm a good nurse— that's important in giving me a lot of the energy I need to keep caring for patients who are sometimes too sick to know—or care—what I'm doing for them.

Involvement

Whether the nurse was under- or overinvolved with the patient-family affected her ability to practice direct and intentional professional nurse caring. Eleven respondents stated that they believed they experienced under and/or overinvolvement when they were new graduates. To illustrate:

> When I was a new grad, it was hard to coordinate being caring with [my] technical skills, so I didn't have as much . . . to give my patient because I was so anxious about getting everything done. . . . I guess I just didn't get much involved with my patients because I was too worried about *me*.

This example contrasts with that of another subject, whose perceived defeat in a recent professional experience can be taken to illustrate caring overinvolvement:

I find what I do in Well Child Clinic frustrating. I give mothers appointments and they don't keep them. I go after them; I call them up; if I see them [in town], I remind them about their having missed an appointment. . . . How much can I do for them? I really worry about this.

Time and Helping

Nine subjects perceived that professional nurse caring required time. "Time" in the professional sphere contrasts with the "time" described as important to subjects' discussion of the natural caring experience. In natural caring, time may not always be available to express caring, but caring's presence is nonetheless still perceived. This appreciation may not carry over to the patient-family's perception of professional caring. One subject asserted:

I have a hectic homelife right now because my husband and I are building our own log house. But even though it seems we're always in a hurry, we still know we love each other. . . . In my nursing, if my patient doesn't think I have time for her, it can really affect my relationship with her, because she doesn't know me . . . how can she know that I care? I *have* to have the time to give emotional and psychological care besides physical care—not just rush in and out of her room. Otherwise I'm a robot, not a nurse.

When the nurse perceives that time is available to become involved, it is also perceived that one can directly and intentionally provide caring that can help the patient–family. Helping did not emerge as a discrete theme of natural caring. As it emerged in professional caring, eight nurses perceived that helping was important to their caring for the patient–family in order to achieve maximum wellness or peaceful death with dignity.

DISCUSSION

All of the foregoing findings provided the basis for creating the fundamental structure of professional nurse caring, which was validated by the three research judges as well as via re-interview of all subjects. Professional nurse caring integrates the lived experience of natural caring with the expression of professional caring. Professional caring is based on natural caring. It is not merely an increased expression of that caring but, rather, is a direct and intentional process in which specific therapeutics transmit professional nurse caring. That is, the nurse's giving of professional caring evolves from natural caring's lived experience, as well as the development of a repertoire of professional intentional actions acquired through both education and professional practice. Professional caring's intentional actions include nursing therapeutics such as physical care modalities as well as psychosocial interventions that provide healing through helping, empathy, and social support. Although the intentionality of professional caring may have the same goal as natural caring, professional caring differs because professional caring's intentionality is professionally therapeutic. This therapeutic derives from nursing education, and depends upon technical competence and professional experience in nursing for its development. It is in this sense that professional nurse caring emerges as different from natural human caring.

Professional caring's reciprocity supports the notion that such caring leads to co-actualization for the nurse as well as the patient. Because its practice appears to be intrinsically satisfying, professional caring may substantively validate the meaning of professional nursing. This meaning does not derive merely from isolated caring actions, rather, it emerges from the entire caring process itself. This finding adds support to Mayeroff's (1971) belief that self-meaning is bestowed not by caring actions but by the caring process itself.

The finding that the nurse must feel technically competent in order to directly and intentionally transmit professional caring can be explained by Benner's (1984) tenets of novice versus expert practice. That is, the expert is more able to practice nursing based on the patient's (rather than the nurse's) needs.

The study's findings indicate that professional nurse caring makes a difference to nurses in their professional lives. That such caring makes a difference suggests that the provision of professional nurse caring must not fall victim to either fiscal constraints or the nursing shortage.

IMPLICATIONS AND RECOMMENDATIONS FOR RESEARCH

The results of this study have implications for the nursing profession in the education, practice, administration, and research arenas. Because the lived experience of natural caring was found to be necessary to the nurse's ability to practice professional caring, it seems logical that educators determine the need for the lived experience of natural caring as early in the education process in nursing as possible. Educators could actively identify student need for natural caring and, if indicated, refer that student to either counseling and/or resources that might provide for natural caring's lived experience. This provision could be used to guide the development of a natural caring action repertoire. That direct and intentional professional nurse caring was not practiced by newly graduated nurses suggests a basis for further research of caring in education. This research should explore methods for developing caring and nursing practice criteria for professional entry.

In the practice arena, nurses could provide for the reciprocity needed for professional caring through developing weekly collegial support activities. These activities might include, for example, unit staff meetings that clearly focus on identifying and responding to nursing concerns and needs, as well as highlighting nursing accomplishments. The support inherent in the reciprocity of professional caring could carry over to administration when used to (1) overcome any communication deficits previously found between staff and administration; and (2) provide a viable basis for administrative practice.

An important recommendation for nursing practice derives from the study's explication of time as important to one's giving of professional caring. The nurses must have time to practice nursing in all its dimensions (not just technical skills) if nursing interventions are to directly and intentionally transmit professional caring.

Several final recommendations relate to research. Additional studies are needed to demonstrate the relationship between professional caring and the nurse's facilitation of patient-family wellness or achievement of peaceful death. Research is also needed to determine what remedies might better facilitate new graduate acquisition of technical competence and professional experience. Investigations must focus on identifying the time frame for this acquisition as a predictor for professional caring capability. In addition, support needs to be gained from patient-families themselves that professional nurse caring does, indeed, make a positive difference in both their satisfaction with health care delivery as well as achieving/maintaining their maximum levels of wellness. Finally, both the study's results as well as the claim that caring is nursing's essence indicate a need for research that will discern similarities and differences in professional caring in nursing compared to other helping professions.

CONCLUSIONS

As it emerged from this study, professional caring can be definitive of nursing's worldview. The *cura* or curing focus of medicine is rooted in healing as a modality, wherein the patient–family receive unidirectional therapeutics from the medical provider. Conversely, nursing's *caritas* or caring centers on the bidirectional transmission of this therapeutic which encompasses healing, yet goes beyond it to include empathy, helping, and social support. As it emerged from this investigation, professional nurse caring affects the human spirit because it is holistically engendered and bidirectionally experienced. It is thus the author's contention that caring defines the profession of nursing.

One final comment relates to the positive effect of the research experience for the investigator. This effect derived from the beauty experienced in literally immersing in the data. This process proved both personally and professionally rewarding. Through the lived experience of using the phenomenological method, the researcher validated her own lived experience of professional nursing.

REFERENCES

Ashbrook, J. B. (1985). *Responding to human pain*. Valley Forge: Judson Press.

Benner, P. (1984). *From novice to expert*. Menlo Park, CA: Addison-Wesley Publishing.

Bevis, E. O. (1978). *Curriculum building in nursing: A process*. St. Louis: C. V. Mosby.

Bogdan, R. C., & Biklen, S. K. (1982). *Qualitative research for education: An introduction to theory and methods*. Boston: Allyn & Bacon.

Colaizzi, P. (1978). Psychological research as the phenomenologist views it. In R. S. Valle & M. King (Eds.), *Existential–phenomenological alternatives for psychology*. New York: Oxford University Press.

Dimond, M., & Jones, S. L. (1983). Social support. In P. L. Chinn (Ed.), *Advances in nursing theory development*. Rockville, MD: Aspen.

Field, P. A., & Morse, J. M. (1985). Nursing research: The application of qualitative approaches. Rockville, MD: Aspen.

Gardner, K. G., & Wheeler, E. (1981). Patients' and staff nurses' perceptions of supportive nursing behaviors: A preliminary analysis. In M. M. Leininger (Ed.), *Caring: An essential human need*. Thorofare, NJ: Slack.

Gaut, D. A. (1979). An application of the Kerr–Soltis model to the concept of caring in nursing education. Unpublished doctoral dissertation, University of Washington.

Gaut, D. A. (1983). Development of a theoretically adequate description of caring. *Western Journal of Nursing Research, 5*(4), 313–324.

Goodwin, L. A., & Goodwin, W. L. (1984). Are validity and reliability "relevant" in qualitative evaluation research? *Evaluation and the Health Professions, 7*(4), 413–426.

Gustafson, D. (1981). Passivity and activity in intentional actions. *Mind, 90,* 41–60.

Harris, M. (1968). *The rise of anthropological theory.* New York: Thomas Y. Crowell.

Haase, J. E. (1985). The components of courage in chronically ill adolescents: A phenomenological study. Unpublished doctoral dissertation, Texas Woman's University.

Henderson, V. (1978). *Principles and practice of nursing,* New York: Macmillan Publishing.

Henry, O. M. M. (1975). Nurse behaviors perceived by patients as indicators of caring. Unpublished doctoral dissertation, The Catholic University of America, Washington, DC.

Hinshaw, A. S. (1979). Planning for logical consistency among three research structures. *Western Journal of Nursing Research, 1,* 250–253.

Hyde, A. (1976). The phenomenon of caring (parts II–IV). *American Nurses Foundation, 11*(1;2;3), 2-3, 18-19.

Kerr, D. H., & Soltis, J. F. (1974). Locating teacher competency: An action description of teaching. *Educational Therapy, 24*(1), 3–16.

Kruger, D. (1981). *An introduction to phenomenological psychology.* Pittsburgh: Duquesne University Press.

Larson, P. J. (1981). Oncology patients' and professional nurses' perceptions of important nurse caring behaviors. Unpublished doctoral dissertation, University of California at San Francisco.

Leininger, M. M. (1977). The phenomenon of caring: The essence and central focus of nursing. *American Nurses Foundation* (Nursing Research Report), *12*(1), 2,14.

Leininger, M. M. (1981). The phenomenon of caring: Importance, research questions, and theoretical considerations. In M. M. Leininger (Ed.), *Caring: An essential human need.* Thorofare, NJ: Slack.

Leininger, M. M. (1984). Caring is nursing: Understanding the meaning, importance, and issues. In M. M. Leininger (Ed.), *Care: The essence of nursing and health.* Thorofare, NJ: Slack.

Leininger, M. M. (1985). Transcultural care diversity and universality: A theory of nursing. *Nursing and Health Care, 6*(4), 202–212.

LeShan, L. (1966). *The medium, the mystic, and the physicist.* New York: Viking.

Mayeroff, M. (1971). *On caring.* New York: Harper and Row.

Nightingale, F. (1969, first published 1860). *Notes on nursing.* New York: Dover Publications.

Noddings, N. (1984). *Caring: A feminine approach to ethics and moral education.* Berkeley: University of California Press.

Norris, C. M. (1982). *Concept clarification in nursing.* Rockville, MD: Aspen.

Nygren, A. (1932). *Agape and eros* (Vol. 1). London: SPCK.

Peplau, H. (1952). *Interpersonal relations in nursing.* New York: G. P. Putnam.

Polkinghorne, D. E. (1989). Phenomenological research methods. In R. S. Valle & S. Halling (Eds.), *Existential–phenomenological perspectives in psychology: Exploring the breadth of human experience.* New York: Plenum Press.

Rogers, C. R. (1961). *On becoming a person.* Boston: Houghton Mifflin.

Thalberg, I. (1984). Do our intentions cause our intentional actions? *American Philosophical Quarterly, 21*(3), 249–260.

Valle, R. S., & King, M. (1978). *Existential–phenomenological alternatives for psychology.* New York: Oxford University Press.

Watson, J. (1979). *Nursing: The philosophy and science of caring.* Boston: Little, Brown.

Watson, J. (1981). Some issues related to a science of caring for nursing practice. In M. M. Leininger (Ed.), *Caring: An essential human need.* Thorofare, NJ: Slack.

Watson, J. (1989). *Nursing: Human science and human care.* New York: National League for Nursing.

Zderad, L. T. (1969). Empathic nursing. *Nursing Clinics of North America, 4*(4), 655–662.

10

The Other Side of the Polished Doors

Phyllis Updike

What a sanctuary it was, the World Health Organization (WHO) building and grounds. The building was a western, modern-looking, four-story structure with satellite communications equipment perched on the roof-top. The entire building was comfortably air conditioned, and large windows overlooked a perfectly kept lawn. The sidewalk leading up to the front door was lined with the flags of the 32 countries which comprise the Western Pacific Region of WHO. Near the entrance were gorgeous palm trees and flowering bougainvillea. Just beside the entrance there was a small pool of beautiful tropical fish. Breezes fanned the spray from the fountains. The pool was kept spotlessly clean—in stark contrast to nearby Manila Bay which had become too polluted to use any longer for swimming. Sometimes I felt almost a schizophrenic experience in walking out of the building and into the street, given the contrast of the two environments.

One day I went out for lunch, and I was quickly reminded that the grounds were not really a sanctuary at all. Outside, the sidewalks were lined with women, sitting on the concrete, obviously situated there for the day. Some kept an eye on small children, some laid their infants, naked, on the bare hot concrete. One held out an empty Coca-Cola cup as a makeshift beggar's receptacle from the only McDonalds in Manila, and another woman bandaged her little girl's sores. No, not with sterile 4×4's or gauze bandages but with yesterday's *Manila Times*. She tore the paper into lengths and wrapped these strips around her daughter's malnourished

133

legs. Although a month had passed since my arrival, I still seemed to reel back when I entered the steamy heat and walked through the crowds of people coupled with the odor of fermenting garbage from side streets.

After lunch, I headed back to the WHO. It felt strange to be alone—thousands of miles away from home, my husband, my son, and anything familiar. I rounded the last corner and came onto United Nations Avenue. Barefooted women were selling "Revolution" T-shirts hanging from branches of a batangas tree. Then I saw him. A small boy lying on his back on the sidewalk. He lay very, very still, and one arm was extended out. One arm clutched his tummy and the other lay outstretched beside him. He had on a bright red shirt and a pair of faded shorts. People walked around his outstretched arm, but paid him no direct attention. To them he was not particularly an unusual sight. To me, however, he had become suddenly important. Beside him the woman who must have been his mother looked away, inattentive, lost in thought.

At that moment I felt the greatest unrelenting urgency. It struck me that he was dead, or if not dead, then ill with a life–threatening illness. I'm not sure, even to this day, what triggered these thoughts or emotional response. Perhaps he was lying too still. Perhaps his chest did not appear to rise and fall with the gentleness of sleeping.

And then, as I looked at him, I saw that he was my own son. It was not that the boy reminded me of my son at that age. No. He had become my son. I looked and saw my own boy. I believed he was mine. I knew he was mine, and I began to run toward him. He would die, I thought if I didn't reach him in time. I had to get to him immediately. I had to get to him now.

I could feel my heart pounding as I ran toward him. I knelt down next to him. My boy, my own. I looked into his face and I understood then that he was asleep. As he lay there on the hot concrete, amidst the flies, vulnerable to the continuous stream of hurrying pedestrians, my son slept. To him the hot concrete sidewalk, in the middle of downtown Manila, had become as real as his own bed, if indeed he had a bed at all, anywhere. Suddenly, I felt the penetration of the experience of motherhood from a global point of view. This boy, all boys, all children, were mine, my responsibility. Anchored in this moment, I reached out to pick him up, to hold him close to me.

But I had attracted the attention of the women nearby, including his mother. Women crowded around me, leaned forward toward me, surrounded me. I felt dizzy with the heat and the power of the experience.

I looked at the faces of these women. I should explain, I thought as I began to re-enter this reality from an altered state of consciousness. They want me to explain. "I'm sorry," I said, "I thought he was sick. I'm sorry to interrupt."

She nodded and seemed to acknowledge my unusual intrusion. "It's all right," she seemed to say. "I'll take care of him. Don't worry." I gathered myself, got to my feet, and continued on back to work. As I walked back, I imagined my son in Denver. There is a 14-hour time difference between Denver and Manila, and I imagined him snuggled under his down comforter and new Martex sheets. Yes, he was back there—safe and living in an affluent cocoon of comfort. You can say "There but for the grace of God . . . ." You can say many, many things. But as the weeks passed and I continued my work at WHO, I realized that for me this had been a profound experience, so intense a shift in consciousness that my perception suddenly exploded and expanded into a realization that, truly, we are all one family. Because of what was happening to me at that time, because for those moments, that boy did become my son in a real and experiential context.

As I neared the WHO grounds, the flowers and tree-lined entrance into that cool, luxurious building, it suddenly occurred to me that the WHO was for me no longer a sanctuary. For there is really no way to keep out, push back, or escape from what exists on the other side of the polished doors. Once you understand the world and its inhabitants as one family, once you pass from under the canopy of luxury, the doors close behind you, and you can never go back again. If the paradigm shift holds significant existential meaning, one does not even wish to return.

Human caring is not merely an emotional state nor concern, for it also requires values, a will to act, and an openness to unpredictable consequences. Caring has re-emerged as a focal underpinning for nursing and other health sciences. It has become a research and practice convergence as well as an epistemic endeavor.

Watson (1985) has articulated the potential for human-to-human connectedness in the caring moment. Each is touched by the human center of the other. In the moment, then, lies the possibility for mutuality. It can be said, however, that mutuality cannot be verified in this account; i.e., the young boy's experience of my presence will never be known. However, this does not detract from the viability of the human connectedness.

Two of Watson's carative factors seem to be exemplified in particular by this experience (1985). One is the sensitivity to self and others. The sensitivity to self became real in the feeling of urgency, dizziness. The sensitivity to others assumes a certain complexity in that a part of it was responding to the boy on the sidewalk and a part was the responding to the boy who was the projected image of my (own) son who was physically 11,000 miles away. This brings to mind the reality of caring which enables the transcendence of specific, local parameters of time and space.

A second carative fact of significance is the one relating to "existential-phenomenological-spiritual forces" (Watson, 1985, p. 75). By way of review, we know that existential refers to being in time and space, and also the condition of a person's awareness of her or his radically free, yet responsible, nature. Phenomenologic refers to knowing an event through the senses rather than by thought. In other words, a process of knowing that is predominately noncognitive. (Spiritual forces will be addressed later in the discussion.) If we reflect on the phenomenological element for a moment, we may center on the vital role of emotion in caring. Several authors have written on this aspect (Watson, 1985; Noddings 1984). The theme of these views is that something critical is missing in a caring relationship if (it) is devoid of any subjective human response or emotion. Rationality or pure cognitive appraisal can override compassion, which may in fact be the drive to respond to the suffering human being. The natural consequence of this would be an apathetic response, which of course, is a nonresponse. Noddings (1984) further argues that we must guard against erecting principles of ethics in advance of an ethic of caring for one who is suffering. She further asserts that one definition of care means an arousal of an emotional state rather than of an analytical, cognitive state. This specific idea translates easily in relation to my own emotional reaction.

Some interesting possibilities emerge from reflecting on worldviews more indigenous to the geographic area of the Western Pacific Region. The East Asian Confucian view maintains that the reality of suffering must be accepted, just as the reality of the world must be accepted. The challenge becomes then, for one to create a daily response to suffering, rather than to alienate it or its meaning from other responses to life (Taylor, 1989). The notion of inclusion, of a gestalt, of larger and more and more unifying wholes, emerges as a theme that pervades not only body–mind–spirit unity, but transpersonal, transcultural, and transspatio-temporal realities. Is it not a provocative thought to realize that this encounter transpired on a street named United Nations Avenue? It almost seems that the street name assumes a metaphor for the experience itself.

Gadow (1984) articulates an aspect of caring that incorporates the role of human touch and human presence. She believes that subjectivity exists at the surface of the body. Touch, physical touch, becomes a dissolution of boundaries between persons. Touch presents considerable risk in an individualistic society, which frequently typifies the Western world. The Philippino people, however, do not insist on this level of autonomy, nor from an expatriate's view, do they even highly value it. In fact, often as I walked the streets, alone or with a companion, I would feel the warmth of small young hands reaching for mine. Human touch can certainly comfort as a medium of caring, as well as deliver one out of self-absorption, and be a delightful consequence of the dissolving of boundaries subjectively. At least, this was my experience of its meaning.

There is an intriguing parallel here between Gadow's assertion and Fowler's (1974) seventh stage of faith which he identifies as universalizing faith. He describes this stage as being beyond paradox and polarities, and that persons in this stage hold visions and commitments which free them for a passionate spending of the self in love, devoted to overcoming division and oppression.

The overcoming of division as described in the encounter may have resulted from the projection of my son onto the boy lying on the sidewalk. What I have often wondered about in the time since the encounter is the Philippino mother's thoughts and internal response to my actions. My hope is that at some level, she felt cared for.

Wang Yang-ming, of the Ming dynasty, illustrates a similar gestalt in responding to those perceived to be in need.

> Heaven and Earth and the myriad things as one body . . . Therefore when he sees a child about to fall into a well he cannot help a feeling of alarm and commiseration. This shows that his humanity forms one body with the child. [Taylor, 1989, 29]

This quote accurately describes my own sense of being at one, or that of "forming one body with the child." This truth I experienced in an organic, literal way as well as metaphorically. This is perhaps another interpretation of Gadow's thought regarding dissolution of boundaries through touch.

Taylor develops this idea further by suggesting that suffering may well serve as a motivating force toward acts of compassion and caring. Awareness of suffering may emerge from our own suffering or from seeing the suffering of others who are close to us. I would add that it may represent physical or emotional proximity. In other words, a compassionate response to suffering creates the potential for creating a bridge from a caring action toward a spiritual engagement of the self. If one accepts this, then one accepts the power as well as the fragility of this bridge. For even though caring assumes a foundation of ethics and emotion, compassion is always vulnerable and tenuous because it invites and requires a personal spiritual involvement.

Let us now shift our attention to some conceptual descriptions of spirituality. Stoll (Carson, 1989) writes of the essence of spirituality, and a few of the summary descriptors of spirit:

- *Imago Dei* (Image of God) within every person, making one a thinking, feeling, moral creative being able to relate meaningfully to God (as defined by the person), self, and others.

- A basic drive for bonding with the transcendent.
- A capacity for God consciousness, however God is defined. [Carson, 1989, p. 6]

Another metaphor for a person's spirit is the literal breath of life. The derivation comes from the Latin *Spiritus*. It is also related to the Greek and Hebrew words for spirit. The word also refers to wind and breath. A very explicit translation of this notion from the encounter with the boy on the sidewalk is that I actually perceived the child as not breathing, "his chest did not appear to rise and fall." What was happening with the *Spiritus*, the breath of life? Was it leaving him? Or me? Or were we both partaking of a *Spiritus* that enfolds us all?

When we reflect on these perspectives, the aspects of both a horizontal and vertical dimension of spirituality become crystallized. The horizontal plane becomes the living human matrix between and among all human beings. The vertical perspective represents a transcendent relationship; that which is outside/beyond the self. The companion experience to this understanding is perhaps the expression, "all sons, all children were mine—and were a part of my/our human family." My hunch is that experience of the horizontal aspect can serve as a vehicle or point of access to the vertical aspect and then empower the comprehension of ever expanding gestalts without fear of losing self. This is part of the inevitable vulnerability of spiritual engagement of the self.

Shelley (1989) reminds us that in order for a nurse to identify a spiritual concept of humanity, and I would add to identify *with* humanity, one must first recognize one's own spiritual needs. One must ask and honestly answer the question, "Are human beings spiritual beings?" If we believe that we are bio-psycho-social-cultural beings, is spiritual just one more compartmentalized linguistic piece to add to the chain of descriptors? Or is *Spiritus* actually the breath of life that permeates, penetrates, indeed perfuses all the other parts of the whole to give it life and integration?

When we remember the history and evolution of nursing, we recall that most nurses were members of religious orders. Throughout the 20th century, nurses have been predominantly employed by secular health care institutions. This is not to imply, however, that cathexis of spiritual care was indicated or preferred (Stuart, Deckro, & Mandle, 1989).

Stallwood & Stoll (1975) contend that the nature of man cannot be limited by culture, faith, orientation, nor time. This philosophic stance is valid from multiple perspectives including physics, the arts, and certainly spirituality.

Let us now return to the context of suffering and recognize that it represents primacy as the center of a spiritual response to the world and its inhabitants. A spiritual and/or religious response is particularly identified with a universe believed to be meaningful and purposeful. (I acknowledge that religion and spirituality may have definitive as well as overlapping boundaries). But on either or both grounds, one must view suffering in some way integral to the projected meanings discovered in the universe. Herein we discover another yearning for the gestalt. A wholeness which fosters increasing diversity within its unity appears to characterize the nature of spiritual engagement of self.

Maslow articulated this inherent human need for a foundation of valuing when he wrote:

> Human beings need a framework of values, a religion or religion-surrogate to live by, in the same sense that they need sunlight, calcium, or love. [Maslow, in Carson, 1989, p. 7]

Caring and compassion play key roles in the response to human need and represent at the very least an implied stance of anyone who maintains the values of a spiritual system. In fact a religious worldview is tenacious in encountering suffering. This is often portrayed in more predominant and explicit paradigms in the developing world today than we may recognize in the developed world. We again discover that religion endeavors to offer meaning to suffering, and at times, to even embrace it. Caring and compassion take on a central unifying focus both from a humanistic response and a spiritual response to the world and its people. The power and significance of this transformation is eloquently expressed by Teilhard de Chardin:

> Someday, after we have mastered the winds, the waves, the tides, and gravity, we shall harness for God the energies of love. Then, for the second time in the history of the world man will have discovered fire.

Perhaps it is so.

REFERENCES

Carson, V. (1989). Spirituality and the nursing process. pp. 150–179. In *Spiritual dimensions of nursing practice.* Philadelphia: Saunders.

Fowler, J. (1974). Toward a developmental perspective of faith. *Religious education, 69*(2), 207–219.

Gadow, S. (1984). Existential advocacy, technology, truth and touch. Paper presented at Research Seminar Series, University of Colorado Health Sciences Center, Denver, CO.

Maslow, A. R. (1968). *Toward a psychology of being* (2nd ed.). New York: D. Van Nostrand.

Mayeroff, M. (1971). *On caring.* New York: Harper & Row.

Noddings, N. (1984). *Caring: A feminine approach to ethics and moral education.* Berkeley: University of California.

Shelly, J. (1989). *The spiritual needs of children.* Downer's Grove, IL: Inter-Varsity.

Stallwood, J., & Stoll, R. (1975). Spiritual dimensions of nursing. In I. Beland & J. Passos (Eds.), *Clinical nursing: Pathophysiological and psychosocial approaches.* New York: Macmillan.

Stuart, E., Deckro, J., & Mandle, C. (1989). Spirituality in health and healing: A clinical program. *Holistic Nursing Practice, 3*(3), 35–46.

Taylor, R. (1989). Compassion, caring, and the religious response to suffering. In R. Taylor & J. Watson (Eds.), *They Shall Not Hurt* (pp. 11–32). Boulder, CO: Associated University.

Watson, J. (1985). *Nursing: Human science and human care, a theory of nursing.* Norwalk, CT: Appleton-Century-Crofts.

Watson, J. (1989). Human caring and suffering: A subjective model for health sciences. In R. Taylor & J. Watson (Eds.), *They shall not hurt* (pp. 125–136). Boulder, CO: Associated University.

11

Elements of Spirituality and Watson's Theory of Transpersonal Caring: Expansion of Focus

Paulette Burns

A respected nurse theorist has raised several questions about the study of caring in nursing (Norris, 1990). She proposes that the current focus of study on caring presents an array of epistemological problems. These problems include the difficulty of interpreting a concept considered to be in the metaphysical realm, the scientific consideration of a concept generally thought of as being in the domain of art, and the possible diminution of the concept by its objectification apart from the human self. Another question ponders whether the focus of study on the nurse as carer is a continuation of our early scientific beginnings when nurses studied nurses rather than addressing phenomena of concern to the science of nursing. Similarly, Conway claims that to conceptualize caring as the central construct in nursing hinders the development of nursing science by "blurring the distinction between the science of nursing and its discipline" (Conway, 1985, p. 78). This article will report a study, on the metaphysical concept of spirituality, that supports the continued investigation of caring from a scientific perspective. It is proposed, however, that the circumscribed study of caring within the context of the nurse-client relationship limits the

This work was partially funded by a grant from Sigma Theta Tau, Beta Delta Chapter. The author acknowledges Rose Nieswiadomy, Helen Bush, Marion Anema, Virginia Smith, and Glen Jennings for their support of this research as a dissertation committee.

141

explication of knowledge about the phenomenon of caring. Instead, this author calls for the expansion of focus of the study of caring to a variety of life relationships including, but not limited to, the nurse-client relationship.

INTERRELATIONSHIP OF MIND, BODY, AND SPIRIT

Watson (1979) describes nursing as the philosophy and science of caring. She posits a metaphysical theory of transpersonal caring that incorporates the spiritual dimension, including the concepts of soul and transcendence (Watson, 1985, 1988). She states that the spiritual dimension includes the degree of harmony among the mind, body, and soul (or between a person and the world), and the person's striving to actualize the self.

Advocates of the holistic health model signal the importance of the spiritual dimension in health (Carlyon, 1984; Guzzeta & Dossey, 1984; Travis, 1981; Tubesing, 1979). Mattson (1982) identifies the major principles of holistic health as unity and interdependence of body, mind, and spirit; involvement of the spiritual domain in healing; and belief in energies that surround all things and beings.

Dunn (1973), the parent of the term high–level wellness, considers the spiritual dimension of the individual as an integral, necessary part of holistic health. He states "the spirit is something very real, that it involves the process of healing . . . (doctors) have frequently observed people with a sick body but a well spirit, and when this is true, such people try to get well and they frequently do get well . . . but we seldom see a person with a sick spirit who has a well body" (Dunn, 1973, p. 11).

The theory of transpersonal caring is differentiated by Watson as going beyond other existential phenomenological theories, such as those proposed by Patterson and Zderad, Parse, or Rogers. The goals of her theory are: "mental-spiritual growth for self and others; finding meaning in one's own existence and experiences; discovering inner power and control, and potentiating instances of transcendence and self-healing" (Watson, 1985, p. 74).

One of the major constructs of her theory is the transpersonal caring process. This process includes the notion of two phenomenal fields, defined as the totality of human experiences, coming together during an actual caring event. Primarily, Watson's interests and studies have focused on the nurse as giver of care and the client as receiver of care, with both being changed by the actual caring event. She defines this event as "a focal point in space and time from which experience and perception are taking place . . . the actual occasion of caring has a field of its own that is greater than the occasion itself and allows for the presence of the geist or spirit of both" (Watson, 1985, p. 58). The intersubjectivity of phenomenal fields is characterized by both persons (nurse and client) being fully present in the moment and feeling a union with the other, a sharing of phenomenological fields.

Watson insists that the individual client is the agent of change, but the nurse can be a coparticipant. Quinn (1989) supports this idea by claiming that all healing is self-healing. She describes the role of the nurse in client-healing as midwife, helping to bring forth new life, relationship, and connection for persons.

The holographic paradigm of science best incorporates the ideas of transpersonal caring according to Watson (1988). She identifies the optimal scientific approach to help discover, explain, and understand transpersonal caring as qualitative in nature and in particular as the methodologies of existential or transcendental phenomenology.

STUDY METHODOLOGY

The importance and significance of the spiritual dimension described by holistic health advocates and specifically identified in Watson's theory of transpersonal caring, and the limited amount of systematic study of the concept, underscored the need to more fully understand spirituality as it is experienced and lived by a person. The phenomenological method was chosen to investigate and identify essential elements of spirituality. The target population of well adults was chosen to uncover the elements of spirituality in persons who labeled themselves as healthy. This was in keeping with the ideas of the holistic health model as the unity of mind, body, and spirit, or wholeness.

Names of well adults between the ages of 23 and 50 and unknown to the investigator were solicited from university faculty colleagues and staff members in a university outreach program serving nursing, public health, and medical students. Sampling criteria included the participant being able to verbally communicate his or her experiences, feelings, and perceptions regarding spirituality, and report being in good health. Ten participants were interviewed.

The ages of the participants ranged from 31 to 48, with a mean age of 38. Six of the participants were male; four were female. Eight were white; two were black. Three of the participants were self-employed, one as an artist, one as a land planner, and one as a clinical social worker. Six were employees in the positions of psychologist, administrative assistant, computer programmer, marriage and family therapist, police officer, and business representative. One was a housewife. Participants' formal education ranged from high school to the doctorate level. Four participants were

Baptist, two were Nazarene, two were transdenominational, and one was interdenominational. One reported being a nonpracticing Catholic who was considering becoming transdenominational. All participants reported good or excellent health. Five participants had two children, two had three children, and three had no children.

An unstructured, audio-recorded interview technique was used to elicit information from participants. Participants were asked to respond to two items: (1) what does spirituality mean to you, and (2) please describe an experience of spirituality. Each recording was transcribed verbatim. Twenty-two experiences of spirituality were shared, with participants sharing from one to four experiences. The experiences chosen for description ranged from an experience that had occurred the day of the interview to lived experiences from early adolescence. Participants provided 102 personal meanings of spirituality.

ESSENTIAL ELEMENTS OF SPIRITUALITY

Data were analyzed using the four-step process set forth by Giorgi:

1. "Read the entire description in order to get a general sense of the whole statement.
2. Re-read the text with the specific aim of discriminating meaning units with a focus on the phenomenon being researched.
3. Reflect on the delineated meaning units and express the insight contained in them more directly.
4. Synthesize the transformed meaning units into a statement regarding the structure of the experience" (Giorgi, 1985, p. 10).

Through synthesis and abstraction of our data, the essential elements of spirituality in the well adult were determined to be: the philosophy of the interrelationship between the Infinite and human, essenergy (essence and energy) permeability, precipitating event, depth experience, human responses, and life–changing.

Philosophy of the Interrelationship Between Infinite and Human

The philosophy of the interrelationship between the Infinite and human was described by all participants, particularly as they discussed their religious upbringing or as they related specifically held beliefs about the transcendent nature of life. All participants described an entity with more power than self and used such terms as God, Spiritual Energy, Unitive Energy, Higher Power, Lord, Jesus Christ, and Holy Spirit. Therefore, the term Infinite was defined as that otherness that an individual believes is vested with more power than self or other humans alone.

Essenergy Permeability

Many of the personal meanings of spirituality used the words essence and energy. These two words were combined, as participants seemed to have difficulty separating the two ideas, to form the term essenergy. This term is defined as the person–specific animating principle, derived from Lane (1987). The element of essenergy permeability indicates an individual's degree of openness to the spiritual dimension.

Precipitating Event

All of the participants reported at least one experience of a crisis event as precipitating an experience of spirituality. Of the 22 experiences, 20 involved maturational, situational, or life–threatening crises in relation to the self or a valued other person. Seven descriptions were related to illnesses of others, three to past illnesses of the participant, three to spontaneous healing experiences, and one to the death of another. The situational crises, other than health related, included two related to supervisors and one to an experience of financial ruin. The four descriptions of maturational crises primarily dealt with adolescent, young adult experiences of professing belief in God and then later questioning that action. Two descriptions did not reflect a crisis event, yet neither were they described as everyday occurrences. The term extraquotidian was coined to reflect these two descriptions and was defined as something more than everyday living.

Depth Experience

Depth experience was a term chosen to reflect the primary substance of the descriptions. Of the 22 descriptions, 11 were described vividly as occurring at a specific moment in time in which the participant knew, without a doubt, that something profound had happened. Participant 3 described her experience of the spontaneous recovery of her premature infant after the infant had been given 24 hours to live by the physicians. She said, "Actually, when they came in and told me that the baby was going to make it and he was all right, I looked at the clock and I realized it was the 24th hour. I mean exactly the 24th hour!"

Participant 4 described his experience with his father in an intensive care unit at the time of his father's death. "And then I went out in the hall, and they said you need to come see your Dad now . . . I was trying to get down the hall and I knew he was dead."

Participant 9 described an experience that had occurred several years earlier involving his unrelenting anguish over the diagnosis of mental retardation of his 18-month-old son. "I didn't hear any whistles. I didn't see any lights. I didn't do anything except, all of a sudden, literally, it was as if it (his own anguish) didn't exist. The problem was still there, but emotionally I wasn't depressed any longer about it. And I'm saying it didn't take two minutes. I got up from my knees and went back to where my wife was sitting and I said, 'It's gone.' And she said, 'Are you sure?' And I said, 'Yes, it's gone. It's gone. I don't hurt.'"

Table 11-1 shows the constituents of the depth experience element of spirituality along with exemplary statements explicated from the participants' transformed meaning units and expressed in the language of the investigator. Giorgi (1985) defined a constituent as a meaning unit that is determined to be meaningful in relation to its context. He described an element as a meaning unit that is determined to be meaningful independent of context. Participants distinguished the depth experience as a moment in time of a visceral knowing, sometimes accompanied by physical sensations, of Infinite care or connectedness as a reality. This was perceived as a personal-intimate episode with the Infinite, different from and more than other experiences, which might be accompanied by propitiary feelings or acts. The individual cannot make or force this experience to happen, but the individual can be open to the experience through such activities as praying, seeking support with friends, and recognizing the limits of individual control.

The depth experiences described by the participants all reflected a sense of harmonious interconnectedness, sometimes described as care, among the self, other human beings, and the Infinite. This is in concert with the findings of Hungelmann, Kenkel-Rossi, Klassen, and Stollenwerk (1985). They conducted a qualitative study using grounded theory to identify indicators of spiritual well-being in persons 65 years of age and older. The basic process of harmonious interconnectedness was determined to be the unifying theoretical construct.

Participants in the present study described their sense of connectedness in a variety of ways including being under the conviction of the Holy Spirit, finding an 'other' to relate to, knowing a distinct ever–present love, asking God for absolution and having it granted, and realizing a couple relationship as one of total connection. Table 11-2 lists the nature of the identified relationship(s) in each description. Most often this experience of harmonious interconnectedness occurred as a consequence of an interaction with, and valuing of, another human being in the context of the relationship.

Human Responses

Participants interpreted and assigned meaning to the depth experience; this meaning was reflected in human responses of feelings and actions after the experience. All of the participants indicated a positive meaning

Table 11-1
Constituents of the Depth Experience Element

Constituent	Example of Statements in Nursing Language
1. Realization of Humanity of Self or Valued Other	Being human to the participant means being able to feel deeply and not always being able to control those feelings.
	He realized, because of her age and the heart attack, that she could die.
2. Event of Non-Human Intervention	The participant was weary of dealing with poison ivy for so many years. The pastor and church prayed, and within 30 minutes he was healed. He has not had another reaction in his life.
	The participant felt something "other" within her body that was making her go to church.
3. Asking for/Receiving Divine Intervention During Event	In communicating with God, he made every effort to share with God how important this job was to him.
	He prayed for God to show him if He had something more for him to experience.
4. Visceral Knowing	There were no miraculous signs that God had taken away his burden, but he knew within him that his anguish was gone.
	The participant discerned a visceral feeling—not from any of his five senses.
5. Willingness to Sacrifice	He was willing to sacrifice his intelligence for his son, to change places with his son's IQ.
	The participant felt totally selfless because she had wanted a baby so very much, yet had been willing, and did, give up that baby for another woman.
6. Physical Sensations	She perceived a physical sensation during the experience.
	He had a sense of perfume in the air.
7. A Personal/Human Experience	The participant found an "other" she could relate to.
	He felt Christ loved him as a parent loves a child.
8. A Reality Experience	The participant experienced within, the fact that something he trusted and hoped for had happened, without a doubt.
	This experience helped to confirm the participant knowing that God was a real, personal Being for him.
9. Not Easily Explained	The participant has difficulty finding the exact words to describe the experience.
	Words cannot describe this feeling of connectedness.
10. Different from/More Than Other Daily Experience	This experience was different from others because he placed a much higher value on this job position than any others in his life.
	She felt like she was in a part of life apart from everyday experience.

Table 11-2
Nature of Connectedness

Experience	Relationship
1	self/Infinite
2	self/Infinite/friend
3	self/Infinite/son
4	self/Infinite/mother
5	self/Infinite
6	self/Infinite/mother
7	self/Infinite/father
8	self/Infinite/supervisor
9	self/Infinite
10	self/Infinite/support group
11	self/Infinite/acquaintance
12	self/fiance
13	self/husband
14	self/Infinite/family
15	self/Infinite
16	self/Infinite
17	self/Infinite
18	self/Infinite/roommate
19	Infinite/father
20	self/Infinite
21	self/Infinite/son
22	self/Infinite

was assigned to the depth experience, even though the outcomes of the precipitating events were not always positive. Participants described having extra energy, feeling whole, elated, totally good, peaceful, encouraged, assured, confident, a deep sense of tranquility, wonderment, reverence, and light. Human action responses included increases in interactions with others and the Infinite and increased abilities to cope with everyday life situations.

Life Changing

The life-changing element incorporated the ideas of positive coping after the experience, finding or recognizing a new purpose in life, and having a sense of personal growth. This element reflects the conversion nature of the depth experience as described by all of the participants.

GENERAL DESCRIPTION OF SPIRITUALITY

The lived experience of spirituality in the well adult was determined to be the process of striving for and/or being infused with the reality of the interconnectedness among the self, other human beings, and the Infinite, that occurs during a depth experience. An individual holds ideas, values, and beliefs—a philosophy—about the interrelationship between the Infinite and human beings. The congruency between these cognitive and affective perceptions and the individual's feelings of rightness or fit for self influences the permeability of the individual's essenergy dimension.

The enhancement of the awareness of an experience of spirituality is precipitated most commonly by a crisis event, but can also be precipitated by an extraquotidian event. The depth experience is characterized as a distinct moment in time when a sense of harmonious interconnectedness among the self, other human beings, and/or the Infinite occurs. Meaning is assigned to the experience and is reflected in human responses and actions. Meaning is overwhelmingly reported as positive. The experience is perceived as life–changing, resulting in a new sense of purpose or a sense of growth for the individual.

Comparison of Essential Elements of Spirituality and Watson's Construct of Transpersonal Caring

Watson (1988, p. 177) describes the human center as "having energy and power of its own," with the potential of expanding through the trans-personal caring process that facilitates healing. The essenergy (essence plus energy) element seems to reflect the human center, and the term permeability relates to the notion of the ability to expand. Examples of this concept reflected in the participants' personal meanings of spirituality are: "energy in the form of love, energy in the form of light, continuing state of change, awareness, process, feeling that comes from within, it comes from your heart, inner nature, essence of a person, real essence, an expression of my soul, it has to be cultivated to be aware of it." Participant 1 expressed the idea as follows: " . . . so I have been trying to tap into the spiritual energy that I feel kind of in an ocean of, and move that through my body to clear the channels that I have been blocking."

The construct of transpersonal caring, proposed by Watson to involve two phenomenal fields (humans with unique life experiences) coming together during an actual caring occasion and experiencing the presence of the spirit of both, was supported in the present study. The process was evident as participants described the precipitating event, the depth experience, and the assignment of meaning to the depth experience. Watson, however, has not proposed that a precipitating event (crisis or extra-quotidian) is part of the actual caring occasion. Also, participants described the depth experience occurring predominantly with some form of Higher Power, usually named God. Eight participants described an experience occurring between the self and the Infinite; 11 occurred among the self, the Infinite, and another human such as a family member, a supervisor, support group, a roommate, or an acquaintance. The depth experience was described as occurring between humans only in two of the descriptions, between a participant and her fiance and between a participant and her husband. Only one experience did not involve the participant, but was described as occurring between the Infinite and the participant's father.

These data suggest that the phenomenal fields of the human and the Infinite can and do join together. The merging of phenomenal fields, implying that there are always at least two phenomenal fields, was supported by all 22 experiences with the possible configurations: human with human, human with God (or whatever label one uses for transcendent being), or human with human with transcendent.

All of the participants described the idea of presence as a part of the depth experience. Watson has posited that presence or intersubjectivity occurs if the event is transpersonal and allows for the spirit of both. Participants richly, albeit with difficulty, described the concept of presence as reflected in Table 11-1 through the constituents and exemplary statements.

Watson stated that if transpersonal caring occurs, "then the event expands the limits of openness and has the ability to expand human capacities" (Watson, 1985, p. 59). Participants unanimously supported this notion. For example, Participant 1 related, "I am sure that the thinking and the knowing about them (spiritual matters) helped to give me a sense of balance." Participant 3 stated, "I just felt full. It was a feeling of joy, but it was a different type of joy. You know, it wasn't a joy like getting a gift or anything like that, it was more fulfilling than that." Participant 6 said, " . . . and I felt physically; my body cavity felt totally good. It felt totally selfless. I felt very light, almost like walking on air."

Participants also described increased capacities in response to the depth experience. Participant 7 related, "My husband had a hospital visit this morning with a man who just had an illiostomy and was devastated by it. He was able to encourage him and his wife, and to share with them that there is life after an illiostomy, and a much more fruitful life for him." Participant 2 described being a closer family unit, "My husband and I, we've talked about death, we've talked about spirituality, we've talked about the Bible, we talk about our innermost feelings with each other, and it's brought us tighter and closer together." Participant 9 talked about his capacities after his depth experience as, "I was able to, and continued to be able to, work with him (his mentally retarded son); at least I can help and guide him." These statements support Watson's (1985) proposition that the actual caring occasion becomes a part of each participant and has the potential to influence each in the present and the future.

REFLECTIVE CONCLUSIONS IN RELATION TO TRANSPERSONAL CARING

The concepts of the metaphysical theory of transpersonal caring were supported in this phenomenological study of spirituality. Of the 22 descriptions, 14 involved a loved one and/or the participant in the health care system. Five experiences related to the hospitalization of a family member for a life-threatening crisis. Another nine of the experiences involved the health care system in some way other than hospitalization. Not one spontaneously elicited description identified a nurse, or any other health care provider, as part of the experience of spirituality, even though the participants had ample opportunity to interact with the providers in the health care system. These descriptions provide evidence that the experience of transpersonal caring can and does occur in a variety of situations and possible configurations other than the nurse-client relationship.

The importance, however, of continuing to describe, explain, and understand caring in the context of the nurse-client relationship remains significant. The data in this study provide support for the idea of transpersonal caring between humans (nurse-client). This is in concert with Sohier's idea that nursing is of the nature of humanness, and therefore, observable in caring human interactions that are either professional or nonprofessional in nature (R. Sohier, personal communication, February 21, 1990).

In light of the findings of this study, the focus of the theory of transpersonal caring needs to be expanded to include the study of the components of spirituality, particularly the depth experience, as it occurs in the everyday living of persons.

Some questions generated for further study might include:

1. What is the experience of spirituality like for persons in different stages of the life cycle?

2. What are the health patterns of persons who have had one or more depth experiences?

3. What life changes result in persons who have had a depth experience?

4. What are the influences of different philosophical orientations on the depth experience?

5. What is the relationship of practices to enhance consciousness (prayer, meditation, visualization) and a person's essenergy permeability?

Quinn (1989) emphasized the fact that our health care system is an illness care system. Persons generally come in contact with professional nurses for care once they enter the illness care system with a medical diagnosis or to receive a medical diagnosis. Transpersonal caring by the professional nurse can potentiate the healing process within this context as proposed by Watson. However, not all persons have access to, or need of, professional nursing care. What are the results of transpersonal caring in contexts other than the nurse–client relationship?

With the emphasis of health care beginning to shift to health promotion and wellness, and cost containment strategies in relation to illness, the importance of developing knowledge about what keeps a person healthy, or non-ill, is imperative. The transpersonal caring process, enriched by the identified components of spirituality in this study, must be investigated as it relates to wellness and health promotion activities of persons in their experiences of everyday living.

Leininger (1981) has long espoused her belief that care, through the history of mankind, has always been essential for human growth, development, and survival. If so, then expanding the study of care and caring to include the interrelationships of persons and the Infinite, as well as nurse–client interactions, will do much to promote a well society.

REFERENCES

Conway, M. (1985). Toward greater specificity in defining nursing's meta-paradigm. *Advances in Nursing Science, 7*(4), 73–81.

Carlyon, W. (1984). Reflections: Disease prevention/health promotion—bridging the gap to wellness. *Health Values: Achieving High Level Wellness, 8*(3), 27–30.

Dunn, H. (1973). *High-level Wellness.* Arlington, VA: Beatty.

Giorgi, A. (1985). Sketch of a psychological phenomenological method. In A. Giorgi (Ed.), *Phenomenology and psychological research* (pp. 8–22). Pittsburg, PA: Duquesne University Press.

Guzzeta, C., & Dossey, B. (1984). *Cardiovascular nursing: Body mind tapestry.* St. Louis: Mosby.

Hungelmann, J., Kenkel-Rossi, E., & Klasson, L. (1985). Spiritual well-being in older adults: Harmonious interconnectedness. *Journal of Religion and Health, 24*(3), 407–418.

Lane, J. (1987). The care of the human spirit. *Journal of Professional Nursing, 3*(16), 332–337.

Leininger, M. (1981). *Caring: An essential human need.* Thorofare, NJ: Charles B. Slack.

Mattson, P. (1982). *Holistic health in perspective.* Palo Alto, CA: Mayfield.

Norris, C. (1990). To care or not care—questions! questions! *Nursing and Health Care, 10*(10), 545–550.

Quinn, J. (1989). On healing, wholeness, and the Haelon effect. *Nursing and Health Care, 10*(10), 553–556.

Travis, J. (1981). *Wellness workbook for helping professionals.* Mill Valley, CA: Wellness Associates.

Tubesing, O. (1979). *Holistic health.* New York: Human Sciences Press.

Watson, J. (1979). *Nursing: The philosophy and science of caring.* Boston: Little, Brown.

Watson, J. (1985). *Nursing: Human science and human care.* Norwalk, CT: Appleton-Century-Crofts.

Watson, J. (1988). New dimensions of human caring theory. *Nursing Science Quarterly, 1*(4), 175–181.

12

Connecting: A Catalyst for Caring

Gloria M. Clayton, Joyce P. Murray, Sharon D. Horner, and Patricia E. Greene

Nursing is distinguished from other health professions by the caring relationship between nurse and patient. Caring has been identified as the "central unique and unifying force of nursing" (Leininger, 1981, p. 133); yet, there is little known about the process of the development of the caring relationship between nurse and patient. While research has identified patients' and nurses' perceptions of caring, little has been done to identify the process involved in the development of the caring relationship. Questions about this unique aspect of the nursing profession abound. What causes some patient-nurse dyads to bond and others to be mechanistic and task oriented? How are the characteristics of caring acquired? Are caring and technical nursing proficiency related? The analysis described in this paper provides some insight into the social-psychological process of the development of a caring relationship between nurse and patient.

The precursor to caring is connecting. Connecting is defined as the transpersonal experiences and feelings that lead to the sense of connection, attachment, or bonding between a nurse and a patient/family. Connecting, within the nurse-patient relationship, is particularly important when

This study was supported by the American Cancer Society through a donation from W. Armin Willig in honor of Lane W. Adams. The authors express appreciation to Sally Hutchinson for assistance with data analysis.

nurses work with cancer patients who may experience the fear and stigma of cancer; often face multiple, devastating medical treatment modalities; and encounter their own mortality.

LITERATURE REVIEW

Research has examined caring by identifying the perceptions of those primarily involved. Nurses rate psychosocial skills, such as listening, comforting, and indicating interest, as the most important caring behaviors. In contrast, studies of patients' perceptions of caring have revealed that technical skills are most highly rated, and are sometimes rated in conjunction with psychosocial skills. Allanach and Golden (1988) found in a study on patients' expectations, that patients rated highly the "amount of time spent" and the technical quality of the care. In the same study, two aspects of caring were identified in patients hospitalized for nonthreatening conditions (Allanach & Golden, 1988). The first aspect was identified as the "demonstration of professional knowledge and skill, [in addition to] surveillance and a reassuring presence" (p. 20). The second aspect of caring involved the nurse recognizing the person's individuality, encouraging independent behavior in the patient, and spending time with the patient.

Other research has examined the impact of the patients' contextual experiences on their reported perception of caring. Research supports the proposition that patients in different medical settings with different diagnoses attend to different qualities in the care they receive. In studies of patient-nurse dyads in which the patient had cancer, Larson (1984, 1986, 1987) found differences in nurses' and patients' rankings of caring behaviors. Nurses ranked listening, touching, and allowing expression of feelings highest, while patients ranked monitoring and technical activities highest. In a study using a population of patients who had recently suffered myocardial infarction, Cronin and Harrison (1988) found patients rated monitoring and teaching as the most important caring behaviors. These differences between nurses' and patients' perceptions of caring were also supported in a study of elderly hospitalized patients. Nurses ranked psychosocial behaviors, including listening and teaching, as most important, while patients ranked treating them as individuals and monitoring as most important (Clayton, 1988).

The differences in perceptions of care also existed among patients. Some patients viewed touching as caring and others viewed it as intrusive and non-caring (Clayton, 1988). The contextual nature of caring identified in the previous research was consistent with the theoretical construct of caring proposed by Watson (1985), Leininger (1981), Benner and Wrubel (1989), and Gardner and Wheeler (1981) which suggests that an infinite number of possibilities exist for the intersubjective caring experience between a nurse and a patient.

Although the existing literature describes nurse and patient perceptions of caring behavior, it does not describe the process by which caring relationships between nurses and patients develop. While it is important to identify nurses' and patients' perceptions of caring behaviors, it is also important to identify how the bonds of a caring relationship are established. The purpose of this paper is to identify and describe variables that affect caring behavior and to describe the proposed stages in the development of a caring relationship between nurse and patient.

The more than 700 pages of narrative data that describe individual instances of outstanding nurse caring behavior support the proposal that connecting is the social–psychological basis for the process of developing a caring relationship between nurse, patient, and the patient's family. Other conditions that affect connecting are also reported and the four proposed stages of connecting are described. Finally, topics for future research are suggested.

METHODOLOGY

The data for this study were acquired from nomination packets for the 1987 and 1988 Lane W. Adams Award for Excellence in Cancer Nursing. This award is offered by the American Cancer Society for excellence in oncological nurse caring. Each nomination packet included a form completed by the nominator and letters written by patients, families, and nurse and physician colleagues of the nurse being nominated. Together these letters and forms provided a detailed description of specific clinical scenarios which demonstrated excellence in nurse caring.

The packets used in this study were drawn from 388 packets received for the 1987 and 1988 awards. During the review processes for the 1987 and 1988 award winners, two independent reviewers attained 100 percent agreement on the final 35 packets for each year. The total of 70 packets from both years ($n = 70$) were used as the sample for this study.

PROCEDURE

Hutchinson (1986) suggests that during the first phase of a qualitative study, the researcher becomes immersed in the data being collected, actively searching for commonalities and contradictory themes. The codes and themes of this study were identified during a pilot study using the nomination packets of ten previous award winners. The substantive codes were identified from the packets. Using the constant comparative method, the researchers sorted these Level I *in vivo* codes into Level II categorical codes. Consensus was achieved among the authors for the sorting of every substantive code after much discussion and frequent forays back to the original sources. A coding sheet was created to assist reviewers in identifying substantive codes. A definition for each category was developed based on the nuances of meanings common to each category (Tables 12-1 and 12-2).

Volunteer nurse reviewers were recruited from the National Nursing Advisory Committee to analyze the sample of 70 packets. The reviewers were trained in the coding process by using nomination packets not included in the sample. Each of the sample packets was analyzed by two reviewers to increase reliability of substantive code identification. Reviewers consistently identified substantive codes identified in the pilot study. Because of the nature of the data, the researchers were unable to verify the data by conferring with participants.

Table 12-1
Level II Categories and Definitions

Environmental Broker
Those things that the nurse can manipulate, control, or influence in the health care setting or community that positively influence the illness experience.

Professional/Expert Knowing
The knowledge, skills, professional activities, "ways of knowing and being" that characterize the expert clinician.

Facilitating Factors
Those behaviors, interactions, or values which are expressed in the human-to-human exchanges between nurse and patient that allow the patient to feel sustained or aided throughout the illness.

Personal Being
Those personality characteristics of the nurse which lead others to view the nurse as special or unique.

Connecting
The transpersonal experiences and feelings which lead to the sense of connection, attachment, or bonding between nurse and patient/family.

Table 12-2
Examples of Behaviors from Level II Categories.

Environmental Broker
Acts as patient advocate.
Attends to details.
Participates in decision-making policies.
Provides administrative leadership through knowledge of system.
Volunteers in community.

Professional/Expert Knowing
Anticipates needs prior to problem occurrence.
Demonstrates expert knowledge (disease and treatment).
Demonstrates competent technical knowledge, i.e., physical care, intravenous access, aspiration, bone marrow.
Maintains high standards

Facilitating Factors
Encourages independence appropriately.
Encourages expression of emotions as a way of coping.
Helps people cope.
Is empathetic, quick to respond, realistic, stern when needed, sympathetic.
Listens.
Prepares patient and family for death.
Provides comfort, emotional support, encouragement, individualized care, spiritual care, and nurturance.
Recognizes unique qualities of each person.
Recognizes whole person.

Personal Being
Balances personal and professional life.
Demonstrates highest moral character.
Has positive attitude.
Is cheerful, compassionate, dedicated, humane, open.
Is assertive, courageous, intuitive.
Shows concern.
Smiles.

Connecting
Awareness of change in relationship (patient).
Exhibits unconditional positive regard.
Involves patient/family in decision-making process.
Participates in the discovery of meaning in illness experience.

FINDINGS

Through constant comparative analysis and conceptual interpretation, the process of connecting emerged from the data. The process of connecting is defined as the transpersonal experiences and feelings that lead to a sense of connection, attachment, or bonding between nurse and patient/family. Connecting may act as a catalyst for changing a potentially overwhelming cancer experience into an empowering experience in which the patient and the patient's family feel supported and in control. Testimony to the positive impact of patients' and families' feelings about nurses can be found throughout the data,

> Our family was thrown into a raging sea when our youngest son was diagnosed with acute lymphoid leukemia. Since that time Annie[1] has been our lifeboat through the storm.

And in another situation,

> From the beginning of our nurse/patient relationship Beth has voiced her support for my physical and emotional well-being. . . . Beth has helped me develop a strength within myself that has enabled me to look beyond the problems I face today to the possibilities I will have tomorrow. She was first my nurse—now she's my friend.

During the next phase of data analysis Glaser's "Cs" (1978) were adopted as the organizing structure. Glaser's "Cs" include (a) antecedent conditions, (b) temporal parameters, (c) causes or accessing mechanisms, (d) context, and (e) consequences. In addition, Hutchinson's (1986) suggestion that the "posing of certain questions during coding enables the researcher to more easily grasp the data and establish theoretical codes" (p. 121) was used to understand the critical properties of connecting.

Antecedent Conditions of Connecting

Antecedent conditions in the patients, their families, and the nurses had an impact on the subsequent caring relationship. Basically, all patients were diagnosed with the "dreaded disease" cancer, and each family member was confronted with the horror of this "disease occurring in a significant other." This threat contributed to the patients' and their families' sense of crisis.

Antecedent conditions for nurses that influenced connecting were an

---

[1]All names in vignettes are pseudonyms.

awareness of, and a sensitivity to, the patients' and their families' needs from moment to moment, and a willingness to respond to supportive behaviors. Additional conditions for nurses included the manipulation of the environment and the utilization of knowledge, skills, and expertise to address the patients' and families' intense feelings. In each situation, intuition was combined with an unconditional positive regard and respect for individuality as the nurse met the patient's needs.

Patients and families described nurses as having various personality characteristics that were important to the caring relationship. Characteristics such as calmness, cheerfulness, compassion, courage, enthusiasm, kindness, openness, and intelligence contributed to the patients' and families' recognition of the nurse as a special or unique person. Along with these characteristics, patients and families described a fit or meshing of personalities that enhanced the "connecting" between nurse and patient.

One condition was repeated frequently throughout the data; it was that "the nurse went above and beyond the call of duty." Examples of behavior that were "above and beyond the call of duty" from the scenarios included descriptions of a nurse who stayed with a family overnight while the patient was dying, of another driving 50 miles to spend Christmas with a family, of another nurse buying a special dress for a child, of a nurse providing support for several years to a family that was continuing to experience grief. The nurses' willingness to go "above and beyond the call of duty" provides evidence for feelings of connectedness between nurse, patient, and the patient's family.

Temporal Aspects of Connecting

The temporal aspects of connecting varied according to the context and the stage of the relationship existing between nurses and patients and their families. Connecting occasionally occurred at the time of diagnosis, or in other scenarios it took days, weeks, or months for this bond to form. Spending time with the patient was frequently stated throughout the data as an important element of connecting. Depending on the circumstances, it was possible for "connecting" to occur immediately or for it to develop over time. A critical or life-threatening event often provided a stimulus for eliciting connectedness or for speeding its progress. In circumstances where death was imminent or threatening, all concerned viewed time as short, and connecting occurred rapidly.

Connectedness may be brief, extend over several years and throughout various events, and it may transcend regular nurse-patient contact. Patients who had reoccurrences after several years, or were treated in other settings and then returned, demonstrated that a previous "connected" relationship between nurse and patient supported a rapid reconnecting of the relationship.

Access to Connecting

Connecting was an individualistic experience with as many avenues to access connecting as there were patients. Connecting took place when experiences that had meaning for the patient were forged between nurse and patient. For some patients, access to connecting with the nurse occurred when the nurse demonstrated proficiency in knowledge and skills that increased the patients' sense of security or control, or reduced their pain. One family described their nurse as a blessing,

> We were scared and baffled as to what was happening, but she answered our questions and sometimes even answered them more than once . . . God has blest *(sic)* us by sending this lady to help.

Another nurse was described by her colleagues as reassuring to families,

> From other families we heard about her help during painful hospitalizations, even coming in on weekends to do an LP or bone marrow aspiration when the child had requested Dawn do it. Dawn's presence always reassures the families.

For other patients, access to connecting began when the nurse was sensitive and responded to the idiosyncratic needs and wishes of individual patients. The thoughtfulness of one nurse was described by the wife of a patient as she explained that,

> Ellen enabled my husband to reach his last goal—going for a ride in our son's new truck. She gave him medication and a reflexology treatment and bundled him in a sleeping bag to stay warm . . . He got to say goodbye to people and places in that last ride . . . (to) go out a winner and not a victim. Somehow she knew how important that ride was to him.

All the nurses in this study developed multiple avenues to facilitate access to connecting with their patients.

Strategies for Connecting

Nurses used many different strategies to facilitate connecting. These strategies incorporated the nurses' personal style along with their professional expertise and experience in caring for patients. Two strategies used by the nurses were identified as facilitating factors and environmental brokering

(Table 12-2). These strategies are mechanisms by which nurses recognized and acknowledged patients' needs and also worked toward meeting those needs. While facilitating factors and environmental brokering involved different activities, they both contributed to the easing of patients' distress.

Facilitating factors reflected the nurses' personal style while working with patients in different situations. One nurse was described as the only person who was able to facilitate humor in a patient's life,

> Mrs. W. was a patient who loved to trade funny stories with Melinda. Despite the terminal nature of her illness, she never discussed her concerns, fears, or problems. Wanting to be sure that the patient was aware that she was available to discuss her needs, Melinda gently brought up the gravity of her situation. Mrs. W. assured her that she could easily discuss her problems with her family or friends. What she needed from Melinda was laughter. 'Everyone is afraid to laugh with me. You are the only one who will.'

The data used in this study were collected on nurses working in many settings including (a) home health agencies, (b) hospice services, (c) clinics, and (d) in-patient units. In every setting, the nurses demonstrated their expertise of the system by acting as environmental brokers for their patients. As brokers, the nurses coordinated the patients' care within the system by establishing and maintaining team networks, and by facilitating links with community agencies or other groups that might meet the patients' or families' needs. The nurses acted as patient advocates to reduce the impact of outside circumstances that could have detrimental effects on the patients' quality of care or daily life.

Context of Connecting

The development or maintenance of connecting was not dependent on context; it occurred wherever the nurse and patient had contact. While most of the data described the occurrence of connecting in traditional nursing settings (i.e., hospitals, clinics, patients' homes, doctors' offices), connecting also occurred in unique settings. For example, nurses accompanied patients to try on wigs and to buy underwear following reconstructive surgery. Other nurses went to grocery stores to teach patients nutrition protocols or to gift shops to buy farewell gifts. Relatives described connecting behavior that transcended context,

> My wife hated being in the hospital. She said it was like jail. She was used to being outside . . . When Robin had to tell her that

she needed more surgery, she put her in a wheelchair and took her to the zoo . . . another one of her good ideas.

Or,

My brother wanted to buy Christmas gifts for his wife and two children . . . seemed impossible . . . he was so weak and in pain. She took him to the hospital gift shop in a wheelchair. He bought his wife a bottle of lotion and coloring books for the kids . . . not much, but he had something for them on Christmas day and he was sure proud. He died December 27.

Consequences of Connecting

The obvious and most important consequence of connecting was higher quality care. While all descriptions of care from the data described in superlative terms the nursing care received by patients, several more specific consequences were also apparent. Once such consequence was reciprocity, which was consistent throughout the data.

Patients who felt connected to a nurse, felt the need for reciprocity. As patients became aware of the nurse as a person and wanted to know more about her or him, the nurse began to share some personal information. The data indicated that patients had intimate knowledge of their nurses.

She brought her only grandchild to see me.

And,

She has two children and she left them on her day off to come see me.

The data provide examples of small gifts and flowers given to the nurses, and many patient letters indicated the need to give something back to the nurse.

We want you to come to the apartment for dinner and we really mean it.

Another consequence of connecting was the inclusion by the nurse of the patient's family, friends, and other significant persons in the connecting process. Relationships that began as dyads expanded through connecting to include those persons important to each patient,

> We were so fortunate to have Linda during my father's illness. She encircled the whole family in her loving arms.

And,

> My daughter was very angry about her father's cancer and death. Helen counseled her even after the funeral.

The connecting process also produced long-term relationships, relationships that were not terminated by the cure or death of the patient. Consistently, and sometimes for years, cured patients remained in contact with their connecting nurse. Likewise, when illness resulted in death, families remained connected to the patient's nurse.

> After my husband's death Susan was, and still is, a terrific support to me.

And,

> On the night my wife died Tony looked across the bed and straight into my eyes and said 'I'm not going to drop you and Johnny, William.' Following Sara's death she helped me and my grandson through the grief process . . . she still checks on us.

STAGES OF CONNECTING

Although analysis of the data revealed multiple variables that affect the process of connecting, the stages of the process of connecting did not clearly emerge from the data. Using descriptions of events contained in the data, the authors proposed the following stages of connecting: (a) presencing, (b) attending, (c) affiliating, and (d) empowering. These stages were supported by other research in which a similar social-psychological process emerged (Hutchinson & Webb, 1988). Table 12-3 presents the stages of connecting.

Presencing, the first stage of connecting, occurred when the nurse and the patient or family encountered each other. The patient or family was experiencing cancer along a continuum of diagnosis, treatment, remission, reoccurrence, or decline and death. The nurse was present as a professional with expertise, knowledge, skill, and personal characteristics which were used to assist patients and families with their needs.

Attending, the second stage, had several characteristics. The focus in

Table 12-3
The Stages of Connecting

Stage 1 Presencing	The patient/family with needs and vulnerabilities comes together with the nurse who is aware and sensitive to their needs, and who has professional knowledge, skills, experiences, and personal characteristics to care for persons in their situation.
Stage 2 Attending	As the patient moves through the clinical scenario dictated by the illness trajectory, the nurse provides evidence of intent and ability to care during the trajectory.
Stage 3 Affiliating	The patient, having experienced the nurse's commitment and abilities, recognizes the uniqueness of their shared experience and not only embraces the nurse's caring, but wishes to reciprocate.
Stage 4 Empowering	Garnering strength and confidence from their shared experience, the nurse and patient/family move toward the final outcome with confidence in self and each other.

this stage was on meeting the immediate needs of the patient and the family. The nurse's sensitivity promoted the identification and meeting of patient and family needs and desires. The nurse was attentive and available. The nurse accepted the patient and the family unconditionally and treated them with dignity and respect.

Affiliating, the third stage, occurred when there was a sense of change in the relationship on the part of the nurse and the patient or family. A bonding occurred in which there was freedom to express affection and to exchange personal information; the nurse was willing to go "above and beyond the call of duty," and a sense of loyalty developed.

Empowering, the last stage, occurred when the patient and the family began to provide more care for themselves with less dependence on the nurse. The nurse facilitated this stage by including the patient and the family in the decision-making process, by promoting growth, and by assisting in the discovery of meaning in the illness experience. Nurses frequently maintained contact with patients or their families to nurture their sense of "power" and to support their feelings of being able to cope.

IMPLICATIONS

The connecting process has implications for nursing practice, education, and research. As the technology and acuity of nursing practice continue to increase, nurses must protect the unique nature of nursing which is caring. The ability to connect successfully with increased numbers of patients will empower nurses. This process is not an additional knowledge or skill we must learn, but rather an opportunity to augment the satisfaction of our practice. As Diekelmann (1990) states, "Nurses don't get burned out from good relationships, but from bad ones."

Educators have the opportunity to explore with students the connecting process. Students will experience connecting if the nursing behaviors involved in the process are reinforced by faculty. Students need the opportunity to experience the process of connecting through clinical experiences. This may require rearrangement of clinical scheduling to allow students to remain with a patient and family until the connecting process is complete.

Several possibilities exist for the continued study of the connecting process. As stated earlier, the process outlined in this paper is a proposed one which needs further validation through research in which it is observed from stage one through stage four. The patients and families in this study were a distinct patient population, i.e., individuals dealing with a cancer diagnosis. The connecting process needs to be investigated with different patient populations and age groups. A final research possibility is suggested by the literature which states some variation may occur in the connecting process based on acuity and the patient's diagnosis.

REFERENCES

Allanach, E.J., & Golden, B.M. (1988). Patient's expectations and values clarification: A service audit. *Nursing Administrative Quarterly, 12,* 17–22.

Benner, P., & Wrubel, J. (1989) *The primacy of caring.* Menlo Park, CA: Addison-Wesley.

Clayton, G. (1988). Research testing Watson's theory: The phenomena of caring in an elderly population. In J. Riehl (Ed.), *Conceptual models in nursing practice* (pp. 245–252). New York: Appleton-Century-Crofts.

Cronin, S.N., & Harrison, B. (1988). Importance of nurse caring behaviors as perceived by patients after myocardial infarction. *Heart & Lung, 17,* 374–380.

Gardner, K.G., & Wheeler, E. (1981). Patients' and staff nurses' perceptions of supportive nursing behaviors: A preliminary analysis. In M. Leininger (Ed.), *Caring: The essential human need* (pp. 109–113). Thorofare, NJ: Charles B. Slack.

Glaser, B. (1978). *Theoretical sensitivity.* Mill Valley, CA: Sociology Press.

Hutchinson, S. (1986). Grounded theory: The method. In P.L. Munhall & C.J. Oiler (Eds.), *Nursing research: A qualitative perspective* (pp. 111–130). Norwalk, CT: Appleton-Century-Crofts.

Hutchinson, S., & Webb, R.B. (1988). Intergenerational geriatric remotivation: Elder's perspectives. *Journal of Cross–Cultural Gerontology, 3,* 273–297.

Larson, P.J. (1984). Important nurse caring behaviors perceived by patients with cancer. *Oncology Nursing Forum, 11,* 46–50.

Larson, P.J. (1986). Cancer nurses' perceptions of caring. *Cancer Nursing, 9,* 86–91.

Larson, P.J. (1987). Comparison of cancer patients' and professional nurses' perceptions of important nurse caring behaviors. *Heart & Lung, 16,* 187–192.

Leininger, M. (1981). Some philosophical, historical and taxonomic aspects of nursing and caring in American culture. In M. Leininger (Ed.), *Caring: The essential human need* (pp. 133–143). Thorofare, NJ: Charles B. Slack.

Watson, J. (1985). *Nursing: Human science and human care.* Norwalk, CT: Appleton-Century-Crofts.

Wolf, Z.R. (1986). The caring concept and nurse identified caring behaviors. *Topics in Clinical Nursing, 8,* 84–93.

13

Exploring Culture and Family Caring Patterns with the Framework of Systemic Organization

Marie-Luise Friedemann

My husband and I are European immigrants and acculturated in most respects. Apart from our slight accents nobody claims to notice any difference in the way we interact with others or react to our surroundings. Why is it then, that our twelve-year-old daughter, an American-born hybrid of two cultures, tells us that our family is weird in the way we take care of each other? She cannot tell us exactly how we differ from other families, but she senses something below the surface—the core of our personality. This core is our identity, a compartment filled with childhood experiences, things our mothers had told us, in short, the truths of our existence. The two cultural cores together form our family identity, our family culture, and we are proud to pass it on. Without realizing it, our daughter has assimilated some of our weirdness into her own personality and some day she will be proud of it too.

Marie-Luise Friedemann

INTRODUCTION

The problem addressed in this paper concerns the frustration nurses experience with clients who are misfits of the health care delivery system, feel misunderstood, and refuse to accept the help offered by well-meaning

169

professionals. This problem is rooted in the great cultural diversity of this country that leaves nurses lost in a complex maze of beliefs and attitudes about health and caring. Cultural differences involve not only variations between ethnic groups, but also among families with homogeneous historic roots who have adapted their style of living in different ways. This process is leading to ever increasing diversity.

There is a need for nurses to understand the relationship between ethnicity and family caring. This understanding is important for nursing, as there are major shifts occurring in the health care delivery system that make a fresh look at caring essential. The most relevant trend is the shift away from hospitalization of the chronically ill to caregiving within families. At the present time, 80 percent of the elderly in the community needing assistance are cared for solely by their families (Gonzales, Steinglass, & Reiss, 1989). Necessarily, there is a parallel shift from nursing of individuals in hospitals to nursing of families in the community that necessitates an understanding of the essence of families and their unique expression of culture.

The statement to be made in this paper concerns the concept of caring in the cultural context as a personal and family experience rather than a cultural group phenomenon. This writer argues that family functioning is the key to cultural understanding since it is the manifestation of the family's culture and consequently the best predictor of caring behaviors.

This position is in agreement with the concepts and definitions advanced by literature and research in caring and transcultural nursing. In contrast, however, the focus on family processes suggests a need for new approaches in educating nurses to provide culturally sensitive care. A look at the present status of the field of caring is needed for clarification.

In recent years, nursing leaders such as Watson, Ray, Leininger, and Travelbee have made significant contributions to the profession by encouraging a nursing focus on caring (Leininger, 1984a). As Leininger postulates, "caring is the essence of and unifying intellectual and practical dimension of professional nursing" (Leininger, 1984b, p. 5) and its full complexity needs to be better understood (Leininger 1978, 1984a). The goal of these pioneers is a strong theoretical description of caring that will serve as a basis for research. Because of this unique knowledge base, Leininger (1984a) claims that nursing ultimately will be awarded its deserved place and stature among the learned professions and in society.

While this dream remains to be dreamed for some time in the future, the field has made significant gains in promoting cultural awareness. Caring, as Leininger describes it, includes two major groups of components, (1) the activities and processes necessary to assist and support a person, and (2) the accompanying attributes or emotions such as empathy and compassion (Leininger, 1978). While these attributes seem to be uniformly present in caring, the patterns of their expression—the actual caring tasks and rituals—are intimately intertwined with the caring person's culture. The transcultural specialists conclude that nurses need to immerse themselves in these cultures and study unique health behaviors and beliefs. In fact, Leininger prides herself on having studied more than 30 cultures in-depth and urges nurses to continue her work in order to cover the world (Leininger, 1984a).

This writer does not dispute the merit of the transculturalists' efforts in informing nurses about the many variations in cultural patterns of caring; however, a word of caution is in place. Two dangers are perceivable, (1) the danger of losing one's self in the details of diversity, and (2) the danger of stereotyping. Referring to the first, Leininger claims that cultural diversity far outweighs common features among cultures (Leininger, 1984a). This is understandable since transcultural researchers explore the outward expressions of humans, their observable behavior patterns. The danger, therefore, exists that the caring practices and rituals become the sole purpose of research at the expense of a broader and more in-depth understanding of culture. This author suggests that there are common factors of the human experience, but they are evident on the level of human striving and motivation, needs and self–preservation, communication and mutual bonding within families and groups.

The second danger is that of neglecting within-group diversity or stereotyping. Stereotyping is ever present when cultural groups are described as holding uniform beliefs and engaging in uniform behavior patterns. An attitude of "they versus us" may counteract all good intentions of caring if the client becomes an oddity to the nurse rather than an object of compassion.

For compassion and caring to take place, there must be a common experience, namely that of humanness. This writer argues that nurses who care in a culturally sensitive way search for sameness while they learn to understand how the conditions of a client's life experience have brought about variations in culture and coping patterns. The remainder of this paper will introduce to the reader the use of a theoretical framework and related literature in formulating theoretical propositions relative to families and culture. These propositions will then be integrated in an interpretation of the differential needs of families who give care to ill members.

CULTURE AND THE FRAMEWORK OF SYSTEMIC ORGANIZATION

The Framework of Systemic Organization (Friedemann, 1989) is based on general systems concepts (Von Bertalanffy, 1968) and draws upon the work of Kantor and Lehr (1975). From this perspective, the family is a system composed of individuals and interpersonal units, all having unique qualities of their own. Family members interact with one another in sequences of acts that take on purposeful recurring patterns. The notion that interactions occur in relatively stable patterns that are constituents of a larger basic family functioning pattern is central to the Framework of Systemic Organization (Friedemann, 1989).

The basic family functioning pattern, in turn, serves as a blueprint for all coping behaviors including caring for ill family members. This pattern is relative to the basic task of all families of weighing against each other family behaviors pertaining to the process dimensions of system maintenance and system change, togetherness, and individuation in order to arrive at a balance of stability and growth of the family system that meets the needs of all members and promotes health (Friedemann, 1989).

The process dimensions have been defined by this writer and are based on her past research (Friedemann, 1988). Likewise, a close look at the family therapy literature reveals that family behavior patterns tend to fall into the same four general dimensions with some consistency.

1. *System maintenance* behaviors involve strategies that families use to organize and structure their system in order to maintain stability. System maintenance strategies are implied in family therapy concepts such as power structure, problem negotiation (Haley, 1976), family structure, generational boundaries (Minuchin, 1974), coalitions, rules, roles (Haley, 1976; Lewis, Beavers, Gossett, & Phillips, 1976), family organization, and control (Moos & Moos, 1984).

2. *Togetherness* behaviors consist of processes that lead family members to bond together and commit time and energy to each other. They include the notions of closeness and empathy (Lewis et al., 1976), cohesion (Moos & Moos, 1984; Olsen et al., 1984), and enmeshment (Minuchin, 1974).

3. *System change* behaviors have been extensively discussed in the literature as necessary strategies to adjust to changes from within the system and the environment (Buckley, 1967). Such strategies are described in discussions of adaptability (Olsen et al., 1984) and family growth and flexibility (Lewis et al., 1976).

4. *Individuation* consists of behaviors that individuals in the family employ to follow their interests and develop their own potential. Individuation also involves the family's accomodating reactions to differences of lifestyle and opinions among family members. Individuation behaviors are implied in concepts such as self-differentiation (Bowen, 1976), self-disclosure, and expressiveness (Lewis et al., 1976).

While the dimensions of system maintenance and togetherness promote stability by passing on values and practices from one generation to the next, system change and individuation lead to system transformation. As new knowledge from the environment is incorporated into the family, the system will eventually change its basic characteristics and become a different system (Friedemann, 1989). Consequently, a model explaining culture with a focus on family functioning seems appropriate since culture and family functioning are a product of both stable inherited patterns and the families' constant attempts to adjust to changing conditions.

Culture is defined as the totality of the human way of life that includes the control of natural forces to meet physical and safety needs of people. Furthermore, culture entails the institutionalization of social, interactional, and spiritual practices in families. According to the Framework of Systemic Organization, culture depends on two processes, acquisition of knowledge and transmission of knowledge. As new knowledge becomes incorporated in a generation's way of life, it becomes culture as it is passed on to the next generation. Culture represents a stable core of beliefs and values and has the capacity for change as new knowledge is added and integrated (Friedemann, 1989).

Like all other family processes, cultural processes occur at various system levels. It is the level of the family system that gives rise to culture as adults pass on their knowledge to the young generation. Culture is reflected in the family's functioning patterns. Many patterns tend to be stable, often over many generations, while others experience change as the family adapts to changes within its environment. The sum of stable and transformed family patterns will then be transmitted as culture to the new generation (Friedemann, 1989).

On the personal level, individuals integrate into their personalities relevant knowledge gained within the family and community systems in order to build up a core of values and principles through which all further information is filtered. This process occurs through behaviors within the process dimension of individuation, and the family system will adjust to the changes in its members through processes of system change. Consequently, the responsibility for knowledge dissemination is shared among individuals, families, and the community, whereas the transformation and transmission of culture over generations occurs primarily in family systems.

Ethnicity represents those stable cultural patterns that are shared by a group of families who have the same historical roots. In the past, the complexity of ethnicity was poorly understood. For example, the variable ethnicity was measured in terms of language skills, insularity, or the country of birth and was found to have little influence on health practices (Alston & Aguire, 1987).

Furthermore, the concepts of ethnicity and race have been treated synonymously. Only recently, mounting evidence of the remarkable diversity within each racial group has led to the realization that racial designations commonly used are artificial labels and preclude the broader ethnocultural distinctions (Valle, in press; Valle, 1989). Deyo and his associates emphasize that there is a great heterogeneity inherent in each culture that is also apparent in family health behaviors and beliefs (Deyo, Diehl, Hazuda, and Stern, 1985). For example, Gelfand and Fandetti (1980) have demonstrated how different segments of the Euro-Anglo families differ in their attitudes and practices of caring for the chronically ill. Blacks also have a heritage of considerable diversity that includes persons from English and French colonies in the Caribbeans, and is evidenced in all facets of family life (Valle, 1989).

Furthermore, in support of the Framework of Systemic Organization, experts in the family field have also recognized that ethnicity is strongly reflected in family functioning and that, in fact, it may be a superficial overlay. That is, ethnicity as a unique variable may be of minor importance compared to the more basic family processes which subsume its effects (Bowen, 1976).

If ethnicity is truly a function of family functioning one may deduce that, on the basis of the family propositions advanced above, ethnicity is maintained in a relatively pure state only if the families' environment encourages system maintenance that allows sustaining long established patterns, and if these established patterns remain functional and beneficial for the families.

This country, however, is marked by an increasing ethnic diversity of historically homogeneous family groups with each new generation. As a rule, families find themselves surrounded by a continuously changing environment. In order to survive and grow the families need to incorporate new knowledge and compromise many of their usual behaviors, a process that inevitably leads to system change and culture transformation. The reason for diversity within cultural groups is the differential rate of system change among families. The rate of change, in turn, is relative to the permeability of the family boundary that permits or prevents the incorporation of new information and change of family operations (Friedemann, 1989).

Furthermore, family systems, in order to become congruent with their environment will adjust to the systems with which they have contact in pursuing their daily business (Friedemann, 1989). As families of differing ethnic origins together contain themselves in the same environment, a blurring of ethnic coping patterns becomes likely, and intercultural differences decrease (Staples & Mirande, 1980). The qualities of environments are largely determined by sociodemographics and geographic factors. On the basis of a healthy family system's capacity to adapt, it seems likely that, over time, environmental qualities become as strong predictors of family coping as the family's ethnic values and traditions.

This process has been described in recent conceptualizations of the black culture. The "Africanity" model was set forth by Staples (1974) and described by Nobles (1978). According to this model, ethnic patterns are played out within the family and are believed to represent African traits that were retained over the years. However, Staples and Mirande (1980) recognize that the cultural fusion with mainstream traits has eliminated uniquely African patterns. The blurring of cultural patterns is also evident from the results of studies of black caring patterns that have revealed a surprising conformity with white health beliefs and practices. Only a few typical black patterns were distinguished. Compared to white families, blacks used a more extensive kin-system for informal help (Cantor, Rosenthal, & Wilker, 1979; Mindel & Wright, 1982; Mitchell & Register, 1984), had a tendency to rely on the eldest daughter (Jackson, 1972), and placed more importance on spirituality in everyday coping as well as decision making (Smerglia, Deimling, & Baresi, 1988).

In summary, the above discussion of the Framework of Systemic Organization and supporting literature should have guided the reader to the proposition that culture is family functioning. Furthermore, there seem to be two processes at work, both taking place at the level of the family. The first is the increasing within-group diversification of culture as families of historically homogeneous groups integrate varying information at differing rates. The second process is the between-group blurring of ethnic uniqueness and cultural specifications as families of differing cultures share environments of common geographic, social, and economic characteristics. These families adapt and compromise their ethnic uniqueness by yielding to the pressures of their common environment. The following section intends to clarify these two processes within the caring context in order to arrive at implications and needs of family nursing.

FAMILY CARING FOR ILL MEMBERS AND THE ROLE OF NURSES

Society's Model for Family Care

The shift from hospitalizing chronically ill to home care has greatly expanded the role of families in providing care for ill, frail, or incapacitated family members. This shift requires that nurses, through their work with outpatient clinics or home care agencies, spend a significant amount of their time teaching and supporting caregiving families.

Families who care for ill members are subjected to certain expectations by the health care delivery system and society at large. They are expected to mobilize their own internal resources and perform the necessary tasks of care. The health care system sees its role as educating families to give care (Aaronson & Lipkowitz, 1981). Furthermore, there is a strong belief among practitioners, which is also reflected in government policies and regulations, that supportive and social services are needed to supplement or augment family assistance. This has led to an increasing interest in developing supportive service programs and policies. Services such as financial assistance, respite services, education and training programs, or support groups are considered essential for families in order to continue providing care over extended periods of time (Brody, 1985; Cantor, 1983; Lebowitz, 1978; Shanas & Sussman, 1977; Sweeny, 1986).

Many families are able and willing to live up to these expectations. They organize the immediate family members in sharing the responsibilities for care and elicit the help of other relatives. In fact, most caregivers seem to be willing to accept help from close kin. Such informal sources of assistance and formal resources such as social and supportive programs traditionally have been considered components of social support in caregiving. Social support has been researched extensively and found to act as a buffer against stress experienced by the caring families (Cleary & Kessler, 1982; Finney, Mitchell, Cronkite, & Moos, 1984). Conversely, the lack of social support has been correlated with high levels of stress and physical illness in caregivers (Bass & Noelker, 1987).

Nursing's Problem—Family Resistance

A breakdown in communication between families and the health care system is evident in that many caring families fail to seek out available services or to use those recommended by well-meaning professionals (Hofer, 1982; Lawton, Brody, & Saperstein, 1989; Montgomery, 1984, 1987; Ory et al., 1985). This longstanding problem has been studied, and the perceived lack of availability and the restricted access to many of these services have been cited as major factors (Aaronson & Lipkowitz, 1981; Ory et al., 1985; Zarit, Gatz, & Zarit, 1982). There is evidence, however, that the problem is considerably broader and more far-reaching. For example, researchers conducting a large longitudinal study had difficulty locating families to participate in a program offering free services and, more important, one-third of the eligible families who were offered both educational and respite services free of charge refused to use them (Montgomery & Borgatta, 1985).

The reason for the reluctance of caregivers to use formal services has not been addressed by previous empirical studies. The issue, however, is most relevant in connection with the above discussion. The Framework of Systemic Organization follows Kantor and Lehr (1975), who have observed that families under stress tend to do more of what they have always done and stay within their traditional restricted repertoire of coping behaviors. Consequently, family functioning is expected to directly influence family caring and accordingly, the use of resources. For example, if the family's functioning pattern subscribes to a strong emphasis on tradition (system maintenance) and an attitude of mistrust toward new resources in caring (system change) the use of certain community services may not be part of the family's coping behaviors.

The issue is of major importance for nurses, who have closer contact with families involved in the care of an ill member than most other professionals. Nurses act as a liaison between families and community agencies or programs in meeting the needs and easing the burden of caregiving families. They are well aware, however, that a great number of families ask for help only when they are at the verge of a severe crisis. Many home care nurses in Horn's study found that family problems were interfering with the effectiveness of treatments and interventions. Excessive demands of caregiving leading to high stress and exhaustion in caregivers had created situations of interpersonal family conflict. In fact, 87.5 percent of the visiting nurses surveyed stated that "managing family problems" was particularly difficult for them. In spite of the families' state of exhaustion, however, the nurses were unable to motivate them to accept help other than medical care (Horn, 1986).

Nursing's Solution—Assessment of Family Diversity

The above discussion supports the power of pre-established family functioning, including the families' repertoire of beliefs and attitudes about caring, in determining what type of actions should be taken for the ill member. Trying to convince families to take an action contrary to the usual way in which they handle their business is a vain effort. Instead, the family's trust can be gained by showing interest in the particularities of their system and by choosing those resources, interventions, and educational approaches that are congruent with the family's perceived needs.

To assess a family's needs is not easy. Needs as families perceive them are often far different from the nurse's perception. Furthermore, nurses and other service providers have observed that many caregivers are too involved in their difficult task to clearly see what their needs are (Brubaker, 1983). In addition, several studies have shown that the caregivers' perception varied with the way they experienced and interpreted their situation. While some reported high levels of stress and great difficulty coping with their tasks, others, in a similar situation, experienced minimal or no burden and appeared to cope effectively with the demands of their role (Cicirelli, 1981; Noelker & Paulshock, 1982).

The solution proposed here involves a twofold focus, a focus on (1) factors of the common human experience, and (2) on family diversity, both inherent in family functioning. Tubman (1986) has noted that caring for the ill is in fact a family phenomenon, but that family variables have been blatantly missing in most research or clinical practice. Contrary to the position taken in transcultural nursing, this writer argues that nurses first need to explore common human cultural factors that transcend ethnic patterns and bridge cultural barriers. Next, the focus is on family diversity and uniqueness.

The initial focus on sameness will create a sense of mutuality that allows the attributes of caring such as empathy and compassion to come into play. The resulting trust leads to sharing and permits the families to voice specific needs, values, and particularities. The subsequent shift of focus on the discussed cultural family propositions will let the nurses minimize value judgments and refrain from imposing on families their own prescriptions for caring.

Consequently, culturally sensitive nurses will—

1. see their clients as equals with needs and aspirations common to all humans,
2. interpret unique qualities of the family in the context of their functioning pattern,
3. see the family as a product of its environment and its behaviors as adaptive,
4. assess and interpret the family's processes of system maintenance and togetherness, system change and individuation in its attempt to achieve stability and growth.
5. will choose those interventions and resources to facilitate caring of the ill member that are congruent with the family's general pattern of functioning, and
6. use communication processes that are based on mutual trust and genuine interest in the family's unique functioning and that will provide honest feedback and cooperation in joint problem solving.

Clinically, the key to cultural family nursing is the accurate assessment of family behaviors within the four discussed family dimensions and the family's emphasis on each of the dimensions. On the basis of its basic pattern, the family's preferred method for providing care and the family's need for a variety of resources can be explored. The planning process is mutual, assisted by the honest feedback of the family that serves as an ongoing validation of the family assessment and its interpretation.

For the benefit of the discipline, the need exists to develop a systemic approach of assessing caregiving families relative to their diverse patterns. Furthermore, nursing interventions and resources need to be categorized into groups that correspond with the various family patterns. The object is the matching of families with nursing interventions and caregiving resources that are tailored to the family's pre-established pattern of functioning.

While the transculturalists are dreaming about exploring and understanding all of the world's cultural health practices (Leininger, 1984a), this writer argues that cultures are dynamic and in a continuous state of change. Therefore, the accurate documentation of ethnic practices is problematic, especially in areas where families' environments are rapidly changing. This author's dream is ambitious as well. It is an instrument that will measure the family's basic pattern objectively, an instrument that is applicable to families of all cultures and developmental stages. Some work has been done (Friedemann, 1988), while much more is waiting.

REFERENCES

Aaronson, M., & Lipkowitz, R. (1981). Senile dementia, Alzheimer's type: The family and the health care delivery system. *Journal of the American Geriatric Society, 24,* 568–571.

Alston, L. T., & Aguire, B. (1987). Elderly Mexican Americans: Nativity and health access. *International Migration Review, 21,* 626–642.

Bass, D. M., & Noelker, L. S. (1987). The influence of family caregivers on elder's use of in-home services: An expanded conceptual framework. *Journal of Health and Social Behavior, 28,* 184–196.

Bowen, M. (1976). Theory in the practice of psychotherapy. In P. J. Guerin (Ed.), *Family therapy: Theory and practice* (pp. 42–90). New York: Gardner Press.

Brody, E. M. (1985). Parent care as a normative family stress. *The Gerontologist, 25*(1), 19–29.

Brubaker, T. H. (1983). *Family relationships in later life.* Beverly Hills, CA: Sage.

Buckley, W. (1967). *Sociology and modern systems theory.* Englewood Cliffs, NJ: Prentice Hall.

Cantor, M. H. (1983). Strain among caregivers: A study of experience in the United States. *The Gerontologist, 23,* 597–604.

Cantor, M. H., Rosenthal, L., & Wilker, L. (1979). Social and family relationships of black, aged women in New York City. *Journal of Minority Aging, 4,* 50–61.

Cicirelli, V. G. (1981). *Helping elderly patients: The role of adult children.* Boston: Auburn House.

Cleary, P. D., & Kessler, R. C. (1982). The estimation and interpretation of modifier effects. *Journal of Health and Social Behavior, 23,* 159–169.

Deyo, R. A., Diehl, A. K., Hazuda, H., & Stern, M. P. (1985). A simple language-based acculturation scale for Mexican Americans: Validation and application to health care research. *American Journal of Public Health, 75*(1), 51–55.

Finney, J. W., Mitchell, R. E., Cronkite, R. C., & Moos, R. W. (1984). Methodological issues in estimating main and interactive effects: Examples from coping/social support and stress field. *Journal of Health and Social Behavior, 25,* 85–98.

Friedemann, M. L. (1988). *Assessment of strategies in families: An instrument to evaluate effectiveness of family functioning.* Unpublished manuscript, Wayne State University, College of Nursing, Detroit, MI.

Friedemann, M. L. (1989). Closing the gap between grand theory and mental health practice with families (Part 1): The Framework of Systemic Organization for nursing of families and family members. *Archives of Psychiatric Nursing, 3*(1), 10–19.

Gelfand, D. Z., & Fandetti, D. V. (1980). Suburban and urban white ethnics: Attitudes toward care of the aged, *The Gerontologist, 20,* 588–595.

Gonzales, S., Steinglass, P., & Reiss, D. (1989). Putting the illness in its place: Discussion groups for families with chronic medical illnesses. *Family Process, 28,* 69–87.

Haley, J. (1976). *Problem solving therapy.* San Francisco: Jossey–Bass.

Hofer, A. (1982). *Strengthening the self capacity of the family caretaker of elderly living at home.* Revision of a paper presented at the 35th Annual Scientific Meeting of the Gerontological Society of America, Boston.

Horn, B. (1986). *The elderly homecare project.* Unpublished preliminary report. Seattle: University of Washington, School of Nursing, Community Health Care Systems.

Jackson, J. J. (1972). Black aged in quest of the Phoenix. In J. J. Jackson (Ed.), *Triple jeopardy: Myth of reality.* Washington DC: National Council on Aging.

Kantor, D., & Lehr, W. (1975). *Inside the family.* San Francisco: Jossey-Bass.

Lawton, M. P., Brody, E. M., & Saperstein, A. R. (1989). A controlled study of respite service for caregivers of Alzheimer's patients. *The Gerontologist, 29*(1), 8–16.

Lebowitz, B. D. (1978). Old age and family functioning. *Journal of Gerontological Social Work, 1,* 111–118.

Leininger, M. M. (1978). *Transcultural Nursing: Concepts, Theories and Practices.* New York: Wiley and Sons.

Leininger, M. M. (1984a). Caring: A central focus of nursing and health care services. In M. M. Leininger (Ed.), *Care: The Essence of Nursing and Health* (pp. 45–59). Detroit, MI: Wayne State University Press.

Leininger, M. M. (1984b). Care: The essence of nursing and health. In M. M. Leininger (Ed.), *Care: The Essence of Nursing and Health* (pp. 3–15). Detroit, MI: Wayne State University Press.

Lewis, J. M., Beavers, W. R., Gossett, J. T., & Phillips, V. A. (1976). *No single thread: Psychological health in family systems.* New York: Brunner/Mazel.

Mindel, C. H., & Wright, R. (1982). The use of social services by black and white elderly: The role of social support systems. *Journal of Gerontological Social Work, 4,* 107–125.

Minuchin, S. (1974). *Families and family therapy.* Cambridge, England: Harvard University Press.

Mitchell, J., & Register, J. C. (1984). An exploration of family interaction with the elderly by race, socioeconomic status, and residence. *The Gerontologist, 24*(1), 48–54.

Montgomery, R. J. (1984). Services for families of the aged: Which ones will work best? *Aging, 3447,* 16–21.

Montgomery, R. J. (1987). Social service utilization. In G. Maddox (Ed.), *Encylopedia of aging.* New York: Springer.

Montgomery, R. J., & Borgotta, E. F. (1985). *Family Support Project.* Final report to the Administration on Aging. Seattle: University of Washington, Institute on Aging/Long–Term Care Center.

Moos, R. H., & Moos, B. S. (1984). *Family Environmental Scale manual* (2nd ed). Palo Alto, CA: Consulting Psychologists Press.

Nobles, W. (1978). Toward an empirical and theoretical framework for defining black families. *Journal of Marriage and the Family, 40,* 679–698.

Noelker, L. S., & Paulshock, S. W. (1982). *The effects on families of caring for impaired elderly in residence.* Final report to the Administration on Aging. Cleveland: Benjamin Rose Institute.

Noelker, L. S., & Wallace, R. W. (1985). The organization of family care for impaired elderly. *Journal of Family Issues, 6*(1), 23–44.

Olsen, D. H., McCubbin, H. I., Barnes, H. L., Larsen, A. S., Muxen, M. J., & Wilson, M. A. (1984). *Families: What makes them work?* Beverly Hills, CA: Sage.

Ory, M. G., Williams, T. F., Emr, M., Lebowitz, B., Rabins, P., Salloway, J., Sluss-Radbaugh, T., Wolff, E., & Zarit, S. (1985). Families, informal supports and Alzheimer's disease: Current research and future agendas. *Research on Aging, 7,* 623–644.

Shanas, E., & Sussman, M. B. (1977). *Family, bureaucracy, and the elderly.* Durham, NC: Duke University Press.

Smerglia, V. L., Deimling, G. T., & Baresi, C. M. (1988). Black/white family comparisons in helping and decision-making networks of impaired elderly. *Family Relations, 37,* 305–309.

Staples, R. (1974). The black family revisited: A review and a preview. *Journal of Social and Behavioral Sciences, 20,* 65–78.

Staples, R., & Mirande, A. (1980). Racial and cultural variations among American families: A dicennial review of the literature on minority families. *Journal of Marriage and the Family, 42,* 887–903.

Sweeney, S. M. (1986). *Family caregiving: A retrospective evaluation—New area of research and demonstrations and policy options.* Report to Office of Policy, Planning and Legislation. Washington, DC: Office of Human Development Services.

Tubman, J. G. (1986). *Family relations in parent care: Moving beyond the primary caregiver.* Paper presented at the 16th Annual National Council on Family Relations, Theory Construction and Research Methodology Workshop, Dearborn, MI.

Valle, R. (1989). U.S. ethnic minority group access to long-term care. In T. Schwab (Ed.), *Caring for an aging world: International models for long-term care, financing, and delivery* (pp. 339–363). New York: McGraw-Hill Information Services Company.

Valle, R. (In press). Cultural and ethnic issues in Alzheimer's disease family research. In E. Light, & B. Lebowitz (Eds.), *Alzheimer's disease treatment and family stress: Directions for research.* Washington, DC: National Institute of Mental Health.

Von Bertalanffy, L. (1968). *General Systems Theory.* New York: George Braziller.

Wheaton, B. (1985). Models for the stress-buffering functions of coping resources. *Journal of Health and Social Behavior, 26,* 352–364.

Zarit, S. H., Gatz, M., Zarit, J. M. (1982). Families under stress: Interventions for caregivers of senile dementia patients. *Psychotherapy: Theory, research, & practice, 19,* 461–471.

14

Clarification of the Unique Role of Caring in Nurse-Patient Relationships

Christine L. Pollack-Latham

Caring is fundamental to the development and survival of mankind (Frankfurt, 1982; Leininger, 1980). However, in this technologic-scientific age, the value society puts on caring is being questioned (Reverby, 1987a; Ropohl, 1983). This is partly reflected in changes apparent in health care, where economic, scientific, and technologic imperatives tend to undermine professional health care providers' inherent value systems (Buerhaus, 1986; Harding, 1980; Moccia, 1988). Caring is central to health care delivery; however, its continued practice in nursing is being threatened (Fry, 1988; Leininger, 1986). The meaning of caring practices used by health care professionals is often confounded by equating social, personal, and professional aspects of caring for patients (Benner, 1984; Noddings, 1984).

These potential threats to caring, its elusive nature, and the technologic-purposive rationality in health care demand that steps be taken to clarify the meaning and importance of caring to professional health care practice, and more specifically, to nurses. A better understanding of critical caring attributes, including the contribution of personal, professional, and social components, may help to delineate aspects of caring that warrant future investigation. An in-depth analysis of this concept, using an expanded version of the dimension–attribute method (Norris, 1982; Rawnsley, 1980), considers the contribution of these three interpersonal components and helps to clarify barriers to the implementation of caring in professional nursing practice. Research efforts that are based on this analysis could then study caring as it is used by the nursing profession, with a goal toward establishing a link to improved patient welfare (Wolf, 1986). This discussion will systematically address two levels of caring. An in-depth analysis of the profession's relationship to three domains of inter-personal caring (personal, social, and professional) is followed by a dis-cussion of historical and social influences in nursing's caring practice. Both micro and macro views of the caring concept, as it relates to the nursing profession, are addressed (Greenleaf, 1980). Finally, the relationship of caring to the discipline of nursing and areas for future research are dis-cussed.

CONTEXT OF CARING

Contemporary meanings of caring that pertain to health care include "in-terest and concern," "liking," and "giving care" (Webster, 1986, p. 207). Interest and concern are often referred to as "caring about"; however, "caring for" signifies a closer, more interpersonally oriented involvement (Noddings, 1984). The term "liking" denotes positive affect (Howard, 1975) rather than love for the other person (Zderad, 1969). Giving care, taking care of someone, and caring are synonymous. For greater clarity and consistency, caring, in the context of this discussion, will signify "caring for" another and will be considered an interactive process occur-ring between two people, which ultimately results in a product, comple-tion of caring in the recipient (Bottorff & D'Cruz, 1984; Fowler, 1987; Noddings, 1984). In this way, caring takes place between the caregiver (the person who is caring for another person) and the recipient (the person to whom caring is directed). The critical attributes of this concept will later be compared to terms that describe similar types of interpersonal encounters. This discussion will emphasize the caregiver's perspective, but will in-clude the recipient's viewpoint as necessary to reflect the relational aspect of caring. The type of caring will be humanistic, adult caring related to health needs, as viewed within the Western culture.

ANALYSIS OF THREE CARING PERSPECTIVES

An analysis of three different interpersonal dimensions of caring, includ-ing personal, social, and professional relationships, was undertaken be-cause of nursing's service-related social purpose and the notion that nurs-ing practice includes both personal and professional domains of caring (Bevis, 1981; Lundh, Soder, & Wareness, 1988). The variables compared within each dimension include participants, caring capacities, motivations, nature of the act, and critical attributes of the caring process. It should be noted that these areas within each domain of caring are not mutually exclusive; overlap is evident since individuals may vary in their approach to caring.

Caring Participants

Noddings (1984) described "circles of caring" which assist in describing participants in each of the domains (pp. 46–48). Personal (or private) caring related to the health of the other is an explicit, close, intimate relationship involving family and friends (de Rivera, 1984). In contrast, social (or public) caring includes caring for strangers and usually involves less intensity and intimacy than personal relationships. The professional caring relationship implies a responsibility on the part of the caregiver to use knowledge and skills to help the recipient after a need is determined (Kitson, 1987). The intensity of this relationship is variable, depending on the continuity and level of involvement of caregivers, as well as their perceived roles (Nowakowski, 1985).

Which of the three domains best reflects caring given by nurses? It is generally accepted that nurse-patient relationships are personal by nature, but this varies depending on the recipient's desire, need for, and acceptance of assistance. Nursing is aligned with the professional caring domain since it entails less intimacy than personal relationships and may not have the amount of continuity present in personal relationships. In addition, this relationship implies that both the caregiver and the recipient are involved in the giving and receiving of caring. This then, assumes that both people have the capacity to care for each other. This component helps to further delineate the concept of caring in nursing.

Caring Capacity

Caring presupposes a human being and self-consciousness (Frankfurt, 1982). The ability to be a caring individual is influenced by previous thoughts, attitudes, and involvement with caring (Gilfillan, 1985; Noddings, 1984). It also includes a self-openness, selflessness, and ability to transcend the self and others (Doona, 1979; Goldsborough, 1969; Kitson, 1987). The recognition and comparison of the recipient's values with one's own caring goals (i.e., who and what to care about) may be most obvious in personal relationships, and least apparent in social relationships (Thoits, 1986). In addition, energy, health, knowledge, empathy, and communication skills influence one's ability to contribute to a caring relationship and provide the necessary level of care (Diers, 1986; Peplau, 1969; Zderad, 1969).

On the adult level, the capacity to care for another also necessitates an in-depth knowledge of one's self, although the need for this varies depending on the caring domain (i.e., personal versus social). Self-knowledge assists complete involvement of the caregiver, including social, psychological, and spiritual realms (Kauffman, 1986). This type of involvement is especially prevalent in the personal caring domain. The need for and use of self-knowledge and complete involvement are influenced by the type of relationship, with social encounters being the least demanding. Wiedenbach, referring to professional caring relationships, indicates that it would be optimal if the caregiver could "recognize thoughts and feelings, respect their importance, and discipline the self to harness them to the purpose and philosophy" of a caring practice (1963, p. 57).

The capacity to be a caring professional is reflected by all three caring domains. Therefore, nurses' capacity to care may involve facets of all three domains. However, if someone has the capacity to care for another, does it then mean that interpersonal caring will ensue? There are a number of other factors influencing the individual's commitment to become involved which must be explored.

Motivation for Caring

Motivation implies a commitment to be a caring individual, as indicated by Johnson's (1973) personal commitment rationale. However, this rationale for caring varies in each domain. Caring of a personal nature is described as an instinctive feeling or natural disposition (Noddings, 1984). On the other hand, social caring's motivation to participate is reflexive and may depend on situational characteristics (Amato & Cook, 1983; Batson, Harris, McCaul, Davis, & Schmidt, 1979; Emmons, Diener, & Larsen, 1985). Social caring for those who are young, weak, or helpless is also an intuitive response which is unconsciously devoted to species survival (e.g., the rescue of the little girl trapped in a well in Texas, or brave attempts to assist those injured in natural or manmade disasters) (Gaylin, 1976).

Caring for others on a social level has been studied with college students to determine underlying motivations. These investigations have attempted to verify whether empathy or compassion, rather than egotistical reasons or the need for social approval, guides altruistic behavior toward others during commonly encountered social situations (Batson et al., 1979; Fultz, Batson, Fortenbach, McCarthy, & Varney, 1986). Generalization of these studies' findings beyond undergraduate psychology students is questionable because college attendance may enhance bonding between students, thereby increasing compassion, empathy, and altruistic behavior. Some of the measurements employed in these studies were indirect, and other conflicting theories (i.e., avoidance of guilt, religious, and positive self–esteem motivations) were not addressed (Lynn & Ol-denquist, 1986; Kemper, 1980; Reddy, 1980). However, these studies lend insight into the complexity inherent in the measurement of motivation to care for others in everyday social situations.

Professionals' commitment to care for another person is based on normative ethics, including theories of value and theories of obligation (Fowler, 1987). The rules and principles of normative ethics are used as guidelines and not as firm behavioral rules or justification for caring actions (Noddings, 1984; Toulmin, 1981). If professional caring behavior is evaluated, professional values and norms must be considered (Newell, 1984). Some of the professional values theorized to support an ethic of caring include formation of a humanistic–altruistic outlook, as well as kindness, concern, love, and respect of self and others (Watson, 1979). Theories of obligation include deontologic and teleologic theories (Fowler, 1987). A humanistic philosophy underlies all of these theories.

Nursing primarily functions within health care institutions. A human-istic philosophy is not always apparent in the highly mechanized, imper-sonal, and complex bureaucratic environment utilized by health care providers (Joseph, 1985; Leininger, 1974); however, it is fundamental to nursing (Watson, 1979). This is reflected in nurses' motivations to care, which include aspects of all three caring domains: an ethical base, a respect for one's self and others, and an intuitive, reflexive response to help those in need.

Therefore, there are a variety of reasons for personal, social, and professional caring. These motivations, together with identification of the participants and their capacities, help to delineate caring within each of the three realms. Other variables, such as the nature of the act and critical attributes of the caring process, also demarcate each domain of caring and assist in determining the type of caring used by nurses.

The Nature of the Interpersonal Caring Act

The level of interpersonal communication, expectations for reciprocity, and asymmetrical relationships are three distinguishing features of the caring act.

Levels of Interpersonal Interaction.   Schutz's description of three levels of interpersonal communication is useful in characterizing the three do-mains of caring (1970). The personal domain of caring emphasizes two of the levels: the "Thou orientation" in which the other is seen as a "living, conscious being" and the "We-relationship," which denotes a simulta-neous, reciprocally oriented participation. This approach does not com-pletely describe personal relationships. Neither initiation of the relation-ship (usually the caregiver is the initiator) (Noddings, 1984) nor emotions within personal relationships (i.e., love or attachment) are addressed by Schutz's theory, but they are evident in personal caring.

Using a similar analogy, social caring may be envisioned as either a "We-relationship" or a "They orientation." Reciprocal acknowledgement is involved at the first level of interpersonal relationship (i.e., the "We-relationship"). However, if the caregiver is not directly involved with, but exhibits caring for the other (e.g., a stranger), a "They orientation" results. This comparison assists in differentiating some forms of social caring from personal caring. The social caring relationship may be short or long-term, and may be initiated by either the provider or the recipient of caring (e.g., charitable relationships). Studies of natural helpers (defined as community volunteers) emphasize that minimal reciprocity is involved in many of their interactions (Kelley & Kelley, 1985). Findings, however, vary according to the types of social or community helper roles studied (Amato, 1985).

The professional caring domain may result in either the "Thou orientation" (seeing the other as a person) or the "We–relationship" (reciprocal involvement of both participants), depending on the reason for the interaction. This relationship is generally recipient-initiated (with the exception of emergency situations), after recognizing that professional knowledge and assistance are needed (Kitson, 1987). The "They orientation" ideally does not exist in direct clinical encounters between patients and professional providers. Gadow's (1980) existential approach to health care relationships indicates that there are equal amounts of involvement by professionals and recipients, but the focus, intensity, and perspective of each participant in the relationship are different.

Nursing includes aspects of all three domains of interpersonal interaction because patient relationships may include personal concern and may be situationally based. However, the professional caring domain best describes the nurse-patient relationship, since it is not based in deep, long-entrenched emotions and personal gratification needs. This overview of interpersonal aspects of caring, however, does not deal with other issues fundamental to the nature of caring, the lack of required reciprocity and the asymmetrical relationship of participants. These factors further distinguish the influence of each of the three caring domains.

Reciprocity Expectations and Nonegalitarian Relationships. Caring for another requires some reciprocity, since it is necessary for a "relation" to occur (Buber, 1970). This level of reciprocity is best explained as an interactive relationship (Bottorff & D'Cruz, 1984; Wolf, 1986). Within caring interactions, there is tacit understanding that the recipient is the beneficiary. In addition, the relation has an inherent inequality, with the caregiver and recipient roles implicitly defined (Gallagher, 1978). Noddings (1984) indicates that there is mutual caring in personal relationships, but other types of relationships may involve "unequal meetings" (pp.

69-70). For example, patients require health care assistance (i.e., knowledge and/or skills), and this gives health care providers an inherent advantage. Benner (1984) suggests that professional nurses' power be used to empower patients. This reinforces the view that the recipient's need for caring should be based in trust, rather than power (such as supervisor-employee roles or paternalistic behavior) (Hall, 1985; Mayeroff, 1971).

In summary, although there is a fundamental interpersonal nature to a two-person caring relationship, it entails minimal reciprocity and usually involves an unequal caregiver and recipient relationship. Caring is facilitated by individuals' awareness of their part in the caring interaction. All of these factors play a role in the process of caring, which will be described next.

Critical Attributes of the Process of Caring

Walker and Avant's (1983) concept analysis approach was used to determine five critical attributes of the caring process. This process includes the caregiver's accurate perception of the entire situation and the whole person (the recipient as well as the self), use of facilitating methods to enhance this perception, methods of demonstrating caring, validation and evaluation of completion of caring in the other, and potential outcomes. Other conceptualizations of caring have been proposed for nursing. Watson's (1979) science of caring theory focuses on the premises and the bases of general types of caring maneuvers. The process-oriented caring concept advocated by Gaut (1986) focuses on implementation of actions, goals, and strategies. The proposed conceptualization of caring is a process focusing on the caregiver and reflects the relational components of caring as well as potential outcomes for both the caregiver and the recipient (Figure 14-1).

A description of each attribute in this conceptual model of the caring process follows. Although this discussion emphasizes the caregiver's perspective, the recipient's role will also be described because of the relational, interactional nature of caring, as depicted in Figure 14-1.

Accurate Perception.   A complete understanding of the recipient of caring involves a complex interplay of subjective, irrational, intuitive components and objective, rational, assimilative, and analytic components within the caregiver (Noddings, 1984). This attempt to "know" the other uses both subjective and objective methods to focus in and understand another person in a holistic sense (Howard, 1975; Peplau, 1969). Becoming acquainted with someone may involve a process of attunement, piecing daily perceptions together to obtain the whole picture (Griffen, 1983). The ultimate goal is an accurate perception of the other's need(s), which facilitates the entire caregiver-recipient interaction (Carter, 1983; Doona, 1979; Wiedenbach, 1963).

Figure 14-1
The Process of Caring:
Critical Attributes and Relational Components

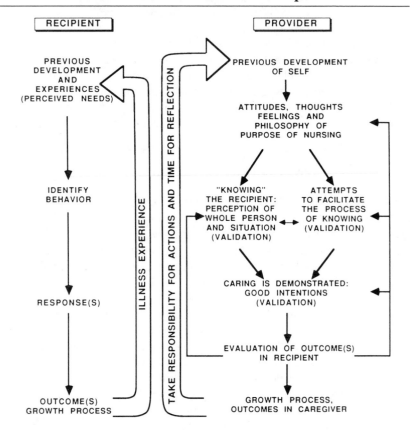

Both the caregiver's and the recipient's perspectives are influenced by sociocultural, psychological, spiritual, and physiological factors (Leininger, 1980). In addition, the caregiver is sensitive to changes or other recipient indicators that caring has been acknowledged in some way (Noddings, 1984). Each attempt to "know" another individual builds the caregiver's experiential base for understanding both the unique and the typical and enhances future understanding of similar encounters (Gadow, 1980).

Each of the caring domains involves some form of "knowing." The personal caring domain emphasizes the caregiver's use of more subjective than objective methods. The limited nature of social encounters usually does not allow opportunities to complete the knowing process, although initial impressions usually form a basis for future comparisons (Poyatos,

1985). The professional's knowledge of a recipient depends on the length and nature of the health-related encounter.

Within the professional caring domain, the knowing phase may be facilitated by the educational process which emphasizes interpersonal communication methods, clinical experiences with different personalities, and methods to understand recipients' needs. Professionals learn how to deal with different types of people who may not share their values. Their knowing process is similar to the personal "receptivity" suggested by Noddings (1984), but is limited by the lack of intense emotional involvement.

While *knowing* the other is important in each of the caring dimensions, there are specific ways to *facilitate* it. Both are believed to be mutually interdependent components of the caring process. Double arrows in Figure 14-1 depict the constant interplay of these two facets of caring.

Use of Facilitating Methods. The four ways to facilitate knowing the other person in a caring relationship are respecting the other (Griffen, 1983; Kitson, 1987), creating an open interpersonal atmosphere (Goldsborough, 1969; Watson, 1979), having a positive feeling toward the other, and offering "true presence" (Doona, 1979; Howard, 1975; Zderad, 1969). Calm, subdued physical surroundings also facilitate recipient expression of feelings and needs.

Although professionals usually do not have control of health care environments, they can alter the environment by using the above facilitating methods. Professionals can also increase their awareness of the recipient's personal space needs and reactions to health care environments. The methods used to facilitate the "knowing" process are highly individualized, depending on the context of the situation and are thus difficult to specify within each caring domain. Other observable caring behaviors are discussed below.

Methods to Demonstrate Caring. This part of the process includes observable behaviors used to indicate caring. Both instrumental and expressive approaches to demonstrate caring should indicate concern and express tenderness (Frankfurt, 1982; Peplau, 1969; Watson, 1979). Caring contributes to, yet is separate from curing (Leininger, 1981). Therefore, not only what is done, but how it is done is important. The implicit assumptions include the intent or desire to see the recipient "grow toward health and wholeness" (Hoffman, 1969, p. 669) by acting (or in some cases, purposefully withholding action in the best interest of the recipient) in a humane manner that aims to protect the inherent personal worth, privacy, and safety of the recipient (Griffen, 1983; Noddings, 1984; Watson, 1979). It is also assumed that these methods protect the recipient's rights of self-determination and freedom of choice and action (Gadow, 1980; Griffen, 1983; Howard, 1975).

These good intentions underlying observable methods to demonstrate caring are evident in each of the three dimensions, but the recipient's response often varies because of health-related circumstances or conflicting perceptions of the other person's behavior. The personal caring realm is more intimate and involves an extended length of interaction, which affords the greatest insight into how caring methods will be interpreted by the recipient. It is more difficult to determine the reaction of a recipient during and following social and professional interventions. Nursing is linked to the professional dimension in this area.

Most of nursing's attention and research on caring has focused on identification of either caregivers' (Fenton, 1987; Paulen & Rapp, 1981) or recipients' (Brown, 1986; Kauffman, 1986; Larson, 1984; Mayer, 1986) perceptions of caring behaviors. Generalization of these studies is somewhat limited because of varying recipient perceptions of past caring experiences, the setting in which caring is delivered, and the type and level of available professional assistance. However, data have uncovered many basic humanistic interventions used by professional nurses. For example, it was discovered that some patients rate instrumental (procedure-oriented) interventions as more important than expressive (interpersonally oriented) nursing behaviors (Larson, 1987). Case studies and interviews with patients indicate that rushed caregivers are perceived to be non–caring (Riemen, 1986a). Phenomenological studies have considered perceptions of the context of the situation surrounding the caring process. These studies have linked professional nurses' interventions (or purposeful deletion of them) to positive health outcomes of recipients and expert levels of professional caring in nursing (Benner, 1984; Drew, 1986; Riemen, 1986a, 1986b).

Caring methodologies can result in a variety of outcomes ranging from preventing dehumanization (by recognizing and respecting the recipient as a person) to having a lasting effect on the other person's lifestyle. Each of the three caring domains could affect outcomes anywhere along this continuum. Some of the final critical attributes of the caring process emphasize validation and evaluation of the intended effect(s) of the caregiver's interventions and other potential outcomes. These two aspects of the process are included in, or influence other, phases of the caring process, as indicated in Figure 14-1.

Validation and Evaluation of Caring Completed in the Recipient. This step in the process is vital to determine if caring has actually taken place, since even the best intentions and actions cannot be considered "caring" unless there is "completion of caring" in the recipient (Noddings, 1984, pp. 68–69). "Completion" means that the recipient has a feeling or inner recognition of being cared for by the caregiver. There may also be tangible evidence, such as verbalization, or other behavioral changes in the recipient which follow caring. The recipient's level of expectation, perceptions, and ability to reason and accept caring influence this stage of the process (Poyatos, 1985).

Personal caregivers are often more successful in validating and evaluating the caring act because of the in-depth knowledge of the other person and the long-term relationship. It should be noted that even if the social or professional caregiver is in a position to evaluate consequences of caring, long-term results are unpredictable (Arendt, 1974). Professional caregivers may be more astute evaluators than those involved with social caring because they are educated to assess the results of their interventions. All other stages of the process are influenced by the validation and evaluation phase. If caring has actually occurred (i.e., it is "completed" or recognized by the other person), it could then lead to a number of consequences for both the provider and recipient of caring, which are discussed in the next section.

Potential Outcomes of Caring. As previously discussed, the nature of caring tends to benefit the recipient. Caregiver involvement may lead to improved recipient health, recognition of feelings associated with illness, or enhanced insight into other aspects of life that could make life more complete (Peplau, 1969). In addition, if stress levels are decreased following caring interactions, the immune response may be enhanced, leading to improved resistance to physiological disorders (Drew, 1986).

There are many potential benefits to the caregiver; however, many are intangible. As a result of enriched insights, the caregiver can function at a higher level in other areas through heightened self-actualization (Mayeroff, 1971; Peplau, 1969). This may include increased "self-discovery," enhanced connectedness to others, or greater appreciation of many other aspects of life (Frankfurt, 1982; Goldsborough, 1969). In addition, the caregiver may feel a great deal of accomplishment as a result of having helped a fellow human being. Noddings (1984) indicates that joy or a sense of euphoria results from involvement with a more personal level of caring, leading to an enhanced commitment to care in the future.

Potentially negative caregiver outcomes, however, must also be addressed because energy is required to sustain the process of caring. This process can be extremely stressful and may lead to feelings of being drained emotionally, depressed, or burned-out. The professional caregiver attempts to deal not only with patients, but also with complex, bureaucratic health care delivery systems, allied health care workers, and social expectations (Bailey, 1985).

It is suggested that reflection is necessary, both during and following the caring process, to cope with potentially negative outcomes and facilitate the positive effects. This, then, improves future caring abilities and ways to deal with one's own vulnerabilities (Noddings, 1984). Support systems, including effective social support, assist in regenerating depleted energy levels following caregiving experiences (Heller, Swindle, & Dusenbury, 1986; Wolf, 1986). Stress related to caregiver responsibilities may also be alleviated by social support and other coping mechanisms (Bailey, 1985). All potential outcomes of caregiving, as outlined in Figure 14-1, create a feedback loop that influences an individual's capacity to care.

Caring outcomes resulting from nursing interventions, however, are not always recognized. As the caring concept is delineated, it must be differentiated from other similar, yet confounding terms. The process of caring (as used by professional nurses) and its outcomes is contrasted with other terms in Figure 14-2.

Figure 14-2 indicates that while many of the terms used to describe caring may have positive recipient outcomes, very few require an in-depth knowledge of the other individual. This summary also indicates that the potential growth of the caregiver is not nearly as prevalent with the other concepts as it is with caring. This may be related to the fact that the complete perception or "knowing" of an individual, together with the

Figure 14-2
Terminology Used to Describe Caring by Professional Nurses

CRITICAL ATTRIBUTES OF CARING	COMPARISON OF SYNONYMS OF CARING									
	CARING	TENDERNESS	CONCERN	KINDNESS	NURTURING	INVOLVEMENT	LOVE	COMFORTING	SUPPORT	EMPATHY
ACCURATE PERCEPTION OF THE WHOLE INDIVIDUAL AND THE ENTIRE SITUATION	X					X				
USE OF METHODS TO FACILITATE AN ACCURATE PERCEPTION	X		X	X						X
METHODS TO DEMONSTRATE CARING	X	X	X	X	X		X	X	X	X
VALIDATION AND EVALUATION OF CARING OUTCOMES	X	X	X	X	X	X	X	X	X	
CONSEQUENCES POTENTIAL FOR GROWTH OF CAREGIVER	X					X	X		X	X
POTENTIAL FOR GROWTH OF RECIPIENT OF CARING	X	?	X	X	X	X	X	?	X	X

other critical attributes of caring, allows greater transferability from one situation to another.

Table 14-1 summarizes the analysis of caring using the three domains of caring in relationship to previously discussed components: participants, motivation to care, nature of the caring act, and critical attributes.

The analysis indicates that both the personal and social caring domains have the greatest influence on nursing practice in three areas, including the capacity and motivation to care and the nature of the caring act. Most of the other variables seem to emphasize nurses' professional commitment. There are a number of other factors which impinge on this ideal conceptualization of professional caring. Attempts to study caring must consider the context of nursing practice and the socio-historical forces that determine the nurse's role. Table 14-2 summarizes the variables pertaining to caring by professional nurses and the potential barriers to the practice of caring for each of the critical attributes and outcomes. These will be discussed after considering other unique working conditions of nurses.

Table 14-1
Comparison Of Three Caring Domains

	Domains		
Variables	**Personal**	**Social**	**Professional**
Participants	Most intense caring by caregiver	Least intensive caring by caregiver	Equal involvement of both caregiver and recipient.
	Mother-child, family members, close friends	Casual acquaintances, strangers	Strangers (generally) or acquaintances from previous encounters.
	(Relationship is established)	(Little or no relationship)	(Relationship is defined.)
Prerequisites	Previous caring relationships	Total involvement not necessary	Previous caring relationships.
	Usually some congruence of value systems	Values not always important	Recognition of each participant's value system.
	Loving attitude		Development of clear, deliberate communication.

(continued on next page)

Table 14-1 *continued*

| Variables | Domains | | |
	Personal	Social	Professional
Motivation for caring	Instinctive Disposition/feeling in caregiver Sense of self-caring Natural	Reflexive Social or distress related	Moral obligation. Commitment. Sense of self-caring. Energy aimed to relieve distress or enhance recipient goals.
Nature of the act of caring	"Thou orientation" "We-relationship" Provider-initiated Long-term	"We-relationship" "They orientation" Provider or recipient-initiated Short or long-term	"Thou orientation." "We-relationship." Provider or recipient-initiated. Short or long-term.
Critical attributes of the process of caring	Well-known recipient; emphasis on subjectivity Demonstration of caring has highly personal implications	Other person not well-known to provider Subjective-objective approach; emphasis on objective Distance may be maintained Caring not as personal	Recipient usually unknown to provider. Continuous validation of caregiving behaviors necessary.
Potential outcomes			
Provider	Enhanced ability to care for self Potential for personal growth Positive (euphoria, joy) or negative (guilt) feelings possible	Feeling of goodwill Feeling of belonging	Feeling of accomplishment vs. frustration.
Recipient	Reciprocity not always expected; able to validate if caring completed in other	Assistance helped relieve distress or social needs	Lack of feelings of depersonalization.

BARRIERS TO CARING WITHIN NURSING

Caring Within the Practice of Nursing

Prior to discussing the barriers to caring by nurses listed in Table 14-2, nurses' unique relationship to patients will be explored. This discussion will focus on hospital nursing (a chief source of employment) and will include the intimate nature of nurse-patient relationships, continuity of care, nurses' subservient relationship to physicians and institutions, and nurses' views of their practice.

While it is generally accepted that nurse-patient relationships are somewhat personal and physically intimate, the caring process is often difficult because of nurses' unique work situation. There is generally a lack of continuity in the nurse–patient relationship. In addition, patients view nurses as nonautonomous and subservient to physicians (Ashley, 1980). Patients are physicians' clients, and the nurses's role is generally not well understood (Bottorff & D'Cruz, 1984; Nowakowski, 1985). The patriarchal-oriented hospital setting leads to nursing frustration and a sense of failure, which may be due to the lack of acknowledgement of nurses' positive qualities (Ashley, 1980). Physicians suggest that nurses have a role as part of the "team," but in actuality nurses are not treated equally. This creates situations where nurses have increased responsibility but limited authority (Lovell, 1980). Not all barriers to caring exist outside of nursing, however; nurses further limit caring by their unique views of their own practice.

Aroskar (1985) attempts to differentiate nursing from medical practice by comparing views held by nurses and physicians in hospital settings. Nurses' views, grouped into six areas, were found to be diametrically opposed to those of physicians. These perspectives further limit the profession's caring practices and inhibit an overall position of equality with other health care providers. These areas are related to the way in which nurses view: time (restricted, rigid, task-oriented), resources (limited, often difficult to obtain), level of analysis (concrete and contextual, lacking in integration), work assignment arrangement (usually inconsistent, lacking in continuity), set of rewards (hourly wage, lack of other rewards), sense of mastery over work (lacking because of inconsistency of patient relationships), and functional division of labor, (task–oriented). In general, the practice realm of nursing is unclear, even for its own members (Engelhardt, 1985). Often, a clear relationship between nursing care and patient outcomes is elusive because of its complex nature (Leininger, 1980). Therefore, both psychological and structural barriers to caring by nurses are present both within and outside of nursing. This unique nurse-patient relationship tends to have high expectations and few tangible rewards. In

Table 14-2

Table 14-2
Professional Nursing's Relationship to the Three Caring Domains

Variables related to caring	Caring domain which reflects professional nursing	Basis of the relationship of professional nursing to the domain	Barriers to professional nursing practice of caring
Participants	Professional	Lacks intensity of personal relationships Need for professional knowledge and skills Limited to time frame of patient need of patient need for professional involvement	Usually confronted by a lack of continuity of professional provider–recipient relationships.
Caring capacity	Personal	Nurse aware of recipient's values Need to be open to the other; empathy Knowledge of self necessary prior to complete involvement	Values may conflict, creating dilemmas. Other professional commitments limit the amount of involvement.
	Professional	Need to identify personal capacity and relate it to professional practice Involvement means clarifying the focus, intensity, and perspective (Gadow, 1980)	Generally, professional involvement is less intense than personal.
	Social	Instinctive nature to help others who are helpless or in need of assistance (Gaylin, 1976)	
Motivation to care	Personal	Ability to respect self and others required Caring disposition	Lack of strong sense of self; early development and later relationships.
	Professional	Basis is normative effects	Ethical components of decision-making process need to be explicit in nursing education; philosophical underpinnings of nursing should be taught (Joseph, 1985; Shapiro, 1985).

Variables related to caring	Caring domain which reflects professional nursing	Basis of the relationship of professional nursing to the domain	Barriers to professional nursing practice of caring
Motivation to care	Social	Intuitive, reflexive nature	Emergencies may limit time with healthier patients.
Nature of the caring act	Personal	May become attached to recipient; not an emotion-based selfless love (eros), but brotherly/sisterly concern(filia)	Strong subjective response limits caregiver's perspective.
	Professional	Reflects the two personal interpersonal relationships as discussed by Schutz (1970)	Situationally based. Conflicting values may be difficult to ascertain and deal with.
		Initiated by caregiver or recipient	Energy-draining; recipient targeted as the beneficiary.
	Social	Influenced by the situation (although professional relationships do not include a "They-orientation")	Bounded by institutional constraints (time, money).
Accurate perception	Professional	Identification of different value systems and the interpersonal process	Length of encounter. Inadequate time to integrate theory and practice related to interpersonal caring processes. Use of both objective and intuitive levels not completely understood (Rew, 1986).
Use of facilitating methods	Professional	Ways to demonstrate respect, positive feelings, and "true presence" in a professional relationship; ambiance crucial to facilitating the knowing process	Constricted by health care rules and regulations; other demands on professional resources.

(continued)

199

Table 14-2 *Continued*

Variables related to caring	Caring domain which reflects professional nursing	Basis of the relationship of professional nursing to the domain	Barriers to professional nursing practice of caring
Use of facilitating methods	Professional	Nurses have insider views and knowledge of health care system	Physical surroundings may hamper process.
Methods to demonstrate caring	Professional	Unable to completely anticipate how participants will interpret actions Curing facilitated by, and linked to, caring process	Lack of in-depth knowledge of what is expected or how the other person likes to be cared for (Thoits, 1986). Short-term interactions and limited continuity may limit caring; outcomes may include decreasing depersonalization. Procedure-related competencies increase responsibility of nurses. Limited theoretical–clinical synthesis/integration of relationship of curing and caring due to inadequate conceptualization of caring.
Validation and evaluation of caring	Professional	Lack of in-depth knowledge of other person Evaluation skills used to a greater degree than the other two caring domains	Ability to evaluate limited by length of relationships, and in some cases, extent of illness/disease process.
Potential outcomes of caring	Professional	Tendency to focus on recipient's improved welfare, and not the continued welfare of the caregiver	Need to identify both nurse and patient support systems. Limited time for reflection due to heavy workloads. Limited institutional or professional reward systems when caregiver attempts to be caring.

addition, nurses often do not see the long-term effects of their caring efforts.

Table 14-2 indicates a number of barriers to nursing's caring practice. These include an inherent lack of control over practice, confusion about educational requirements, lack of support for caring practice, and inattention to the profession's socialization process (which can influence an individual's level of caring). The origins of many of these barriers are illuminated by examining current and past influences on the practice of nursing.

Historical and Social Influences on Nurses as a Caring Group

The five major issues from nursing's history that influence its current dilemmas regarding caring include its religious and Victorian roots (Hughes, 1980), woman-worker base in a patriarchal health care system (Chinn, 1980; Melosh, 1982; Reverby, 1987a), ineffective use of interpersonal skills and lack of communication strategies (Benner, 1984; Carter, 1983; Menikheim & Meyer, 1986), educational disunity and lack of consistency in instruction of caring (possibly related to confusion concerning nursing's definition of practice) (Christman, 1983; Reverby, 1987b), and lack of autonomy resulting in an inability to control its own practice (Reverby, 1987a, 1987b). Other current factors are categorized in Table 14-3.

Table 14-3 indicates that nurses need to become involved at a number of levels (nurse-to-nurse, with other health care providers, and community/society) to avoid threats related to the undervaluing and potential discontinuance of their caring practices.

CARING'S RELATIONSHIP TO THE DISCIPLINE OF NURSING

Caring reflects all four of nursing's metaparadigm concepts (health, person, environment, and nursing), and two of the three themes of nursing inquiry (behavior patterning and adaptation) (Donaldson & Crowley, 1978; Fawcett, 1984). Caring is also reflected by all four patterns of knowing discussed by Carper (1978), knowledge of caring as a science for nursing (the observable aspects of caring methodologies), its esthetic meanings (including the "knowing" of an individual), personal knowledge related to caring (the unique, contextual, situational aspects), and ethical knowledge (relating to the commitment to care). To date, classifications of caring are too broad to assist with delineating pertinent aspects within the discipline of nursing (Leininger, 1981). Because of its broad focus and in view of this detailed analysis of its professional basis, it appears that caring by nurses could be best defined by studying its

Table 14-3
Social Goals for Continued Caring Within the Nursing Profession

Nurses' relationships with each other
Provide more effective support for each other (Carter, 1983; Cronin-Stubbs & Brophy, 1985; Heller, et al., 1986; Kaufman & Beehr, 1986).
Support caring by nurses, health care institutions, and professional nursing organizations (Constable & Russel, 1986; Leninger, 1986; Reimen, 1986).
Unify, regardless of specialty area (Brickhead, 1978); incorporate technology into practice (Braillier, 1978).
Cope with stress related to caring for others (Bailey, 1985).

Nurses' relationships with other health care providers
Address medical dominance/deceptive tactics that increase nurses' responsibilities, but not their autonomy (Connors, 1980; Harding, 1980; Lovell, 1980).
Address decisions between the health care team and the patient (Pelligrino, 1985).
Address rights related to resources needed for caring (Griffen, 1983).
Prove economic worth of caring by nurses (Leininger, 1980).

Nurses' relationships with community/society
Publicly acknowledge nurses' work responsibilities and practice goals (Kalisch & Kalisch, 1986).
Empower patients (through expert caring); this will result in improved patient relations and increased nursing power (Benner, 1984).
Address low prestige ratings as compared to other health care professionals (Greenleaf, 1980).
Gain understanding of other perspectives and political maneuvering (Schraeder, 1986).
Become involved with policymaking (Moccia, 1988).
Enforce postmodern technological perspective; become involved with assessment of technology (Pacey, 1983; Winner, 1986).
Study community needs and folk-caring methods (Buerhaus, 1986; Leininger, 1980).

---

relationship to various types of nursing practice (Dunlop, 1986). This focus could emphasize nurse-patient dyad descriptions of the caring process or its outcomes, giving due consideration to the barriers discussed earlier.

Considerations for Research of Caring by Nurses

The context in which caring takes place is important. In addition, both expectations and perceptions need to be considered (Miller & Turnbull, 1986). Either the process or product component of caring can be studied. Caring is only present if it is "completed" in the recipient (Noddings, 1984). Therefore, the patient's feelings about being cared for, or other indicators that caring has been received, are important to establish its presence. There are a number of factors influencing this pattern in nurse–patient relationships.

The caring process seems to be contextually bound and may best be studied by qualitative research methods such as the phenomenological approach (Dunlop, 1986). On the other hand, one could focus on more basic caring product(s) or outcomes. It is generally understood these outcomes are wide-ranging; quantitative studies could build on previous nursing research which has identified patient and nurse feelings and behaviors related to caring interactions (Brown, 1986; Larson, 1984, 1987). The level of caring (i.e., preventing depersonalization versus changing the recipient's life outlook) must be identified if a quantitative outcome approach is used. Both qualitative and quantitative research approaches would assist in uncovering caring's complete meaning for nurses.

In summary, an expanded version of the dimension-attribute method suggests that nursing practice is primarily described by the professional caring domain. Caring is reflected in many of the themes and concepts characterizing the discipline of nursing, indicating that it is the "essence of nursing" (Leininger, 1980). It is suggested that research dealing with the process or outcomes of caring within the nursing profession should consider broader socio-historical factors and the context of the interaction. Further definition and study of caring would help to maintain it as nursing's unshakable foundation.

REFERENCES

Amato, P.R. (1985). An investigation of planned helping behavior. *Journal of Research in Personality, 19*(2), 232–252.

Amato, P.R., & Cook, J. (1983). The helpfulness of urbanites and small town dwellers: A test between two broad theoretical positions. *Australian Journal of Psychology, 35*(2), 233–243.

Arendt, H. (1974). *The human condition.* Chicago: University of Chicago Press.

Aroskar, M.A. (1985). Ethical relationships between nurses and physicians. In A.H. Bishop & J.R. Scudder (Eds.), *Caring, curing, coping: Nurses, physicians, and patient relationships* (pp. 44–61). Alabama: University of Alabama Press.

Ashley, J.A. (1980). Power in structured misogyny: Implications for the politics of care. *Advances in Nursing Science, 2*(3), 3–22.

Bailey, R.D. (1985). *Coping with stress in caring.* Boston: Blackwell Scientific Publications.

Batson, C.D., Harris, A.C., McCaul, K.D., Davis, M., & Schmidt, T. (1979). Compassion or compliance: Alternative dispositional attributions for one's helping behavior. *Social Psychology Quarterly, 42*(4), 405–409.

Benner, P. (1984). *From novice to expert: Excellence and power in clinical nursing practice*. Menlo Park: Addison-Wesley.

Bevis, E.O. (1981). Caring: A life force. In M. Leininger (Ed.), *Caring: An essential human need* (pp. 49–60). Thorofare, NJ: Charles B. Slack, Inc.

Birckhead, L.M. (1978). Nursing and the technetronic age. *Journal of Nursing Administration, 7*(2), 16–19.

Bottorff, J.L., & D'Cruz, J.V. (1984). Towards inclusive notions of "patient" and "nurse." *Journal of Advanced Nursing, 9*, 549–553.

Braillier, L.W. (1978). The nurse as holistic health practitioner. *Nursing Clinics of North America, 13*(4), 643–655.

Brown, L. (1986). The experience of care: Patient perspectives. *Topics in Clinical Nursing, 8*(2), 56–62.

Buber, M. (1970). *I and thou*. (W. Kaufmann, Trans.). New York: Charles Scribner's Sons.

Buerhaus, P.I. (1986). The economics of caring: Challenges and new opportunities for nursing. *Topics in Clinical Nursing, 8*(2), 13–21.

Carper, B.A. (1978). Fundamental patterns of knowing in nursing. *Advances in Nursing Science, 1*(1), 13–23.

Carter, S.L. (1983). Rehumanizing the nursing role: A question of love. *Topics in Clinical Nursing, 5*(3), 11–17.

Chinn, P.L. (1980). From the editor. *Advances in Nursing Science, 2*(3), viii–xvi.

Christman, L.P. (1983). The future of nursing is predicted by the state of science and technology. In N.L. Chaska (Ed.), *The nursing profession: A time to speak* (pp. 802–805). San Francisco: McGraw-Hill.

Connors, D.D. (1980). Sickness unto death: Medicine as myth, necrophilic, iatrogenic. *Advances in Nursing Science, 2*(3), 39–54.

Constable, J.F., & Russel, D.W. (1986). The effect of social support and the work environment upon burnout among nurses. *Journal of Human Stress, 12*(1), 20–26.

Cronin-Stubbs, D., & Brophy, E.B. (1985). Burnout: Can social support save the psych nurse? *Journal of Psychosocial Nursing and Mental Health Services, 23*(7), 8–13.

de Rivera, J. (1984). The structure of emotional relationships. *Review of Personality and Social Psychology, 5*, 116–145.

Diers, D. (1986). To profess to be a professional. *Journal of Nursing Administration, 16*(3), 25–30.

Donaldson, S.K. & Crowley, D.M. (1978). The discipline of nursing. *Nursing Outlook, 26*(2), 113–120.

Doona, M.E. (1979). *Travelbee's intervention in psychiatric nursing.* Philadelphia: F.A. Davis.

Drew, N. (1986). Exclusion and confirmation: A phenomenology of patients' experiences with caregivers. *Image, 18*(2), 39–43.

Dunlop, M.J. (1986). Is a science of caring possible? *Journal of Advanced Nursing, 11*(6), 661–670.

Emmons, R.A., Diener, E., & Larsen, R.J. (1985). Choice of situations and congruence models of interactionism. *Personality and Individual Differences, 6*(6), 693–702.

Engelhardt, H.T. (1985). Physicians, patients, health care institutions, and the people in between: Nurses. In A.H. Bishop & J.R. Scudder (Eds.), *Caring, curing, coping: Nurse, physician, and patient relationships.* Alabama: University of Alabama Press.

Fawcett, J. (1984). *Analysis and evaluation of conceptual models of nursing.* Philadelphia: F.A. Davis.

Fenton, M.V. (1987). Development of the scale of humanistic nursing behaviors, *Nursing Research, 36*(2), 82–87.

Fowler, M.D.M. (1987). Introduction to ethics and ethical theory: A road map to the discipline. In M.D.M. Fowler and J. Levine-Ariff (Eds.), *Ethics at the bedside* (pp. 24–38). Philadelphia: J.B. Lippincott.

Frankfurt, H. (1982). The importance of what we care about. *Synthese, 53*(2), 257–272.

Fry, S.T. (1988). The ethic of caring: Can it survive in nursing? *Nursing Outlook, 36*(1), 48.

Fultz, J., Batson, C.D., Fortenbach, V.A., McCarthy, P.M., & Varney, L.L. (1986). Social evaluation and the empathy–altruism hypothesis. *Journal of Personality and Social Psychology, 50*(4), 761–769.

Gadow, S. (1980). Existential advocacy: Philosophical foundation of nursing. In S.F. Spicker & S. Gadow (Eds.), *Nursing Images and Labels* (pp. 79–101), New York: Springer.

Gallagher, E.B. (1978, April). *The doctor-patient relationship in the changing health scene.* Paper presented at the International Conference sponsored by John E. Fogarty Center for Advanced Study in Health Sciences, Bethesda, MD.

Gaut, D.A. (1986). Evaluating caring competencies in nursing practice. *Topics in Clinical Nursing, 8*(2), 77–83.

Gaylin, W. (1976). *Caring*. New York: Alfred A. Knopf.

Gilfillan, S.S. (1985). Adult intimate love relationships as new editions of symbiosis and the separation–individuation process. *Smith College Studies in Social Work, 55*(3), 183–196.

Goldsborough, J. (1969). Involvement. *American Journal of Nursing, 69*(1), 66–68.

Greenleaf, N.P. (1980). Sex-segregated occupations: Relevance for nursing. *Advances in Nursing Science, 2*(3), 23–38.

Griffen, A.P. (1983). A philosophical analysis of caring in nursing. *Journal of Advanced Nursing, 8*, 289–295.

Hall, P.M. (1985). Asymmetric relationships and processes of power. *Studies in Symbolic Interaction* (Suppl. 1), 309–344.

Harding, S. (1980). Value-laden technologies and the politics of nursing. In S.F. Spiker & S. Gadow (Eds.), *Nursing: Images and labels* (pp. 49–75). New York: Springer.

Heller, K., Swindle, R.W., & Dusenbury, L. (1986). Component social support processes: Comments and integration. *Journal of Consulting & Clinical Psychology, 54*(4), 466–470.

Hoffman, G.S. (1969). The concept of love. *Nursing Clinics of North America, 4*(4), 663–671.

Howard, J. (1975). Humanization and dehumanization of health care: A conceptual view. In J. Howard & A. Strauss (Eds.), *Humanizing health care* (pp. 57–102). New York: John Wiley & Sons.

Hughes, L. (1980). The public image of the nurse. *Advances in Nursing Science, 2*(3), 55–72.

Johnson, M.P. (1973). Commitment: A conceptual structure and empirical application. *The Sociological Quarterly, 14*, 395–406.

Joseph, D. (1985). Humanism as a philosophy for nursing. *Nursing Forum, 22*(4), 135–138.

Kalisch, P.A., & Kalisch, B.J. (1986). *The advance of American nursing*. Boston: Little, Brown.

Kauffmann, K.M.S. (1986). Caring in the instance of unexpected pregnancy loss. *Topics in Clinical Nursing, 8*(2), 37–46.

Kaufman, G.M., & Beehr, T.A. (1986). Interactions between job stressors and social support: Some counterintuitive results. *Journal of Applied Psychology, 71*(3), 522–526.

Kelley, P., & Kelley, V.R. (1985). Supporting natural helpers: A cross-cultural study. *Social Casework: The Journal of Contemporary Social Work, 66*(6), 358–366.

Kemper, T.D. (1980). Altruism and voluntary action. In D.H. Smith & J. Macaulay (Eds.), *Participation in social and political activities* (pp. 306–338). San Francisco: Jossey Bass.

Kitson, A.L. (1987). A comparative analysis of lay-caring and professional (nursing) caring relationships. *International Journal of Nursing Studies, 24*(2), 155–165.

Larson, P. (1984). Important nurse caring behaviors perceived by patients with cancer. *Oncology Nursing Forum, 11*(6), 46–50.

Larson, P. (1987). Comparison of cancer patients' and professional nurses' perceptions of important nurse caring behaviors. *Heart and Lung, 16*(2), 187–193.

Leininger, M. (1974). Humanism, health, and cultural values. In M. Leininger & G. Buck (Eds.), *Health care issues* (pp. 1–43). Philadelphia: F.A. Davis.

Leininger, M. (1980). Caring: A central focus of nursing and health care services. *Nursing and Health Care, 1,* 135–143.

Leininger, M.M. (1981). Some philosophical, historical, and taxonomic aspects of nursing and caring in American culture. In M. Leininger (Ed.), *Caring: An essential human need* (pp. 133–144). Thorofare, NY: Charles B. Slack.

Leininger, M. (1986). Care facilitators and resistance factors in the culture of nursing. *Topics in Clinical Nursing, 8*(2), 1–12.

Lovell, M.C. (1980). The politics of medical deception: Challenging the trajectory of history. *Advances in Nursing Science, 2*(3), 73–95.

Lundh, U., Soder, M., & Wareness, K. (1988). Nursing theories: A critical view. *Image, 20*(1), 36–40.

Lynn, M., & Oldenquist, A. (1986). Egoistic and nonegoistic motives in social dilemmas. *American Psychologist, 41*(5), 529–534.

Mayer, D.K. (1986). Cancer patients and families' perceptions of nurse caring behaviors. *Topics in Clinical Nursing, 8*(2), 63–69.

Mayeroff, M. (1971). *On caring.* San Francisco: Harper and Row.

Melosh, B. (1982). *"The physician's hand:" Work culture and conflict in American nursing.* Philadelphia: Temple University Press.

Menikheim, M.L., & Meyer, M.W. (1986). Communication pattern of women and nurses. *Women in health and illness.* Philadelphia: W.B. Saunders.

Miller, D.T., & Turnbull, W. (1986). Expectancies and interpersonal processes. *Annual Review of Psychology, 37*, 233–256.

Moccia, P. (1988). At the faultline: Social activism and caring. *Nursing Outlook, 36*(1), 30–33.

Morris, C. (1956). *Varieties of human value.* Chicago: University of Chicago Press.

Newell, J.D. (1984). The justification of a professional ethic for physicians. In D.H. Smith (Ed.), *Respect and care in medical ethics* (pp. 131–150). New York: University Press of America.

Noddings, N. (1984). *Caring: A feminine approach to ethics and moral education.* Berkeley: University of California Press.

Norris, C.M. (1982). Concept clarification: Evolving methods in nursing. In C.M. Norris (Ed.), *Concept clarification in nursing* (pp. 37–47). Rockville, MD: Aspen.

Nowakowski, L. (1985). Complexities and clarity in nurse–client and nurse-patient relationships. *Journal of Professional Nursing, 1*, 212–216.

Pacey, A. (1983). *The culture of technology.* Cambridge, MA: MIT Press.

Paulen, A., & Rapp, C. (1981). Person-centered caring. *Nursing Management, 12*(9), 17–21.

Pellegrino, E.D. (1985). The caring ethic: The relation of physician to patient. In A.H. Bishop & J.R. Scudder (Eds.), *Caring, curing, and coping* (pp. 8–30). Alabama: Alabama University Press.

Peplau, H.E. (1969). Professional closeness. *Nursing Forum, 8*,(4), 342–359.

Poyotas, F. (1985). The deeper levels of face-to-face interaction. *Language and Communication, 5*(2), 111–113.

Rawnsley, M.M. (1980). The concept of privacy. *Advances in Nursing Science, 2*(2), 25–31.

Reddy, R.D. (1980). Individual philanthropy and giving behavior. In D.H. Smith & J. Macaulay (Eds.), *Participation in social and political activities* (pp. 370–399). San Francisco: Jossey Bass.

Reverby, S. (1987a). *Ordered to care: The dilemma of American nursing.* New York: Cambridge University Press.

Reverby, S. (1987b). A caring dilemma: Womanhood and nursing in historical perspective. *Nursing Research, 36*(1), 5–11.

Rew, L. (1986). Concept analysis of a group phenomenon. *Advances in Nursing Science, 8*(2), 21–28.

Riemen, D.J. (1986a). Noncaring and caring in the clinical setting: Patients' descriptions. *Topics in Clinical Nursing, 8*(2), 30–36.

Riemen, D.J. (1986b). The essential structure of a caring interaction: Doing phenomenology. In P.L. Munhall & C.J. Oiler (Eds.), *Nursing research: A qualitative perspective* (85–108). Norwalk: Appleton-Century-Crofts.

Ropohl, G. (1983). A critique of technological determinism. In P.T. Durbin & F. Rapp (Eds.), *Philosophy and technology* (pp. 83–90). Boston: D. Reidel Publishing.

Schraeder, B.D. (1986). Caring for low birth weight infants beyond the intensive care nursery: Developing public policy. *Topics in Clinical Nursing, 8*(2), 22–29.

Schutz, A. (1970). *On phenomenology and social relations.* Chicago: University of Chicago Press.

Shapiro, S.B. (1985). An empirical analysis of operating values in humanistic education. *Journal of Humanistic Psychology, 25*(1), 94–108.

Thoits, P.A. (1986). Social support as coping assistance. *Journal of Consulting and Clinical Psychology, 54*(4), 416–423.

Toulmin, S. (1981). The tyranny of principles. *The Hastings Center Report, 11*(6), 31–39.

Walker, L.O., & Avant, K.C. (1983). *Strategies for theory construction in nursing.* Norwalk: Appleton-Century–Crofts.

Watson, J. (1979). *The philosophy and science of caring.* Boston: Little, Brown.

Webster's Ninth New Collegiate Dictionary. (1986). Springfield, MA: Merriam-Webster.

Wiedenbach, E. (1963). The helping art of nursing. *American Journal of Nursing, 63*(11), 54–57.

Winner, L. (1986). *The whale and the reactor.* Chicago: University of Chicago Press.

Wolf, Z.R. (1986). The caring concept and nurse-identified behaviors. *Topics in Clinical Nursing, 8*(2), 84–93.

Zderad, L.T. (1969). Empathic nursing. *Nursing Clinics of North America, 4*(4), 655–661.

15

An Assessment of the Concept of Expectation: Its Usefulness in Nursing Practice

Andrea M. Barsevick and Diane Lauver

Popular wisdom and best-seller publications suggest that recovery from physical illnesses is affected by people's expectation about the prospect of recovery (Browne, 1989). Siegel (1986, 1989), Simonton (1978), and Cousins (1979) all have asserted in best-seller publications that positive expectations—positive outlook, confidence, optimism, or "fighting spirit" about one's chances for recovery—are associated with cure or increased longevity after a diagnosis of cancer or other chronic disease. Only recently has research supported this assertion, although not to the extent claimed by these authors.

It is important for nurses caring for patients to have a current scientific understanding of the concept of expectation for several reasons. First, nurses could influence expectation about illness by providing people with information, by modeling attitudes about illness, and possibly by what they do not say. Second, health care professionals are likely to be asked by patients to evaluate books, pamphlets, and educational programs designed to alter expectation in hopes of improving outcomes of illness. A current understanding of this concept would enhance the professional's ability to deal with these clinical issues. Third, health care professionals are

The comments of Jacqueline Fawcett and Jean Johnson during the development of this manuscript are gratefully acknowledged.

in a position to contribute to our scientific understanding of the effects of expectation on health care outcomes. The identification of areas in need of research could provide a focus for clinical research efforts.

This paper assesses current understanding of the concept of expectation and identifies areas for further research. The paper focuses on the usefulness of the concept as described in several different theories, the influence of expectation on health care outcomes, and how expectation can be modified in clinically meaningful ways.

THEORIES OF EXPECTATION

Self-Efficacy Theory

Expectation has been discussed within many psychological perspectives, one of which is self-efficacy theory (Bandura 1977, 1982; O'Leary, 1985). In this theory, expectation is viewed as the belief that one can successfully perform specific recommended behaviors in a difficult or novel situation. The expectation of self-efficacy is quite specific, referring to judgments about how well one will perform in a specific setting. The expectation of self-efficacy is distinguished from expectation about outcome, which refers to the judgment that performance of specific behaviors will result in a desired outcome. For example, a person judges that regular aerobic exercise reduces the risk of heart disease (expectation about outcome); the individual also judges his or her ability to perform this exercise (expectation of self-efficacy). According to the theory, the expectation of self-efficacy determines whether or not the individual engages in this health behavior. A person may judge that aerobic exercise reduces risk, but only if the person makes a positive judgment of his or her ability to do the exercise will the individual engage in this health behavior.

A problem with this theory is that expectation of self–efficacy and expectation about outcome are confounded. For example, people recovering from myocardial infarctions (Ewart, Taylor, Reese, & DeBusk, 1983) and persons with chronic obstructive pulmonary disease (Kaplan & Atkins, 1984) judged their ability to walk distances ranging from one block to three miles and to climb stairs for distances from a few steps to several flights. They made judgments of self-efficacy, that is, judgments about whether or not they could perform this behavior. However, they also made judgments about the likelihood that they could achieve a goal of aerobic exercise, to walk a specific distance in a specific time period. This confounding of type of expectation raises the question of whether expectation of self–efficacy, expectation about outcome, or both influence outcomes.

Personal Control Theory

Personal control theory provides another perspective of expectation (Rotter, 1954, 1966; Averill, 1977; Thompson, 1981). Personal control theory views expectation as beliefs about the availability of situational responses, including internal and external resources that could reduce the aversiveness of an event or situation. Increasing the responses available to the individual in a difficult situation is thought to increase perception of control and, therefore, result in more positive outcomes.

This definition of expectation is similar to that advanced in self-efficacy theory in that it focuses on ability to engage in specific behaviors. However, the definition has been broadened to include another dimension of responses: beliefs about the availability of external responses. For example, individuals with cancer judged their personal ability to avoid a recurrence of cancer (internal resource); they also judged the success of their surgery in removing all the cancer (external resource) (Timko & Janoff-Bulman, 1985). In fact, the definition put forth in personal control theory may be closer to the reality of health care situations in which individuals make judgments about the availability of both internal and external resources.

A problem with personal control theory is that its propositions have not been supported consistently (Thompson, 1981; Burger, 1989). Many studies, some in health care situations, have documented that increasing personal control sometimes has negative effects such as negative emotional responses (Mills & Krantz, 1979), relinquishment of the control offered (King, Norsen, Robertson, & Hicks, 1987), or poor performance (Burger, 1989). These contrary findings have led theorists to propose alternative explanations (Thompson, 1981). One alternative is that expectation about outcome rather than expectation about available situational responses may be the critical determinant of outcomes (Thompson, 1981; Burger, 1989). If an individual expects that having personal control will result in a poor outcome, that person, if given control, will experience negative affect, poor performance, or will relinquish control. However, if the individual expects a positive outcome by having personal control, he or she will initiate and persist in behaviors directed toward the achievement of that outcome.

Self-Regulation Theory

An alternative theory that may have utility for the study of expectation about health care is self-regulation theory (Carver, 1979). Within self-regulation theory, expectation is viewed as a judgment about the likelihood of achieving a desired goal or standard. This definition of expectation is very similar to the reinterpretation of personal control as expectation about outcome. It also incorporates both types of expectation described in self-efficacy theory, judgments about personal ability (expectation of self-efficacy) and judgments about achieving a desired outcome (expectation about outcome).

A feedback system guiding behavior engages when a person notices a discrepancy between his or her present state and a desired goal (Scheier & Carver, 1985). When faced with a discrepancy that appears manageable, a person focuses attention inward and takes action to reduce the discrepancy. However, in a difficult or novel situation, the person first judges the likelihood of attaining the goal. This judgment, the expectation about the likelihood of achieving the desired outcome, determines whether or not the individual initiates and persists in behaviors to reduce the discrepancy between present state and desired goal.

As the concept of expectation has evolved within each of these theories, expectation about outcome—that is, the judgment about one's ability to achieve a desired goal or outcome—has emerged as a critical element because this type of expectation has found the greatest empirical support (Scheier & Carver, 1987). The self-regulation theory of expectation is based on this definition and thus may have the greatest utility for nurses seeking a theoretical understanding of the concept.

HEALTH CARE OUTCOMES AND EXPECTATIONS

It is important to consider the types of health care outcomes that can be influenced by expectation. The popular but controversial writings of Siegel (1986, 1989), Simonton (1978), and Cousins (1979) suggest that a variety of outcomes, including both psychological well-being and physical well-being, can be influenced by expectation. A review of studies that involved people dealing with a variety of health care problems is provided here to assess the degree to which different types of health care outcomes are influenced by expectation.

There is strong evidence linking expectation with psychological well-being. Reker and Wong (1985) studied expectation about outcome among elderly people, half living in the community and half in institutions. During an initial interview, respondents verbalized events they looked forward to and rated their level of confidence that each event would occur. This measure of confidence reflects the concept of expectation advanced in self-regulation theory describing global positive beliefs about outcome. During the initial interview and a second interview two months later, depression and well-being were measured. Confidence was related positively to perceived physical well-being, number of activities to which the individual devoted time and effort, and sense of life purpose, but was negatively related to depression at the initial interview. Confidence at the initial interview was positively related to psychological well–being and happiness two months later. This last finding must be interpreted cautiously because changes over time in the relationship of expectation and well-being did not take into account differences in the level of well-being that existed at the initial time of measurement. Despite the limitation, this study is important because it demonstrates that the concept of expectation is relevant to the elderly, a population for whom health care problems are especially prevalent.

Global positive beliefs about the future have also been associated with psychological well-being among women in the third trimester of pregnancy and early postpartum period (Carver & Gaines, 1987). Controlling for initial symptoms of depression, the researchers found that positive expectation was inversely correlated with postpartum depressive symptoms. This concept of expectation reflects generalized beliefs about outcome as described in self-regulation theory.

Research on persons with cancer indicates that expectation influences psychological state. Much of this research was based on personal control theory using the concept of expectation as beliefs about internal and external resources. For example, women with breast cancer who had positive expectations about treatment efficacy expressed fewer depressive symptoms, feelings of worry or displeasure with self, and feelings of shame (Timko & Janoff-Bulman, 1985). The expectation that cancer recurrence was unlikely was associated with feelings of serenity and was inversely associated with depression. Also, the relationship between expectation about illness severity and depression was markedly lower among women with breast cancer who held positive expectations about treatment efficacy and about their ability to control their health (Taylor, Lichtman, & Wood, 1984). Conversely, negative expectation about the future has been associated with emotional distress among cancer patients with a variety of cancer diagnoses (Weisman & Worden, 1976). Among patients with hematologic malignancies, the expectation that one's actions influence health and the expectation that medication would control or cure the disease diminished the relationship between perceived severity of illness and psychological depression (Marks, Richardson, Graham, & Levine, 1986).

These findings, taken together, demonstrate that expectation is related to psychological well-being in a variety of adult populations, including young and elderly, with a variety of acute and chronic health care problems. It is important to note that expectation both about internal and external resources as well as expectation about outcome have been found to influence psychological well-being. But what about the link between expectation and physical well-being that is advanced in the popular literature?

The evidence supporting a link between expectation and physical well-being is less consistent than that linking expectation with psychological well-being. Among persons recovering from coronary artery bypass surgery, global positive expectations about the future were related to decreased incidence of elevated SGOT levels and new Q waves on EKG, both of which are physiological indicators of myocardial infarction (Scheier & Carver, 1987). In this study, expectation was viewed from a self-regulation perspective.

People with arthritis judged their ability to cope with pain and activities of daily living (Schoor & Holman, 1984). In this study, expectation was viewed from the perspective of self–efficacy theory. Positive expectation was negatively associated with pain and perceived disability four weeks later. This study controlled for baseline pain and functional status, as well as type and duration of arthritis. Although the findings of this study suggest that heightened perception of coping ability can reduce the degree of discomfort and disability experienced, it must be noted that the outcome measured was perception of physical well-being and there was no objective indicator of physical well-being.

Other research also suggests a link between expectation and physical well-being. Among women undergoing first trimester abortions, those who reported positive expectations about their ability to cope with the experience reported fewer physical complaints (abdominal cramps, nausea, dizziness, and back pain) than women with negative expectations (Major, Mueller, & Hildebrandt, 1985). This study adopted a view of expectation which is congruent with that advanced in self-regulation theory.

Among women with stage 1 cervical cancer, cervical intraepithelial neoplasia (CIN I, CIN II, and CIN III), and a control group with leiomyoma (a benign uterine tumor), a moderate relationship was observed between negative life events and cancer progression (Goodkin, Antoni, & Blaney, 1986). This relationship, however, was stronger among women with global negative expectations and weaker among women without these negative expectations. This measure of expectation reflects the concept of expectation advanced in self-regulation theory. Although the findings suggest that chronic negative expectations can promote the development of illness, the study is limited in that it was not prospective. These women were studied during the process of being evaluated for gynecologic symptoms. Because the physical abnormality was present at the time of testing (although unknown to investigator or subject), it is possible that negative expectations resulted from or occurred concurrently with stressors and illness.

A study of people with newly diagnosed malignant diseases followed for three to eight years after diagnosis suggests that expectation is not related to survival (Cassileth, Lusk, Miller, Brown, & Miller, 1985; Cassileth, Walsh, & Lusk, 1988). A number of psychosocial factors were assessed including hopelessness and helplessness. Measures of hopelessness and helplessness are analogous to global generalized expectations about outcomes. Neither hopelessness nor any of the other psychosocial factors was associated with survival.

Taken together, the findings of these studies provide some support for a relationship, although somewhat tenuous, between expectation and physical well-being in health care situations. Perhaps one of the difficulties in establishing this link lies in finding good indicators of physical well-being that are likely to be influenced by psychosocial factors.

MODIFICATION OF EXPECTATION IN CLINICALLY MEANINGFUL WAYS

It is important for health care professionals to understand how expectation can be altered in clinically meaningful ways. This is important in planning care for patients so that interventions can be tailored for individuals with different expectations. It is also critical for professionals to understand that the way they present information about anticipated outcomes can influence peoples' expectations, their choices regarding different aspects of care, and their health care outcomes. Professionals need to be aware of this so they don't inadvertently undermine appropriate expectations.

Expectation has been modified by providing concrete objective information in preparation for health care procedures (Leventhal & Johnson, 1983; McHugh, Christman, & Johnson, 1982). This type of information has been found to increase positive expectation and result in positive outcomes. Concrete objective information includes a description of when an event is expected, how long it is expected to last, and what sensations are likely to occur. Women receiving this type of information about hysterectomies reported changes in expectation including lower perception of difficulties, higher perception of ability to deal with difficulties, and a better match between the expected and actual experience than women who received no information or instruction in cognitive and behavioral coping strategies (Johnson, Christman, & Stitt, 1985). This study demonstrated that providing concrete objective information about what to expect during a health care experience is an effective means of enhancing peoples' expectations about their ability to cope with the experience. Although this study did not demonstrate a significant effect of preparatory information on desirable health outcomes (e.g., length of hospital stay and time to resumption of usual activities), previous research has repeatedly demonstrated significant positive effects of concrete objective information on these outcomes (Johnson, Fuller, Endress, & Rice, 1978; Johnson, Rice, Fuller, & Endress, 1978; Johnson, Morrissey, & Leventhal, 1973).

Johnson (1984) has suggested that concrete objective information influences the individual's cognitive image or schema of an impending experience. A cognitive schema consists of the objective and detailed perceptual elements of an experience. This information is at a low level of logical complexity or abstraction. The maplike schema provided via concrete objective information could be used by people in health care situations in much the same way that a road map is used by a traveler on an unfamiliar road. A road map contains information about the characteristics of roads and about spatial relationships of objects in the environment. A good road map provides the individual with a cognitive schema for processing the stimuli encountered during a journey and allows the traveler to respond as if in a familiar environment. Concrete objective information could provide a similar structure for the individual in a health care situation to predict and monitor a new experience and to respond to it in familiar ways.

Instruction in specific coping strategies has also been found to influence expectation and outcomes (Johnson, 1984). Cognitive coping strategies include the use of relaxation techniques, attention to favorable aspects of the experience, and techniques for reducing negative thoughts. Behavioral coping strategies include specific skills appropriate to a particular situation, such as techniques for smoking cessation or the prevention of surgical complications (ambulation, coughing, and deep breathing).

Instruction in coping strategies has had mixed effects on health care outcomes. It has been associated with shortened hospitalization (Wilson, 1981), reduced negative emotions after surgery (Langer, Janis, & Wolfer, 1975; Johnson, et al., 1978), increased exercise tolerance for persons with chronic obstructive pulmonary disease (Kaplan & Atkins, 1984), and better compliance during endoscopy when combined with concrete objective information (Johnson et al., 1973). However, instruction has also been associated with poor outcomes. Blood donors who were encouraged to cope by choosing the arm from which blood was drawn reported more pain, discomfort, and anxiety than persons who were not encouraged to use this strategy (Mills & Krantz, 1979). Women instructed in a cognitive coping strategy after hysterectomies had longer hospital stays than control patients (Johnson et al., 1985). Furthermore, only 17 percent of these women reported using this coping strategy after surgery, suggesting that this coping strategy lacked credibility.

In all of the situations in which instruction in coping strategies was effective, there was the possibility of active participation and self-control. The situations in which it was ineffective were ones in which there was limited opportunity for active coping, or in which the coping strategy taught was not credible for that situation. Thus, clinical health care professionals are cautioned to evaluate carefully the appropriateness of coping strategies for particular situations (Leventhal & Johnson, 1983; Burger, 1989). Instructing people in coping strategies that are inappropriate to a situation could undermine their confidence in their existing coping abilities, resulting in poor outcomes (Johnson et al., 1985).

FUTURE CHALLENGES

The concept of expectation has relevance both for nursing clinical practice and research. The claims of the popular writers (Simonton, 1978; Cousins, 1979; Siegel, 1986, 1989) about the influence of expectation on outcomes have received some support in clinical research of health care problems. Available evidence suggests that psychological well-being is influenced by expectation in health care situations. Little evidence, however, is available linking physical well-being with expectation. Until we have more evidence linking these two factors, nurses cannot advise patients that improving their outlook will improve their physical condition.

Recent evidence, however, does suggest that continued interest in the effect of expectation on physical well-being is warranted (Temoshok, 1985, 1987). Clinical studies are needed to identify physiological factors that are sensitive to changes in psychological state. Recent interest in immune response (Greer, Pettingale, Morris, & Haybittle, 1985; Levy, Herberman, Maluish, Schlien, & Lippman, 1985; Temoshok, 1985) and in beta receptor response to stress (Williams & Lefkowitz, 1984) may have promise for future investigations. Clinical studies are also needed to further delineate how clinical interventions influence expectations and outcomes for patients. Although it is known that teaching people active coping strategies in situations where there is the possibility of active participation is effective, it is not known whether teaching passive strategies in situations where there is little possibility for control is effective. The key to improved health for the population is the ability of nurses and other health care professionals to identify actions and interventions that improve people's health.

REFERENCES

Averill, J.R. (1977). Personal control over aversive stimuli and its relationship to stress. *Psychological Bulletin, 45*, 395–418.

Bandura, A. (1977). Self-efficacy: Toward a unifying theory of behavior change. *Psychology Review, 84*, 191–215.

Bandura, A. (1982). Self-efficacy mechanism in human energy. *American Psychologist, 37*(2), 122–147.

Browne, M.W. (1989, January 16). Research hints at link between patient's attitude and progress of AIDS. *New York Times*, p. A6.

Burger, J.M. (1989). Negative reactions to increases in perceived personal control. *Journal of Personality and Social Psychology, 56*(2), 246–256.

Carver, C.S. (1979). A cybernetic model of self-attention processes. *Journal of Personality and Social Psychology, 37*(8), 1251–1280.

Carver, C.S., & Gaines, J.G. (1987). Optimism, pessimism, and postpartum depression. *Cognitive Therapy and Research, 11*(4), 449–462.

Cassileth, B.R., Lusk, E.J., Miller, D.S., Brown, L.L., & Miller, C. (1985). Psychological correlates of survival in advanced malignant disease. *New England Journal of Medicine, 312*(24), 1551–1555.

Cassileth, B.R., Walsh, W.P., & Lusk, E.J. (1988). Psychosocial correlates of cancer survival: A subsequent report three to eight years after cancer diagnosis. *Journal of Clinical Oncology, 6*(11), 1753–1759.

Cousins, N. (1979). *Anatomy of an illness as perceived by the patients: Reflections of healing and regeneration.* New York & London: W.W. Norton & Company.

Ewart, C.K., Taylor, C.B., Reese, L.B., & DeBusk, R.F. (1983). Effects of early postmyocardial infarction exercise testing on self–perception and subsequent physical activity. *The American Journal of Cardiology, 51*, 1076–1080.

Goodkin, K., Antoni, M.H., & Blaney, P.H. (1986). Stress and hopelessness in the promotion of cervical intraepithelial neoplasia to invasive squamous cell carcinoma of the cervix. *Journal of Psychosomatic Research, 30*(1), 67–76.

Greer, S., Pettingale, K.W., Morris, T., & Haybittle, J. (1985). Mental attitudes to cancer: An additional prognostic factor. *Lancet, 1*, 750.

Johnson, J.E. (1984). Psychological interventions and coping with surgery. In A. Baum, S.E. Taylor, & J.E. Singer (Eds.), *Handbook of health and psychology: Social Psychological aspects of health.* Hillsdale, NJ: Laurence Erlbaum Associates.

Johnson, J.E., Christman, N.J., & Stitt, C. (1985). Personal control interventions: Short-and long-term effects on surgical patients. *Research in Nursing and Health, 8*, 131–145.

Johnson, J.E., Fuller, S.S., Endress, M.P., & Rice, V.H. (1978). Altering patients' response to surgery: An extension and replication. *Research in Nursing and Health, 1*, 111–121.

Johnson, J.E., Morrissey, J.F., & Leventhal, H. (1973). Psychological preparation for an endoscopic examination. *Gastrointestinal Endoscopy, 19,* 180–182.

Johnson, J.E., Rice, V.H., Fuller, S.S., & Endress, M.P. (1978). Sensory information, instruction in a coping strategy, and recovery from surgery. *Research in Nursing and Health, 1,* 4–17.

Kaplan, R.M., & Atkins, C.J. (1984). Specify efficacy expectations mediate exercise compliance in patients with COPD. *Health Psychology, 3*(3), 233–242.

King, K.B., Norsen, L.H., Robertson, R.K., & Hicks, G.L. (1987). Patient management of pain medication after cardiac surgery. *Nursing Research, 36*(3), 145–150.

Langer, E.J., Janis, I.L., & Wolfer, J.A. (1975). Reduction of psychological stress in surgical patients. *Journal of Experimental Social Psychology, 11,* 155–165.

Leventhal, H., & Johnson, J.E. (1983). Laboratory and field experimentation: Development of a theory of self regulation. In P.J. Woolridge, M.H. Schmidt, J.K. Skipper, & R.C. Leonard (Eds.), *Behavioral science and nursing theory.* St. Louis: C.V. Mosby.

Levy, S., Herberman, R., Maluish, A., Schlien, B., & Lippman, M. (1985). Prognostic reassessment in primary breast cancer by behavioral and immunological parameters. *Health Psychology, 4,* 99–113.

Major, B., Mueller, P., & Hildebrandt, K. (1985). Attributions, expectations and coping with abortion. *Journal of Personality and Social Psychology, 48*(30), 585–599.

Marks, G., Richardson, G.L., Graham, J.W., & Levine, A. (1986). Role of health locus of control beliefs and expectations of treatment efficacy in adjustments to cancer. *Journal of Personality and Social Psychology, 51*(2), 443–450.

McHugh, N.G., Christman, N.J., Johnson, J.E. (1982). Preparatory information: What helps and why. *American Journal of Nursing, 82*(5), 780–782.

Mills, R.T., & Krantz, D.S. (1979). Information, choice, and reactions to stress: A field experiment in a blood bank with laboratory analogue. *Journal of Personality and Social Psychology, 37,* 608–620.

O'Leary, A. (1985). Self-efficacy and health. *Behavioral Research and Therapy, 23*(4), 437–451.

Reker, G.T., & Wong, P.T.P. (1985). Personal optimism, physical and mental health. In J.E. Birren & J. Livingston (Eds.), *Cognition, Stress, and Aging.* New Jersey: Prentice-Hall.

Rotter, J.B. (1954). *Social Learning and Clinical Psychology*. Englewood Cliffs, NJ: Prentice-Hall.

Rotter, J.B. (1966). Generalized expectancies for internal versus external control of reinforcement. *Psychological Monographs, 80*(1, No. 609).

Scheier, M.F., & Carver, C.S. (1985). Optimism, coping and health: Assessment and implications of generalized outcome expectancies. *Health Psychology, 4*(3), 219–247.

Scheier, M.F., & Carver, C.S. (1987). Dispositional optimism and physical well-being: The influence of generalized outcome expectancies on health. *Journal of Personality, 55*, 169–210.

Schoor, S.M., & Holman, H.R. (1984). Development of an instrument to explore psychological mediators of outcome in chronic arthritis. *Transactions of the Association of American Physicians, 97*, 325–331.

Siegel, B.S. (1986). *Love, medicine, & miracles: Lessons learned about self-healing from a surgeon's experience with exceptional patients*. New York: Harper & Row.

Siegel, B.S. (1989). How to heal yourself: The curing power of hope, joy and inner peace. *Redbook*, 110–111.

Simonton, O.C. (1978). *Getting well again: A step-by-step, self help guide to overcoming cancer of patients and their families*. New York: St. Martin's Press.

Taylor, S.E., Lichtman, R.R., & Wood, J.V. (1984). Attributions, beliefs about control, and adjustment to breast cancer. *Journal of Personality and Social Psychology, 46*,(1), 489–502.

Temoshok, L. (1985). Biopsychosocial studies on cutaneous malignant melanoma; psychosocial factors associated with prognostic indicators, progression, psychophysiology and tumor-host response. *Social Science and Medicine, 20*, 833–840.

Temoshok, L. (1987). Personality, coping style, emotions, and cancer: Toward an integrative model. *Cancer surveys, 6*(3), 545–567.

Thompson, S.C. (1981). Will it hurt less if I can control it? A complex answer to a simple question. *Psychological Bulletin, 90*(1), 89–101.

Timko, C., & Janoff-Bulman, R. (1985). Attributions, vulnerability and psychological adjustment: The case of breast cancer. *Health Psychology, 4*(6), 521–544.

Weisman, A.D., & Worden, J.W. (1976). The existential plight in cancer: Significance of the first 100 days. *International Journal of Psychiatry and Medicine, 7*, 1–15.

Williams, L.T., & Lefkowitz, R.J. (1984). *Receptor binding studies in adrenergic pharmacology.* New York: Raven Press.

Wilson, J.F. (1981). Behavioral preparation for surgery: Benefit or harm? *Journal of Behavioral Medicine, 4,* 79–102.

16

An Interactive Model for Finding Meaning through Caregiving

Carol J. Farran and Eleanora Keane-Hagerty

INTRODUCTION

In order to advance scientific knowledge, professionals are being challenged to combine the critical elements of theory, research, and clinical practice (Chinn & Jacobs, 1987). The relationships among theory, research, and clinical practice are reciprocal, but complex. Simply stated, theory serves to guide research, while at the same time research adds to the body of theoretical knowledge. Both theory and research guide effective clinical practice, but it is often in the clinical practice arena that the most interesting and critical research questions and empirical observations emerge.

In recent years, increased research has been conducted with family caregivers of the elderly. Many of these studies have used theoretical frameworks of stress and coping, family systems, and crisis intervention (Boss, 1988; Brubaker, 1987; McCubbin & Thompson, 1987). To date, no theoretical frameworks exclusively devoted to family caregiving have emerged. Research concerning family caregivers of the elderly has tended

This project was funded by the National Institute of Mental Health, Geriatric Mental Health Academic Award, 1 K07 MH 00612; Alzheimer's Disease and Related Disorder's Association, Inc., PRG 86-199, PRG 87-153, and IIRG 88-004; and Rush University College of Nursing, Research Resource Fund.

to describe this experience in negative terms—as stressful or burdensome (George & Gwyther, 1986; Poulshock & Deimling, 1984; Zarit, Orr, & Zarit, 1985). However, educational support interventions with family caregivers of persons with dementia, suggest that caregivers work hard to make sense of, or find meaning in, these difficult experiences (Farran & Keane-Hagerty, 1986; Keane-Hagerty, Farran, & Salloway, 1990).

These more subtle clinical nuances prompted researchers to design open-ended qualitative questions that comprehensively tapped the caregiving phenomena (Keane-Hagerty & Farran, 1986). When these qualitative data from 94 caregivers of persons with dementia were evaluated within the usual theoretical frameworks of stress and coping, family systems, and crisis intervention, a "theoretical vacuum" was apparent (Farran, Keane-Hagerty, Salloway, Kupferer, & Wilken, 1990). That is, the data went beyond the more familiar theoretical perspectives. In an effort to further understand these data, the loss and grief literature was examined. These theoretical formulations, however, focused on specific responses of persons to the grief experience observed when a loved one dies; they did not describe how persons make sense or find meaning through difficult experiences which may extend for years (Farran, Monbrod-Framburg, & Russell, in press). The existential literature provided a more comprehensive understanding of how persons may find meaning through suffering or difficult experiences.

It is out of these subtle clinical observations, research data, and existential theoretical formulations, that an Interactive Model for Finding Meaning through Caregiving (IMFMC) is being proposed. The major goal of this model is to explain how caregivers of persons with dementia find meaning through the experience of caregiving. In so doing, it is assumed that four major components or concepts are vital to the potential outcome of finding meaning through caregiving: (1) critical antecedents to caregiving, (2) stages of caregiving, (3) responses to caregiving and, (4) phases of suffering. Interactive relationships exist within and amongst each of these major components of the model, as shown in Figure 16-1. The structure of the model rests on the assumption that the first component, critical antecedents to caregiving, is in place before family members begin providing care for a family member. It is also assumed that the first component of the model shapes the other three components, as well as the potential caregiving outcome. The four major components are each experienced in a simultaneous and reciprocal manner, and they work interactively to shape the potential caregiving outcome.

It is hypothesized that the development of the IMFMC will assist in: (1) clarifying our understanding of how persons may find meaning through caring for others, and (2) specifying recommendations for future model testing. The following paragraphs define essential terms related to

Figure 16-1
An Interactive Model for Finding Meaning Through Caregiving

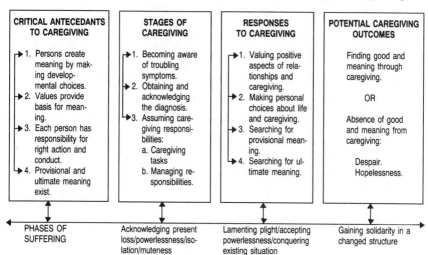

CRITICAL ANTECEDANTS TO CAREGIVING	STAGES OF CAREGIVING	RESPONSES TO CAREGIVING	POTENTIAL CAREGIVING OUTCOMES
1. Persons create meaning by making developmental choices. 2. Values provide basis for meaning. 3. Each person has responsibility for right action and conduct. 4. Provisional and ultimate meaning exist.	1. Becoming aware of troubling symptoms. 2. Obtaining and acknowledging the diagnosis. 3. Assuming caregiving responsibilities: a. Caregiving tasks b. Managing responsibilities.	1. Valuing positive aspects of relationships and caregiving. 2. Making personal choices about life and caregiving. 3. Searching for provisional meaning. 4. Searching for ultimate meaning.	Finding good and meaning through caregiving. OR Absence of good and meaning from caregiving: Despair. Hopelessness.
PHASES OF SUFFERING	Acknowledging present loss/powerlessness/isolation/muteness	Lamenting plight/accepting powerlessness/conquering existing situation	Gaining solidarity in a changed structure

this model, discuss relevant assumptions, and specify relationships and structures which exist amongst the model's major components.

Definition of Terms

Caregiving. The process of caring for the physical, psychosocial, environmental, and/or spiritual needs of another person who cannot independently meet these needs because of functional disability.

Caregiver. The person, usually a family member, who provides care to the impaired person.

Care-receiver. The impaired person who requires physical, psychosocial, environmental, and/or spiritual care from another person because functional disability prevents him or her from meeting these needs.

Existentialism. A theoretical perspective which has roots in philosophy, theology, literature, and psychology and which generally addresses individuals' uniqueness and isolation in a hostile or indifferent universe. Common themes include freedom of choice, responsibility, consequences of actions, and meaning (Nauman, 1971; Yalom, 1980).

Suffering. A sense of powerlessness or inability to change one's external circumstances. It involves afflictions in four areas: physical, psychosocial, environmental, and spiritual. Afflictions at one or two levels are easier to overcome and forget, whereas afflictions in all four areas constitute suffering in its truest sense (Frankl, 1978; Missine, 1984; Soelle, 1975).

General Assumptions Underlying the Model

The general assumptions underlying this model evolve primarily out of the framework of existentialism:

1. Finding meaning is an option for persons who provide care to others.
2. Finding meaning is phenomenologically based. Events cannot be considered outside of their context; they are unique and ever-changing (Nauman, 1971; Yalom, 1980).
3. Finding meaning is individually determined. Persons can be assisted in the process of finding meaning through caregiving, but each person has responsibility for developing his or her own unique perspective.
4. Finding meaning through caregiving is not a quick or easy process but involves a combination of time, effort, and chance.
5. Finding meaning does not answer the question of why, but rather, answers the question of what can I make out of this situation (Missine, 1984).
6. The potential outcome of finding meaning through caregiving involves an interactive and ongoing process amongst the components of this model: critical antecedents, stages of caregiving, responses to caregiving, and phases of suffering.

OVERVIEW OF THE MODEL

Critical Antecedents to Caregiving

Critical antecedents comprise one of the four major components of the model and include those characteristics that must be present before the family assumes caregiving responsibilities. These critical antecedents are derived primarily from existential literature and are empirically supported by qualitative data from caregivers (Farran et al., 1990). Four specific, interactive assumptions about critical antecedents are drawn from Frankl's work (1963, 1967, 1978) which evolved out of his concentration camp experiences: (1) persons create meaning by making choices; (2) values provide basis for meaning; (3) each person has responsibility for right action and conduct; and (4) there are two levels of meaning—provisional and ultimate.

1. *Persons create meaning by making choices.* Throughout their lives, caregivers have been confronted with various developmental choices. These choices have been made as a result of their pre-existing values, goals, and internal and external circumstances. Ironically, when it comes

to caregiving, persons often perceive that they do not have a choice as to whether or not they will become caregivers. In reality, choosing the caregiving role is influenced by both societal conditioning (especially for women) and by unconscious psychodynamic forces (Levine et al., 1984; Sommers & Shields, 1987). Levine et al. (1984) suggest that caregivers are confronted with the conflict between existential freedom and existential guilt. On the one hand, caregivers have the freedom to make a conscious choice about caregiving. If caregivers can confront the idea that they have choices and even entertain the possibility of *not* becoming a caregiver, then the fact that they have considered this as a plausible option opens up a whole new range of choices which the caregiver has never heretofore considered. One of the problems, however, is that caregivers are often constricted in their thinking and feel guilty even considering *not* caregiving as an option. Therefore, this "terrifying new series of choices" may reflect "a fear of unwelcome possibility," resulting in caregivers making the choice to provide care out of fear as opposed to "true choice" (Levine et al., 1984, p. 220).

2. *Values provide basis for meaning.* Frankl suggests that values fall into three categories: creative, experiential, and life belief or attitudinal (1963). Values can be expressed through creative means such as jobs or hobbies; they can be experientially based in attitudes and feelings persons have toward others; or they can be based upon one's life or attitudinal beliefs. Each of these values can be expressed through the experience of caring for others. Caregivers use their creative expression when they devise novel ways to care for their impaired family members. Caregivers act upon their experiential values through enjoyment of their impaired family members. One family member said, "We still enjoy our little tickling games." Finally, caregivers express their attitudinal values in reports about making conscious choices in interpreting their caregiving experiences (Farran et al., 1990).

3. *Each person has responsibility for right action and conduct.* From his concentration camp experiences, Frankl suggests "that life ultimately means taking responsibility to find the right answer to its problems and to fulfill the tasks which it constantly sets for each individual" (1963, p. 122). This assumption holds both responsibility and choice in tandem. Caregivers have the responsibility to make choices as to whether or not they will provide care, as well as the responsibility for choosing how they will carry out their caregiving tasks.

4. *There are two levels of meaning—provisional and ultimate.* Frankl (1963) and others (Missine, 1984) suggest that provisional meaning refers to more short-term or transitory experiences which assist persons to find meaning, while ultimate meaning refers to deeper life experiences often associated with one's spiritual nature, beliefs, or practices. Caregivers find provi-

sional meaning from such things as their relationship with their impaired family members, or their personal satisfaction with the care they provide. They find ultimate meaning through their spiritual/religious beliefs and rituals such as knowing they have a Higher Power, or relying on such rituals as prayer, meditation, and/or spiritually oriented written materials (Farran et al., 1990).

Stages of Caregiving

The second major component of the model evolves primarily out of clinical experiences and qualitative data from caregivers of persons with dementia. It describes three different stages or crisis points that caregivers experience in the process of becoming caregivers (Chenowith & Spencer, 1986; Farran et al., 1990; Levine et al., 1984; Mace & Rabins, 1981; Missine & Willeke-Kay, 1985): (1) becoming aware of troubling symptoms, (2) obtaining and acknowledging the diagnosis, and (3) assuming caregiving responsibilities.

1. *Becoming aware of troubling symptoms.* Kuhn (1990) identifies the first stage or crisis point in the process of providing care for persons with dementia as the occurrence of "troubling symptoms." Symptoms of dementia develop insidiously and care-receivers' responses to the disease and their environment may be inconsistent. Because of these vague changes, family members often begin to subtly compensate for some of the impaired family member's deficits. Often, it may take several years before a family clearly identifies that "something is wrong."

2. *Obtaining and acknowledging the diagnosis.* This generally constitutes the second stage or crisis of caregiving (Kuhn, 1990). During the period of "troubling symptoms," family members may be told by physicians that the impaired person is just "getting old" or is "senile." Even when dementia is diagnosed, it is a differential diagnosis. The lack of diagnosis certainty and fluctuation of the patient's symptoms leave room for a protracted time of denial, in what eventually becomes an extended mourning process (Levine et al., 1984; Russell, 1988).

3. *Assuming caregiving responsibilities.* This third stage of caregiving often begins gradually with a progressive, deteriorating disease, such as dementia. Early caregiving tasks may include gentle reminders and careful structuring of the environment so as to maintain the impaired family member's functioning. As the impaired relative continues to deteriorate, caregiving tasks become more complex and time-consuming. In addition to implementing the more immediate caregiving tasks, such as instrumental and personal activities of daily living, caregivers report that caregiving responsibilities also incorporate management types of responsibilities (Farran et al., 1990). Management responsibilities include such things

as being accountable for the care, whether provided by the caregiver or someone else, planning for and obtaining supplies and equipment necessary for providing care, and anticipating future concerns such as institutionalization.

Responses to Caregiving

The third major component of this model is defined as those responses that caregivers make to their caregiving experience. These responses include the following: (1) valuing positive aspects of relationships and caregiving, (2) making personal choices about life and caregiving, (3) searching for provisional meaning, and (4) searching for ultimate meaning (Farran et al., 1990). Assumptions specifically related to this major component of the model suggest that each caregiver's response to the caregiving experience is individually determined and may change over the course of caregiving.

1. *Valuing positive aspects of relationships and caregiving.* Caregivers reported that family and social relationships were vital to their continuing to provide care, as were their feelings of love toward and companionship with the care-receiver and their ability to see positive aspects of the current caregiver—care-receiver relationship. Another positive aspect of caregiving was their own sense of, and the care-receivers' satisfaction with, the type of care they were providing, as well as their ability to recall and cherish past positive life experiences. It is hypothesized that relationships with others and individual perceptions may provide caregivers with a sense of provisional or more immediate meaning in their caregiving experiences (Frankl, 1963).

2. *Making personal choices about life and caregiving.* This category of responses focused on caregivers' personal choices about life and caregiving which reportedly assisted them in dealing with the caregiving experience. Caregivers discussed the process of using personal and/or situational fortitude, using a sense of humor and paradox in defining their situation, maintaining a future orientation, making a conscious choice about how to look at caregiving, seeing others as worse off, and taking one day at a time (Lazarus & Folkman, 1984).

3. *Searching for provisional meaning.* Caregivers made some direct comments about finding purpose and meaning through their experiences. Some reported that they were providing care for a greater good, and that they found meaning and personal growth through this experience. As one caregiver said, "There's some reason I'm doing this, something good will come out of it."

4. *Searching for ultimate meaning.* Numerous caregivers reported that they called upon an external philosophy to help them through this caregiving experience. Most responses centered on the reassuring presence of

spiritual or religious structure, while a few responses focused on the reassuring presence of nature (Farran et al., 1990). Existential formulations support these findings and suggest that events and/or cosmic sources facilitate the process of finding meaning in life (Frankl, 1963, 1967, 1978; Missinne & Willeke-Kay, 1985; Yalom, 1980).

Specific responses to caregiving do not occur in lock-step fashion, but rather they are elicited by the changing demands of caregiving. They are also shaped by caregivers' values, choices, and conduct, as well as by the stages of caregiving and phases of suffering experienced by the caregiver.

Phases of Suffering

The fourth major component of the model, as noted at the bottom of Figure 16-1, hypothesizes that caregivers encounter three phases of suffering throughout the process of caregiving: (1) acknowledging present loss/powerlessness/isolation/muteness; (2) lamenting/accepting powerlessness/conquering existing situation; and (3) gaining solidarity in a changed structure. It is hypothesized that the concept of burden, commonly associated with caregiving (George & Gwyther, 1986; Poulshock & Deimling, 1984; Zarit, Orr, & Zarit 1985), may have some relationship to these phases of suffering. However, the concept of suffering is preferentially selected because of its broader theoretical base which suggests that in spite of difficult experiences, persons can find meaning.

This component of the model rests on the assumption that persons have experienced aspects of suffering in the general course of living, prior to assuming the caregiving role. Indeed, their previous suffering may have already shaped the first component, critical antecedents to caregiving. The onset of dementia in a relative, however, sets off an almost continual process of suffering as the disease progresses, and caregivers begin working through the stages of caregiving and their responses to caregiving. Caregivers do not move through the phases of suffering in a sequential progression, but rather, may re-experience and respond to suffering at each stage of caregiving. Suffering, like finding meaning, is an individual experience. Similar events, in this case caregiving, have different meanings for different people; it is up to each caregiver to create meaning through his or her own suffering.

Soelle (1973), a German theologian, suggests that there are three interactive phases of suffering: (1) acknowledging present loss/powerlessness/isolation/muteness; (2) lamenting plight/accepting powerlessness/conquering existing situation; and (3) gaining solidarity in a changed structure.

1. *Acknowledging present loss/powerlessness/isolation/muteness.* Initially the individual experiences pain or loss at physical, psychological, en-

vironmental, and spiritual levels. This pain often results in feelings of powerlessness, isolation, and muteness. Caregivers validated this pain when they expressed their feelings of grief for both themselves and their family members. They mourned the loss of their intimate relationship with the care-receivers and the loss of the care-receivers' physical capabilities and ability to communicate. Caregivers' powerlessness was also apparent. Some described their caregiving situation as being constricted, hopeless, and/or endless; a number of them expressed that there was nothing pleasant about caregiving (Farran et al., 1990).

Soelle (1973) suggests that initially persons may be mute and unable to express their feelings of suffering. If they remain mute, their suffering may move into a deep sense of despair. Persons helped to "lament" their suffering are more likely to accept their powerlessness and move into the second phase of suffering.

2. *Lamenting plight/accepting powerlessness/conquering existing situation.* In this second phase, caregivers lament their plight and begin to accept and conquer their existing situation. Lamenting their plight may take many different forms. The positive response of caregivers to the interview process has been interpreted as an opportunity which allows caregivers to lament (Farran et al., 1990). Lamenting may also occur as caregivers express their feelings to friends and other family members or to persons in similar circumstances such as support group members. Caregivers often report that their ability to eventually accept or conquer their powerlessness is embodied in expressions such as the Alcoholic Anonymous' Serenity Prayer:

> God grant me the serenity to accept the things I cannot change, courage to change things I can, and wisdom to know the difference (1976).

3. *Gaining solidarity in a changed structure.* This third phase of suffering involves a process of changing, and gaining a sense of solidarity with oneself and one's situation, within a changed structure. That is, the caregivers' situations may not have changed, but they begin to experience and respond to their situations in new ways (Soelle, 1973). They have assumed responsibility for making active choices, and as a result of their values and choices, they begin to find both provisional and ultimate meaning in their caregiving experiences.

Potential Outcomes

The potential outcomes of this model evolve out of a culmination of the four components: critical antecedents to caregiving, stages of caregiving, responses to caregiving, and phases of suffering. Potential outcomes include finding or not finding good and meaning through caregiving. The assumptions that support the model as a whole are key to determining whether persons will find meaning through caregiving. That is—caregivers must perceive that finding meaning is a contextual option; that meaning is individually determined; that it is not quick or easy; that it focuses on answering the question of "what can I make out of this situation"; and that finding meaning can occur at a number of levels and through a variety of experiences. What must be underscored is that finding meaning through caregiving is an individual process, and as such, will be different for each caregiver and in each caregiving situation.

It is assumed, however, that when persons do not find good or meaning through caregiving, both they and the care-receivers will suffer. For the caregiver, it may mean a pervading sense of despair or hopelessness, suggesting not only a compromise in emotional health but also in physical health (Frankl, 1978). For the care-receiver, anecdotal clinical observations suggest that when the caregiver is more emotionally distressed, the care-receiver tends to exhibit more disruptive behaviors. It is assumed that when meaning is not found through caregiving, premature or inappropriate institutionalization or care-receiver abuse may result (Phillips & Rempusheski, 1986). This is not to say, however, that institutionalization is automatically associated with the inability of the caregiver to find meaning through caregiving, as appropriate institutionalization may also contribute to the experience of finding meaning through caregiving.

RECOMMENDATIONS FOR FUTURE MODEL TESTING

As previously noted, this IMFMC was derived from theoretical literature which articulates how persons find meaning through suffering, from qualitative data reported by caregivers of persons with dementia, from clinical literature which reports various aspects of the caregiving process, and from clinical experiences with caregivers. Several approaches may be taken for testing the proposed IMFMC. One approach would triangulate or combine these qualitative data with other quantitative data so that the following questions could be addressed:

1. What association do such variables as gender, caregiver relationships (spouse versus child), and socioeconomic status have with each of the major components of the model?

2. What relationship does the stage of caregiving have upon caregivers' responses to caregiving, phase of suffering, and potential outcome?

3. Are phases of suffering associated with physiological and psychological health outcomes?

4. Do caregivers who report finding good and meaning have differing physiological and psychological health outcomes from caregivers who report an absence of good and meaning?

5. Do different caregiving situations (adult versus child, acute disease versus chronic disability) affect caregiver's ability to find meaning through caregiving.

A second approach for testing the IMFMC would be to use quantitative instruments which measure the major components of the proposed model, such as the critical antecedents to caregiving, stages of caregiving, responses to caregiving, phases of suffering, and finding meaning (Reker, Peacock, & Wong, 1987). An inherent difficulty with using this approach to model testing would rest on the ability to find or develop research instruments that measure obscure concepts such as choices, values, responsibility, right action and conduct, and provisional and ultimate meaning. Whether qualitative or quantitative approaches are taken, future research of caregivers should focus on the potential for finding meaning through caregiving as an important aspect of the total caregiving experience.

REFERENCES

Alcoholic Anonymous. (1976). (3rd ed.). New York, Alcoholics Anonymous World Services, Inc.

Boss, P. (1988). *Family stress management.* Newbury Park, CA: Sage Publications.

Brubaker, T. (1987). *Aging, health, and family: Long term care.* Newbury Park, CA: Sage Publications.

Chenowith, B., & Spencer, B. (1986). The experience of family caregivers. *The Gerontologist, 26*(3), 267–272.

Chinn, P.L., & Jacobs, M.K. (1987). *Theory and nursing: A systematic approach.* St. Louis: C.V. Mosby.

Farran, C.J., & Keane-Hagerty, E. (1986). *A study of caregivers of persons with dementia.* Unpublished manuscript, Rush University College of Nursing, Chicago.

Farran, C.J., Keane-Hagerty, E., Salloway, S., Kupferer, S., & Wilken, C. (1990). *A qualitative study of caregivers of persons with dementia: Finding meaning through caregiving.* Proceedings of the 1990 Gerontological Society of America (Abstract), Boston, MA.

Farran, C.J., Monbrod-Framburg, G., & Russell, C. (In press). *Loss, mourning and suffering: Caregivers' daily fare.* N. Hollywood CA: Charles Press.

Frankl, V.E. (1963). *Man's search for meaning.* New York: Washington Square Press.

Frankl, V.E. (1967). *Psychotherapy and existentialism.* New York: Washington Square Press.

Frankl, V.E. (1978). *The unheard cry for meaning.* New York: Washington Square Press.

George, L.K., & Gwyther, L.P. (1986). Caregiver well-being: A multidimensional examination of family caregivers of demented adults. *The Gerontologist, 26*(3), 253–259.

Keane-Hagerty, E., & Farran, C.J. (1986). *Caregiver questionnaire.* Unpublished manuscript, Rush University College of Nursing, Chicago.

Keane-Hagerty, E., Farran, C.J., & Salloway, S. (1990). *Dementia educational support group manual.* Chicago: Rush Alzheimer's Disease Center.

Kuhn, D. (1990). The normative crises of families confronting dementia, *Families in Society, 71*(10), 451–460.

Lazarus, R.S., & Folkman, S. (1984). *Stress, appraisal, and coping.* New York: Springer Publishing Co.

Levine, N.B., Gendron, C.E., Dastoor, D.P., Poitras, L.R., Sirota, S.E., Barza, S.L., & Davis, J.C. (1984). Existential issues in the management of the demented elderly patient. *American Journal of Psychotherapy, 38*(2), 215–223.

Mace, N.L., & Rabins, P.V. (1981). *The 36-hour day.* Baltimore: Johns Hopkins University Press.

McCubbin, H.I., & Thompson, A.I. (1987). *Family assessment inventories for research and practice.* Madison, WI: University of Wisconsin-Madison.

Missinne, L.E. (1984, March). Reflections on the meaning of suffering. *The Priest,* 11–13.

Missinne, L.E., & Willeke-Kay, J. (1985). Reflections on the meaning of life in older age. *Journal of Religion and Aging, 1*(4), 43–58.

Nauman, St. E. (1971). *The new dictionary of existentialism.* New York: Philosophical Library.

Phillips, L.R., & Rempusheski, V.F. (1986). Caring for the frail elderly at home: Toward a theoretical explanation of the dynamics of poor quality family caregiving. *Advances in Nursing Science, 8*(4), 62–76.

Poulshock, S.W., & Deimling, G.T. (1984). Families caring for elders in residence: Issues in the measurement of burden. *Journal of Gerontology, 39*(2), 230–239.

Reker, G.T., Peacock, E.J., & Wong, P.T.P. (1987). Meaning and purpose in life and well-being: A life-span perspective. *Journal of Gerontology, 42*(1), 44–49.

Russell, C. (1988). *Loss, grief and depression: An analysis of caregivers of persons with dementia.* Unpublished manuscript, Rush University College of Nursing, Chicago.

Soelle, D. (1975). *Suffering.* (E.R. Kalin, Trans.). Philadelphia: Fortress Press. (Original work published 1973).

Sommers, T., & Shields, L. (1987). *Women take care: Consequences of caregiving in today's society.* Gainesville: Triad Publishing Company.

Yalom, I.D. (1980). *Existential psychotherapy.* New York: Basic Books.

Zarit, S.H., Orr, N.K., & Zarit, J.M. (1985). *The hidden victims of Alzheimer's disease.* New York: New York University Press.

17

Cesareans and Care

Lynn McCreery Schimmel

In response to the threefold increase in cesarean delivery during the 1970s, from 5.5% to 15.2% by 1978, a National Institutes of Health (NIH) Consensus Development Conference was held in 1980. The report issued (NIH, 1981) recommended the use of specific management practices (such as vaginal birth after a previous cesarean and vaginal delivery of the term breech infant under certain circumstances) to help reverse the increase. Among other findings was the recommendation for future research to focus on the effects of medical training and economic, legal, and ethical concerns upon the method of delivery, as these were still unexamined variables potentially associated with the problem.

Despite the findings of the Consensus Development Conference, cesarean birth rates have continued to climb not only in the United States, but in other countries as well. The rate of cesarean births in the United States had risen to 24% by 1986 (Placek, Taffel, & Moien, 1988). In 1978, 510,000 women had cesareans (Placek & Taffel, 1983); in 1987, the number

This work, done while the author was a student at University of California, San Francisco (UCSF), was supported in part by a March of Dimes grant for integrating ethics into clinical nurse specialist study at the UCSF Perinatal Clinical Nurse Specialist Program. The author thanks Dyanne Affonso, Patricia Benner, and Jeanne DeJoseph for being models of caring and its articulation.

239

rose to 959,000 (National Center for Health Statistics, 1989). Anderson and Lomas (1985) have expressed concern about Canada's rapidly increasing surgical birth rate, as have Notzon, Placek, and Taffel for countries world-wide (1987). Wide variations have been noted in the procedure's incidence; for example, a rate of less than 5% was reported during 1984 in Dublin's National Maternity Hospital (O'Driscoll, Foley, MacDonald, & Stronge, 1988), while the rate for Blue Shield subscribers in California during 1985 was 41% (R.W. Schaffarzick, MD, personal communication, August, 4, 1986). Clearly, there has been a "short-term failure" of the 1980 Consensus Conference (Gleicher, 1984, p. 3273); two years later, Gleicher (1986, p. 563) termed the problem an "epidemic."

The overall justification for the continued rise in the cesarean birth rate has been a presumed causal relationship between declining perinatal morbidity and mortality rates and the incidence of cesarean birth (Bottoms, Rosen, & Sokol, 1980). Although this inverse relationship has been disputed (Haynes de Regt, Minkoff, Feldman, & Schwarz, 1986; Myers & Gleicher, 1988; O'Driscoll & Foley, 1983; Porreco, 1985), and the significant economic, physical, and emotional costs of cesarean birth have been published, the problem persists.

ECONOMIC COSTS

For economic reasons alone, it is important that each cesarean be a necessary procedure. Gleicher (1984) calculated that each 1% increase in the cesarean rate amounted to an additional cost of $63 million to the U.S. health industry. Using a decision analysis model, Shy, LoGerfo, and Karp computed that $5 million per 10,000 women would be saved if appropriate trials of labor were offered to women instead of routine repeat cesareans (1981). It is noteworthy that in 1988, Placek et al. found, as they had in 1983, that the expected source of payment was closely related to cesarean rates, with Blue Cross and other private insurance clients, as well as proprietary hospitals, having the highest rates. In 1988, the California Health Policy and Data Advisory Commission reported that if the ratio of actual to observed admissions for cesareans were reduced only to the state's average ("expected") rate of 24.6%, a savings of $5 million per year would be realized.

PHYSICAL COSTS

The mortality rate for the mother who has a cesarean is two to five times greater than for one who has a vaginal delivery (Danforth, 1985; NIH, 1981;

Petitti, Cefalo, Shapiro, & Whalley, 1982); the NIH report also stresses that maternal mortality rates are under-reported. If the 1981 statistics from the Centers for Disease Control (Rubin, Peterson, Rochat, McCarthy, & Terry) are extrapolated to present numbers of cesareans and corrected for confounding associated conditions, then over 500 mothers die as a direct result of this mode of birth annually. If one-half to two-thirds of the cesarean procedures are unnecessary, as claimed by those who advocate safer alternatives to abdominal delivery when possible (Bottoms, Hirsch, & Sokol, 1987; Myers & Gleicher, 1988; O'Driscoll & Meagher, 1986; Phelan, Clark, Diaz, & Paul, 1987; Pettiti, 1989), many women die unnecessarily each year. Increased infection rates constitute the greatest part of maternal morbidity (NIH, 1981), although long-term complications may include bowel obstruction from adhesions and placenta accreta in future pregnancies (Bowes, 1989). Problems of cesarean-related infant morbidity and mortality include iatrogenic prematurity and transient or severe respiratory distress (Danforth, 1985; NIH, 1981). There are also reported incidents of fetal morbidity and mortality from scalpel accidents (Bowes, 1989).

EMOTIONAL COSTS

Emotional reactions to cesarean birth include distorted body and time perceptions, feelings of being unable to breathe, fear of dying, and a sense of powerlessness (Affonso & Stichler, 1978); insults to self-esteem and body image (Marut & Mercer, 1981); depression (Hobfoll & Leiberman, 1987); difficulties coping physically, anger, long-term grief, and repression of some of the experience's negative aspects (Lipson & Tilden, 1980); fears in the postpartum period regarding ability to recover physically (Arizmendi & Affonso, 1987); feelings of indifference toward and of being in too much pain to enjoy the baby (Garel, Lelong, & Kaminski, 1987); and an excess of psychosomatic symptoms during the first year postpartum (Garel, Lelong, & Kaminski, 1988).

In contrast, Sargent and Stark conclude that their findings "clearly reflect an acceptance of the medicalization of birth and expectation for technological intervention at delivery" (1987, p. 1275). A phenomenologic view of their data, however, challenges this conclusion: 33% of the women interviewed felt negatively, offering such statements as "I just wanted a vaginal delivery," "I'll never know what it feels like for her body to come through," and "like breastfeeding, you just can't replace it." Although Sargent and Stark report 67% of the women were "neutral" regarding their method of giving birth, they note that 41% felt that some significant aspect of the experience was "missing" (see also Affonso, 1977), that 49% felt feeding their infants was more difficult, and that, according to the women,

55% of their husbands were dissatisfied with the course of events. Since the cesarean rate at the hospital where they interviewed clients was reported to be 30%, and since 80% of the vaginal births there involved epidural anaesthesia, it is proposed that "an expectation for technological intervention" on the part of the women was not inappropriate. However, the authors demonstrated an unawareness of the psychological phenomena of "la belle indifférence" (whereby symptoms experienced are diminished in significance), at best, and identification with the aggressor, at worst. The question remains: if a percentage of these cesareans could have been safely avoided by alternative management strategies, does the relative safety of the procedure and the ability of humans to adapt to, and rationalize, distressing events outweigh the significance of the real physiological and psychological pain reported by many women? Efforts to justify the use of excessive surgical intervention constitute an example of Lazarus' concept of the "trivialization of distress"—the societal and professional tendency to downplay the negative and accentuate the positive, thus "undermining [the] legitimacy and challenging the reality of the circumstances that generate" the distress (1986, p. 36).

RATE VARIATIONS: MORE QUESTIONS THAN ANSWERS

Several authors, in response to the NIH task force recommendations and their own concerns, have either assessed the observed variations in rates of cesarean birth or attempted to lower their own rates in accordance with the NIH recommendations. The resulting publications have an underlying assumption that cesarean rates in the United States are excessive, and that there is variance unaccounted for in the observed rates.

There is agreement in the literature concerning the major variables that account for 90% of the cesareans performed: repeat cesareans, dystocia, fetal distress, and malpresentation (NIH, 1981). Women with increased maternal age (over 34), who are nulliparous (no previous birth), and/or are delivering a low or high birthweight infant are more likely to undergo a cesarean birth (Bottoms, Rosen, & Sokol, 1980; Taffel, Placek, & Liss, 1987; U.S. Bureau of the Census, 1989; Williams & Chen, 1983). These variables are generally normally distributed throughout populations with the exception of repeat cesareans, which are markedly increased when a provider's primary cesarean rate is high and vaginal birth after cesarean (VBAC) is not practiced.

National Variations

The only attempt at a comprehensive look at national cesarean rates comes from the National Center for Health Statistics. Notzon, Placek, and Taffel have contributed to the recording of the persistence of the cesarean rate problem over the last two decades (Placek & Taffel, 1980; Taffel & Placek, 1983; Taffel, Placek, & Liss, 1987; Placek, Taffel, & Moien, 1988). The 1987 study was done to "improve our understanding of this rapid and apparently widespread transformation in obstetrical practice," (Notzon, Placek, & Taffel, p. 386), and because previous comparative studies have been limited to very few countries.

Notzon, Placek, & Taffel obtained a convenience sample of births between 1980 and 1983 by creating a questionnaire that addressed trends, rates of various characteristics, and limitations of the data collected and sending it to government statistical offices and university researchers in 25 countries of Europe, North America, and the Pacific. Nineteen countries responded.

The United States cesarean rate, the highest rate of all, was 50–200% higher than that of all the other countries except Australia and Canada. Notzon et al. confirmed that highest rates of cesareans are found among first births and women over 35, but noted that the U.S. rates were sharply higher for women of younger ages. They also found that the largest difference between countries concerned the practice of VBACs—5% in the U.S. compared to 43% in Norway. A high U.S. rate for six other surgical procedures has been previously noted, in comparison to Norway and England (McPherson, Wennberg, Hovind, & Clifford, 1982). It is of interest, for reasons that will be addressed below, that the highest rate variation of all the procedures McPherson et al. studied was for the only female-specific one, hysterectomy.

Notzon et al. commented that, although data were given for cesarean rates per 100 hospital deliveries, if the Netherlands' rate had been calculated on the basis of all deliveries (since one–third of births there occur at home) five rather than nine per 100 births were surgical. Relevant information omitted, however, is that over 40% of Netherlands births are by midwives (Treffers, 1989). The NIH report (1981) states that there is an observed correlation between increasing cesarean rates and increasing use of obstetricians over other providers for birthing. Rates in the Netherlands have been thought difficult to duplicate because of the relatively homogeneous, economically well-off population, yet the correlate middle to upper class white population in the United States has the highest observed rates (Williams & Chen, 1983).

Because of the Netherlands' traditionally heavy reliance upon midwives, it is worth considering some U.S. data regarding cesarean birth rates in certified nurse midwives' practices. In one of the few studies employing a quasi-experimental design, investigators found a significant cesarean rate difference ($p < .001$) when comparing a stratified random sample of 800 women delivering at a nurse-midwifery birthing center, where the cesarean rate was 7.3%, to a frequency matched sample of the same size at a tertiary teaching hospital, where the rate was 19.3% (Strombino, Baruffi, Dellinger, & Ross, 1988). Similarly, a retrospective analysis of a rural certified nurse midwife (CNM) practice, co-managed by physicians in case complications arose, had a rate of 9.9% of 730 births (Wingeier, Bloch, & Kvale, 1988). The 1989 National Birth Center Study investigators (Rooks et al.), analyzing the outcomes of 11,815 low-risk women delivering at 84 free-standing birth centers in the United States, found a total cesarean birth rate of 4.4% and a primary rate of 9.9%. The cesarean rate of less than 5% at Dublin's National Maternity Hospital is also at a site where "the delivery suite is in the hands of a senior midwife," and each mother has one-on-one care (Garcia, Corry, MacDonald, Elbourne, & Grant, 1985, p. 80).

Socioeconomic Variations

Cesarean birth rates have also been correlated with socioeconomic status. Gould, Davey, and Stafford (1989), studying a cohort of 245,854 singleton infants, >500 g, born in Los Angeles County in 1982 and 1983, found a consistent and statistically significant relationship between socioeconomic status and use of surgical delivery even when controlling for age and parity of mothers. The cesarean rate was 76% higher in the group with median family incomes over $30,000 than in the group with median family incomes under $11,000. In all four birth weight categories assessed, increasing income was associated with increased birth-weight-specific cesarean rates ($p < .003$).

The Gould et al. findings are supported by a 1986 study in which investigators found lower cesarean rates in clinic patients when 65,647 women receiving clinic or private care were evaluated (Haynes de Regt, Minkoff, Feldman, & Schwarz). Their retrospective analysis attributed these rate variations to management differences. Among women with a single complication giving birth to their first child, private patients were 2.48 times more likely ($p < .001$) to have a cesarean birth than clinic patients, yet significantly more infants of private patients were found to have low Apgar scores and birth injuries ($p < .001$) than infants of clinic patients. In Porreco's 1985 study, management criteria changes in a clinic resulted in a clinic cesarean rate of 5.7%, while the corresponding private service's rate during the two years of the study was 17.6%. Perinatal mortality rates and low five-minute Apgar scores were not significantly different, despite stringent changes in management of cephalopelvic disproportion (CPD), breech presentation, fetal distress, and previous cesareans. Porreco concluded that cesarean rates in excess of 10% are unnecessarily high. Higher cesarean rates for private clients than clinic clients also persisted without apparent justification in a later study in which he and colleagues confined their investigation to women presenting at full term with singleton fetuses in vertex position (Neuhoff, Burke, & Porreco, 1989). These publications also provide support for the next variable under consideration.

Practice Style Variations

Goyert, Bottoms, Treadwell, & Nehra (1989) concluded that something other than birth weight, maternal age, socioeconomic level, degree of obstetrical risk, or recent medical-legal experience determined a woman's chance for a cesarean. They cited Haynes de Regt, Minkoff, Feldman, and Schwarz (1986) and Anderson and Lomas (1984) who referred to the feeling commonly expressed by obstetricians that the "malpractice problem" is responsible for defensive medicine and the resulting high cesarean rates; it was unprecedented to include this factor as a variable. "Medical-legal factors" were defined as recent medical-legal experiences and subjective perception of the influence of the current legal climate on obstetrical decision making. A self-designed medical-legal survey, though not accompanied in the article by any information on validity or reliability, was an attempt to control for contemporaneous events in this category.

Goyert et al. prospectively analyzed the cesarean birth rates of the 11 attending obstetricians in the community hospital of an affluent suburb of Detroit for a 12-month period, 1986–1987. The study was done in a setting in which the patient population, the health care delivery system, and the method of physician reimbursement were relatively homogeneous. The primary cesarean birth rates among these eleven physicians varied from 9.6% to 31.8%. It was determined that only nulliparity had a greater effect (X^2 = 106.4 with 1 df; $p < .0001$) on the primary cesarean rate than identity of the physician (X^2 = 30.7 with 10 df; p = <.001), even when controlling for perception of medical-legal risk. Birth weight and age had no significant effect. Goyert et al. named this variable "physician factor," using the term interchangeably with "practice style."

The findings of Goyert et al. regarding the importance of "practice style" are corroborated by Myers and Gleicher (1988). Myers and Gleicher implemented a program to affect "practice style," in the form of management recommendations, in a Level III perinatal center that served both private and clinic clients. The investigators found, after reviewing 4,402 births, that although the cesarean birth rate among clients of the private staff was 20% in 1985 before the study began, two years later it was 12.4%. The faculty rates fell from 15% to 11.5% in the same time period, also without neonatal compromise. "Neonatal outcome" was stringently defined by both one- and five-minute Apgar scores, as well as neonatal mortality rates per 1,000. Additionally, the Green Bay cesarean study investigators, when studying 2,106 women with singleton fetuses, also reported variations in cesarean rates (5.6% to 19.7%) not attributable to obstetric risk factors, socioeconomic status, or duration of physician practice, but, rather, individual management decisions (DeMott & Sandmire, 1990).

The question of what underlies the observed variations remains. Lowenburg (1989) has implicated economic motivations, decrying the lucrative pull of technologically based medical approaches. Thomas Burke, former Health and Human Services chief of staff and health policy analyst, also sums up the problem as monetary in origin. Burke states there is a need to hold down doctors' propensity to give extra treatments to make money: "Medicine is a business. There's a billion-dollar industry out there taking out uteruses and 60-70% of it is unnecessary. Cesareans . . . are also big business, but very few are done under Medicaid—it doesn't pay (*San Francisco Examiner*, Aug. 29, 1989). Bruce Hilton, director of the National Center for Bioethics, relates the unjustifiably high rates of both hysterectomies and cesarean births to a systematic devaluing and dehumanizing of women as patients ("Bioethics," 1989).

In a publication entitled: "How can we translate good science into good perinatal care?", David Grimes, then at the Centers for Disease Control, called for "a reestablishment of the primacy of the patient" whom he notes is "far more than an elaborate Tupperware container temporarily housing a fetus" (Grimes, 1986, p. 88). Given the present economic disincentives for cognitive rather than procedural interventions and attitudes toward female clients defined by bioethicist Hilton, why do some nurses and doctors choose to use management practices that result in exemplary rates of cesarean births? I propose that their basic ethical, conceptual orientation is one of care rather than cure.

CURE, OR CARE AND CURE?

In *The Task of Medicine*, K.L. White admonishes:

> We do not seem to understand that not only other physicians, but also many other scholars and scientists with diverse interests, have . . . considered the problems and issues we still ponder and have advanced rather different formulations for understanding and appreciating them. [1988, p. 18]

It is argued that our present dilemma of unacceptably high cesarean rates is, as the philosopher Alasdair MacIntyre says, a result of our "lost . . . theoretical and practical comprehension of morality" (1984, p. 2). What is the historical basis for that view of the present problem?

Historical Background

In his study of the history of moral theory, *After Virtue*, MacIntyre (1984) writes that the central theme of the heroic age was an understanding and respect for the fragility and vulnerability inherent in life. It was also during this period that important themes emerged to which I will return: one's actions and the excellence thereof defining who one is as a person, accountability for one's actions, and the particular, contextual importance of community and its relationships.

Aristotle, in later centuries, did not ground his thought historically yet shared a similar philosophy that human connection was a major virtue. Aristotle stressed, however, the interrelatedness of all virtues and, in fact, all morality and law, with excellence of character, practice, and intelligence necessarily intertwined. This was also the first era to articulate the virtue of *sôphrosunê*—the virtue of a man (for ethical discourse was confined to male citizens) who could, but does not, abuse his power. Later medieval views of morality, MacIntyre continues, though pluralistic, were the first to link virtues to a particular notion of the narrative of life's journey, using them to deal with the problems of self and society. Persons were seen as moving toward good in time, with a *telos* as previously, but with a life of good possible for anyone whose actions were morally grounded.

During the Enlightenment period of the 17th and 18th centuries, the dominant Northern European culture "repudiated the classical view of human nature, and with it a great deal central to morality" (MacIntyre, 1984, p. 165). The moral was separated in thought from the logical and legal, and the study of ethics was relegated to a subspecialty of philosophy unrelated to science. Although empiricism sought to close the gap between what seems and what is, the natural sciences were enlarging this gap while thoughts of self-knowledge and the goods associated with purposes were eliminated from discourse. Reason was transcendent; bodily, social, and historical experiences were irrelevant (Flax, 1987); and life's fragility and vulnerability were foreseen as conquerable. The germ theory strengthened the Cartesian notion of mind/body dualism (Allan & Hall, 1988), and the truth and primacy of objectivity reigned essentially unquestioned. Objectivity found autonomy central, connectedness irrelevant, and specifically, physician care superior to, not complementary of, midwifery (Rich, 1986).

Regarding current views of our Enlightenment-derived sciences, Keller feels that an impulse toward power and domination has been evident since Francis Bacon, citing Bacon's thought that science is "leading you to Nature with all her children to bind her to your service, and make her your slave" (1982, p. 598). Keller argues that these impulses, rather than being seen as objective, should be viewed as a projection of an alienated masculine self that needs to deny its relatedness to others (including its field of inquiry); with this object/subject dualism, there is no need for ethical self-examination (as the self is the objectivist ideal) or for a moral theory that embraces the reality of human connection and its implications.

Medicine Today

Although White mourns the current notion that "the development of technology based on scientific understanding and the deployment of that technology constitutes science" (1988, p. 12), that association is flourishing especially in regard to women's birthing. Sandelowski argues that current childbearing experiences are being reinvented "within a conceptual system emphasizing separation and distance" (1988, p. 43) with the increased use of cesareans, epidurals, and other birthing technologies. There is a "progressive severing of women's connection to maternity" (p. 36), with women becoming the raw material from which the product is scientifically extracted. Given the pain associated with the inherent fragility and vulnerability of life that the heroic age understood, it is not surprising that there is some appeal to medicine to attempt to transcend this with technology. Yet as early at 1960, Guttentag warned that "medicine has become so impressed with its own . . . progress that it has forgotten to examine the theoretical limitations of its pursuit" (p. 903), and referring to the "discontent from without and disquietude from within" the medical profession (p. 904), called for an ontological analysis of the very theoretical premises of medicine. Regarding that disquietude, however, nurse ethicist Benner reminds us that "a disillusioned self accompanies a disengaged self" (1989a, p. 6).

Disengaged, technology-oriented doctors are comparable to MacIntyre's "central characters:" those who are the unofficial moral representatives of the culture and embody the obliteration of the distinction between manipulative and nonmanipulative social relations. A character such as this purports to restrict himself to realms of rational agreement, and his claims to effectiveness rest on "the existence of a domain of morally neutral fact about which he is an expert" (p. 77). MacIntyre argues that this believed-in reality disguises certain other realities (especially the chance of knowledge being located elsewhere in the network), and that this posture of power is really meant to disguise the reality of one's impotence. The power seems, however, real enough to the women who watched the cesarean birth rate begin to soar as soon as their insistence for non-alienated birthing became audible. Abuses of power have also been evident by the use of legal intimidation and political action aimed at restriction of licensure of less disease-oriented professions such a midwifery (Allan &

Hall, 1988) and the virtual control of health care and its economy in favor of physicians, despite evidence that such care is not best in all cases (Institute of Medicine, 1988).

Besides the alleged self-interest of medicine, what else may underlie its cure/control paradigm? The impotence just alluded to is an important factor, given the culture's enormous fear of death and uncertainty (Sarah, 1987) and the general discomfort with vulnerability and connection that birth and embodiment entail (Ruddick, 1989). We have seen that the rationalist thinker prizes autonomy and transcendence of the body, yet nothing more than birthing represents the antithesis to "Reason's" values, according to philospher Ruddick in her book *Maternal Thinking*. Birthing's intimacy "foreshadows a . . . lifeshaping tie to a particular, dependent person" while, "most troubling of all its social aspects, birthing labor is uniquely female" (1989, p. 191). Men's fear and envy of labor "and the female bodies responsible for it" (p. 192) are seen in the persistent minimalization of birthing from Plato's works on, as "they claim for themselves a higher creativity" (p. 192). That this is a form of psychic defense against such envy is traced in the work of Kittay (1984); only Ruddick, though, characterizes birth as "incontinent, insufficiently individuated, and vulnerable to pain, confinement, and onerous responsibility" as opposed to Reason, which is "active, autonomous, controlling, progressive, and socially powerful yet exempt from unwanted social responsibilities" (p. 196).

Ruddick characterizes laboring as "repetitiously irregular," countering current obstetrical discomfort with non-normative labor. It is difficult, however, for a woman to have the trust in her body that successful birthing demands when even her health care provider is conflicted regarding its capacity. This doubt can lead to the rationalizing of an intentional rupture of her body, often to theoretically save a potential uterine rupture. Yet, since humans are embodied, in the phenomenologic view (Benner & Wrubel, 1989), the body's powers or lacerations are empowerings or rendings of the very self. Likewise, a woman's baby is embodied and thus dependent on her well-being for the totality of its own. The "sturdy dependencies" (Ruddick, 1989, p. 211) that birthing presupposes are ideally comparable to those that a woman will have in her birth attendant. These dependencies are of an extremely risky nature, however, if the attendant's actions are not first ethically grounded.

This need for a centrally guiding force has been alluded to by others. "The health care system has become an organism guided by misguided choices; it is unstable, confused, and desperately in need of a central nervous system that can help it cope" (Ellwood, 1988, p. 1550). That central nervous system, it is proposed, should be the paradigm of care rather than cure.

Care

The definition of care used, "commitment to alleviation of vulnerability," is taken from Gadow's work in the book, *The Ethics of Care and The Ethics of Cure* (1988). Gadow points out that treatment measures that might come to mind as the most dramatic measures to alleviate vulnerability—surgical interventions—are actually the *least* consistent with the concept of care as "they achieve their effect through the exercise of power by one person over another, and the exercise of power always *increases* the vulnerability of the one over whom it is exercised, no matter what benevolent purpose the power serves. . . . Only in the context of care can the overpowering of one person by another that cure entails be redeemable (from the realm of torture)" (p. 7).

The Enlightenment rupture that separated moral thought from human action has allowed untenable cesarean rates to continue nearly unquestioned. MacIntyre states that a lack of relevant intellectual virtues corrupts tradition and one's judgment; nowhere is this more relevant than in the tradition of women's birthing labor. Rather than being part of action that affirms the body's capabilities and trustworthiness (Benner, 1989c), physicians have contributed to a rupture in the disciplinary matrix of mothering worse than the uterine rupture they purport to fear, causing unredeemable amounts of excess vulnerability in women's lived experience.

Since nursing is the paradigmatic public caring profession (Benner, 1988), it is not surprising that literature regarding nurses' birthing practices has demonstrated low rates of induced vulnerability in the form of surgical delivery. Women do know most intimately, as Ruddick says, the history and cost of human flesh. Yet doctoring too, although limited by scientism, reductionism, commercialism, and a biotechnical orientation (Benner, 1989c), traditionally has been a caring practice and is often still demonstrated to be so, as Gleicher (1984, 1986), White (1988), and others have modeled. What then constitutes a "practice" in the morally grounded ethical tradition?

MacIntyre defines a practice as an organized, coherent, complex form of social activity through which goods internal to that activity are realized in the course of achieving evolving excellence. Benner calls this distinction of ethics as skilled practical knowledge "skillful ethical comportment" (1989b), and declares that we know it in our hearts when we see it. Although bereft of a scientific obstetrical language, a birthing woman knows when she has been cared for with such comportment, and she has the embodied knowledge to know when she has not (see examples of this in Cohen & Estner, 1983). It is important to note that the concept of skillful ethical comportment includes not only the usual quandary or breakdown ethics questions (such as the appropriateness of court-ordered cesareans), but also illuminates the larger but heretofore invisible part of the ethics iceberg—the consequences of the trivialization of distress, of disregard of the literature, of discounting the midwifery knowledge base, and of power abuses inherent in unnecessarily high rates of surgical or instrumental intervention. The engaged nature of excellent practice, whereby a woman is viewed as a person whose life's story will be positively or negatively affected by the caregiver's actions, makes disengaged objectified "care" amoral.

As caregivers live out the narrative that is the story of their lives, they have a basis for evaluating the ethics of their caregiving. As each answers, "what sort of person am I to become?" by the excellence or lack of same in the action of their lives, a reflection is seen of the heroic tradition that reminds us that people *are* what they do. Does one act honorably, displaying *sôphrosunê*, or is one a woman-rupturer unnecessarily? Does one contribute to a woman's confidence at this important juncture by caring enough to choose the least vulnerability-producing management practices for enabling her (Benner & Wrubel, 1989), or does one consciously or unconsciously choose to honor time, economic, and other incentives, disregarding the long shadow that this brief time of birth will cast? A disengaged view of the potential vulnerability inherent in those few hours negates how the birth will unavoidably help constitute the woman's future life in unfortellable ways. If outcome is the only issue, human concerns of comfort, hope, dignity, vulnerability, shame, good, and evil are irrelevant (Benner, 1988). Listening to clients in years subsequent to the births of their offspring teaches us that they are not.

CONCLUSION

MacIntyre warns us that our practice of morality is in grave danger, and that "the barbarians are not waiting at the frontiers" but rather have been in control for some time (1984, p. 263). Many women from whom the power of birth has been wrested and the many nurses and doctors who do care agree that our lack of consciousness about this is, as MacIntyre says, our predicament.

No one argues that the ability to safely perform necessary cesarean births is anything but blessed. Benner reminds us, though, that "excellence and its absence can guide us, because moral outrage over the failure of care practices can point to what we consider to be essential and minimal as well as what we consider to be excellent" (1988, p. 8). With care being the complex, cognitive, ethically grounded skill that it is, the continued antithesis of this, in the form of nonadherence to the NIH consensus statement suggestions, is amoral. In the midst of our present opportunity-providing instability of cultural thought (Flax, 1987; Tronto, 1987), attention to care may be most fruitful; and nursing, for framing current dilemmas in ways which embrace all of what matters, may be seen as the paradigm of ethically grounded health care that it is.

REFERENCES

Affonso, D.D. (1977). Missing pieces: A study of postpartum feelings. *Birth and the Family Journal, 4*, 159–164.

Affonso, D.D., & Stichler, J.F. (1978). Exploratory study of women's reactions to having a cesarean birth. *Birth and the Family Journal, 5*(2), 88–94.

Allan, J.D., & Hall, B.A. (1988). Challenging the focus on technology: A critique of the medical model in a changing health care system. *Advances in Nursing Science, 10*(3), 22–34.

Anderson, G.M., & Lomas, J. (1984). Determinants of the increasing cesarean birth rate. *New England Journal of Medicine, 311*, 887–892.

Anderson, G.M., & Lomas, J. (1985). Explaining variations in cesarean section rates: Patients, facilities or policies? *Canadian Medical Association Journal, 132*, 253–259.

Arizmendi, T.G., & Affonso, D.D. (1987). Stressful events related to pregnancy and postpartum. *Journal of Psychosomatic Research, 31*, 743–756.

Benner, P. (1988, October). *Nursing as a caring profession.* Paper presented at the meeting of the American Academy of Nursing, Kansas City, MO.

Benner, P. (1989a, February). The moral dimensions of caring. In American Academy of Nursing (Ed.), *Proceedings of the Wingspread Invitational Conference of Knowledge About Care and Caring, State of the Art and Future Developments.*

Benner, P. (1989b, September). The quest for control and the possibilities of care. Paper presented at the Applied Heidegger Conference.

Benner, P. (1989c, October). *Nursing as caring: Can there be a science of caring?* Lecture, University of California, San Francisco.

Benner, P., & Wrubel, J. (1989). *The primacy of caring.* Menlo Park, CA: Addison-Wesley.

Bioethics. (1989, October 15). *San Francisco Examiner*, p. E–15.

Bottoms, S.F., Hirsch, B.S., & Sokol, R.J. (1987). Medical management of arrest disorders of labor: A current overview. *American Journal of Obstetrics and Gynecology, 156*, 935–939.

Bottoms, S.F., Rosen, M.G., & Sokol, R.J. (1980). The increase in the cesarean birth rate. *New England Journal of Medicine, 302,* 559–563.

Bowes, W.A., Jr. (1989). Clinical aspects of normal and abnormal labor. In R.K. Creasy & R. Resnick (Eds.), *Maternal-fetal medicine* (pp. 449–489). Philadelphia: Saunders.

California Health Policy and Data Advisory Commission. (1988). *Analysis of small-area variations in California hospital admissions: Biennial report on cost containment.* CA: Office of Statewide Health Planning and Development.

Cohen, N.W., & Estner, L.J. (1983). *Silent knife.* South Hadley, MA: Bergin & Garvey.

Danforth, D.N. (1985). Cesarean section. *Journal of the American Medical Association, 253,* 811–817.

Demott, R.K., & Sandmire, H.F. (1990). The Green Bay cesarean section study. *American Journal of Obstetrics and Gynecology, 162,* 1593–1602.

Ellwood, P.M. (1988). Outcomes management—a technology of patient experience. *New England Journal of Medicine, 318,* 1549–1556.

Flax, J. (1987). Postmodernism and gender relations in feminist theory. *Signs: Journal of Women in Culture and Society, 12,* 621–643.

Gadow, S. (1988). Covenant without cure. In J. Watson & M.A. Ray (Eds.), *The ethics of care and the ethics of cure* (pp. 5–14). New York: National League for Nursing.

Garcia, J., Corry, M., MacDonald, D., Elbourne, D., & Grant, A. (1985). Mothers' views of continuous electronic fetal heart monitoring and intermittent ausculation in a randomized controlled trial. *Birth, 12*(2), 79–85.

Garel, M., Lelong, N., & Kaminski, M. (1987). Psychological consequences of caesarean childbirth in primiparas. *Journal of Psychosomatic Obstetrics and Gynaecology, 6,* 197–209.

Garel, M., Lelong, N., & Kaminski, M. (1988). Follow-up study of psychological consequences of caesarean childbirth. *Early Human Development, 16,* 271–282.

Gleicher, N. (1984). Cesarean section rates in the United States: The short-term failure of the National Consensus Development Conference in 1980. *Journal of the American Medical Association, 252,* 3273–3276.

Gleicher, N. (1986). The cesarean-section epidemic. *Mount Sinai Journal of Medicine, 53,* 563–565.

Gould, J.B., Davey, B., & Stafford, R.S. (1989). Socioeconomic differences in rates of cesarean section. *New England Journal of Medicine, 321,* 233–239.

Goyert, G.L., Bottoms, S.F., Treadwell, M.C., & Nehra, P.C. (1989). The physician factor in cesarean birth rates. *New England Journal of Medicine, 320,* 706–709.

Grimes, D.A. (1986). How can we translate good science into good perinatal care? *Birth, 13,* 83–90.

Guttentag, O.E. (1960). A course entitled "the medical attitude": An orientation in the foundations of medical thought. *Journal of Medical Education, 35,* 903–907.

Haynes de Regt, R., Minkoff, H.L., Feldman, J., & Schwarz, R.H. (1986). Relation of private or clinic care to the cesarean birth rate. *New England Journal of Medicine, 315,* 619–624.

Health analyst wants doctors to be salaried. (1989, August 29). *San Francisco Examiner,* p. A–11.

Hobfoll, S.E., & Leiberman, J.R. (1987). Personality and social resources in immediate and continued stress resistance among women. *Journal of Personality and Social Psychology, 52,* 18–26.

Institute of Medicine. (1988). *Prenatal care: Reaching mothers, reaching infants.* Washington, DC: National Academy Press.

Keller, E.F. (1982). Feminism and science. *Signs: Journal of Women in Culture and Society, 7,* 589–602.

Kittay, E.F. (1984). Womb envy: An explanatory concept. In J. Trebilcot (Ed.), *Mothering: Essays in feminist theory* (pp. 94–127). Totowa, NJ: Rowman & Allanheld.

Lazarus, R.S. (1986). The trivialization of distress. In P.I. Ahmed & N. Ahmed (Eds.), *Coping with juvenile diabetes* (pp. 33–60). Springfield, IL: Charles C. Thomas.

Lipson, J.G., & Tilden, V.P. (1980). Psychological integration of the cesarean birth experience. *American Journal of Orthopsychiatry, 50,* 598–609.

Lowenberg, J. (1989). *Caring and responsibility.* Philadelphia: University of Pennsylvania.

MacIntyre, A. (1984). *After virtue: A study in moral theory* (2nd ed.). Notre Dame: University of Notre Dame Press.

Marut, J., & Mercer, R.T. (1981). The cesarean birth experience: Implications for nursing. *Birth Defects, 17,* 129–152.

McPherson, K., Wennberg, J.E., Hovind, O.B., & Clifford, P. (1982). Small-area variations in the use of common surgical procedures: An international comparision of New England, England, and Norway. *New England Journal of Medicine, 307,* 1310–1314.

Myers, S.A., & Gleicher, N. (1988). A successful program to lower cesarean-section rates. *New England Journal of Medicine, 319,* 1511–1516.

National Center for Health Statistics. (1989). *Vital and health statistics: Detailed diagnoses and procedures, NHDS, 1987* (DHHS Publication No. (PHS) 89–1761). Hyattsville, MD: Department of Health and Human Services.

National Institutes of Health. (1981). *Cesarean childbirth: Report of a consensus development conference* (NIH Publication No. 82–2067). Bethesda, MD: Department of Health and Human Services.

Neuhoff, D., Burke, M.S., & Porreco, R.P. (1989). Cesarean birth for failed progress in labor. *Obstetrics and Gynecology, 73,* 915–920.

Notzen, F.C., Placek, P.J., & Taffel, S.M. (1987). Comparison of national cesarean–section rates. *New England Journal of Medicine, 316,* 386–389.

O'Driscoll, K., & Foley, M. (1983). Correlation of decrease in perinatal mortality and increase in cesarean section rates. *Obstetrics and Gynecology, 61,* 1–5.

O'Driscoll, K., & Meagher, D. (1986). *Active management of labour* (2nd ed.). London: Bailliere-Tindall.

O'Driscoll, K., Foley, M., MacDonald, D., & Stronge, J. (1988). Cesarean section and perinatal outcome: Response from the House of Horne. *American Journal of Obstetrics and Gynecology, 158,* 449–452.

Pettiti, D. (1989). Commentaries: The cesarean section rate is 25 percent and rising. Why? What can be done about it? *Birth, 16,* 120–121.

Petitti, D.B., Cefalo, R.C., Shapiro, S., & Whalley, P. (1982). In-hospital maternal mortality in the United States: Time trends and relation to method of delivery. *Obstetrics and Gynecology, 59,* 6–12.

Phelan, J.P., Clark, S.L., Diaz, F., & Paul, R.H. (1987). Vaginal birth after cesarean. *American Journal of Obstetrics and Gynecology, 157,* 1510–1515.

Placek, P.J., & Taffel, S.M. (1980). Trends in cesarean section rates for the United States, 1970–1978. *Public Health Report, 95,* 540–548.

Placek, P.J., & Taffel, S.M. (1983). The frequency of complications in cesarean and noncesarean deliveries, 1970 and 1978. *Public Health Report, 98,* 396–400.

Placek, P.J., Taffel, S.M., & Moien, M. (1983). Cesarean section delivery rates: United States, 1981. *American Journal of Public Health, 73,* 861–862.

Placek, P.J., Taffel, S.M., & Moien, M. (1988). 1986 C–sections rise; VBACS inch upward. *American Journal of Public Health, 78,* 562–563.

Porreco, R.P. (1985). High cesarean section rate: A new perspective. *Obstetrics and Gynecology, 65,* 307–311.

Rich, A. (1986). *Of woman born: Motherhood as experience and institution* (10th anniversary ed.). New York: W.W. Norton.

Rooks, J.P., Weatherby, N.L., Ernst, E.K., Stapleton, S., Rosen, D., & Rosenfield, A. (1989). Outcomes of care in birth centers: The national birth center study. *New England Journal of Medicine, 321,* 1804–1811.

Rubin, G.L., Peterson, H.B., Rochat, R.W., McCarthy, B.J., & Terry, J.S. (1981). Maternal death after cesarean section in Georgia. *American Journal of Obstetrics and Gynecology, 139,* 681–685.

Ruddick, S. (1989). *Maternal thinking.* Boston: Beacon Press.

Sandelowski, M. (1988). A case of conflicting paradigms: Nursing and reproductive technology. *Advances in Nursing Science, 10*(3), 35–44.

Sarah, R. (1987). Power, certainty, and the fear of death. *Woman and Health, 13,* 59–71.

Sargent, C., & Stark, N. (1987). Surgical birth: Interpretations of cesarean delivery among private hospital patients and nursing staff. *Social Science and Medicine, 25,* 1269–1276.

Shy, K.K., LoGerfo, J.P., Karp, L.E. (1981). Evaluation of elective repeat cesarean section as a standard of care: An application of decision analysis. *American Journal of Obstetrics and Gynecology, 139,* 123–129.

Strombino, D.M., Baruffi, G., Dellinger, W.S., & Ross, A. (1988). Variations in pregnancy outcomes and use of obstetric procedures in two institutions with divergent philosophies of maternity care. *Medical Care, 26,* 333–347.

Taffel, S.M., & Placek, P.J. (1983). Complications in cesarean and non-cesarean deliveries: United States, 1980. *American Journal of Public Health, 73,* 856–860.

Taffel, S.M., Placek, P.J., & Liss, T. (1987). Trends in the United States cesarean section rate and reasons for the 1980–85 rise. *American Journal of Public Health, 77,* 955–959.

Treffers, P.E. (1989). Obstetrical care in the Netherlands: Home and hospital deliveries. In E.V. van Hall & W. Everaerd (Eds.), *The free woman: Women's health in the 1990s. Invited papers of the 9th International Congress of Psychosomatic Obstetrics and Gynaecology* (pp. 62–68). Park Ridge, NJ: Parthenon.

Tronto, J.C. (1987). Beyond gender difference to a theory of care. *Signs: Journal of Women in Culture and Society, 12,* 644–663.

U.S. Bureau of the Census. (1989). Statistical abstract of the United States: 1989 (109th ed.). Washington, DC: U.S. National Center for Health Statistics.

White, K.L. (1988). *The task of medicine: The dialogue at Wickenburg*. Menlo Park, CA: Henry J. Kaiser Family Foundation.

Williams, R.L., & Chen, P.M. (1983). Controlling the rise in cesarean section rates by the dissemination of information from vital records. *American Journal of Public Health, 73*, 863–867.

Wingeier, R., Bloch, S., & Kvale, J.K. (1988). A description of a CNM-family physician joint practice in a rural setting. *Journal of Nurse-Midwifery, 33*(2), 86–92.

18

The Importance of Knowing What to Care About: A Phenomenological Inquiry Using Laughing at Oneself as a Clue

Francelyn Reeder

The nursing profession has been at the forefront of caring by recognizing the empowering quality of personal strengths and creative potential in people. Currently there are a number of nursing theories of a transcendent nature (Rogers, 1970; Watson, 1985; Newman, 1986; Paterson & Zderad, 1971; Barrett, 1989). The purpose of these theories is not solely to focus on the immediate consequences of human caring related to health and healing. Going beyond immediacy, these scholars focus on the enlarged purposes and meanings of caring moments in the lives of people. One example of the experience of the transcendent is recognized in the nature of human laughter.

LITERATURE ON LAUGHTER

The transcendent nature of laughter, in addition to being appreciated as a positive emotion (Cousins, 1979) is taken seriously as an unexplored human potential for health (Eastman, 1966; Grotjahn, 1957; Mindess, 1971a; Robinson, 1983; Schaier & Cicirelli, 1976). After centuries of contradictory theories to explain the origin, characteristics, and consequences of laughter (Freud, 1960; Fry, 1963; Greig, 1923; Holland, 1983; McDougall, 1960; Mindess, 1971b; Morreall, 1983; Lorenz, 1936; Plessner, 1970; Ziv, 1984), 20th century researchers admit of its elusive nature and much to their dismay, continue to leave a trail of inconclusive findings (Coser, 1959; Fry, 1977; Goldstein, 1956; Hertzler, 1970; Jackson, 1982; Peterson & Pollio, 1982; Piddington, 1963; Scogin, 1983; Prerost, 1983). Asking one-sided questions of an objective nature was cited as a limitation in nearly all of the research reports. Recommendations were made for future studies to address the subjective aspects of laughter and to explore the perspective of the one laughing (McGhee & Goldstein, 1983).

PURPOSE AND DESIGN OF STUDY

The purpose of the study discussed in this article was to explore the human strengths of persons who laugh at themselves and to understand the meaning this experience has had for them in their lives. Previous studies on the antecedents and consequences of laughter did not address the transcendent nature of laughter, nor the potential life orientation that could be enlarged by individuals for the benefit not only of daily living, but also for a sense of solidarity with generations to come.

Several conclusions identified in the research literature influenced the design of this inquiry. Because mirthful laughter (Grotjahn, 1957) and laughing at oneself have been associated with maturity (Goodman, 1983) and described as having an intellectual quality (Eble, 1966) individuals with many years of life experience were sought for this study. Senior citizens were favored even more as subjects of this study as it became evident that studies on laughter have been limited to the periods of early childhood and school age. A developmental perspective beyond childhood including adolescence, adulthood, and aging, has the potential to effectively gather the fragments of these phases of life into a whole that can represent the continuity of a life orientation (Luce, 1979; Brady, 1986; Hultsch & Deitsch, 1981). Thus the eminent and transcendent features of life could be studied more readily with a senior citizen population.

The knowledge of human strengths available through the study of healthy, active persons, which was recognized by Maslow three decades ago, is also a hallmark of nursing's propensity to consider and mobilize the strengths of persons seeking health. Doing so enlarges our personal attention to the surprises and paradoxes of people's lives, an important complement to attention given to deficiencies, a common practice of the medical profession (American Nurses' Association, 1980; Clark, 1981; Henry & Moody, 1985; Hill & Smith, 1985; Chapman, 1983). Therefore, sampling among senior citizens who were active in society and living in noninstitutional settings was consistent with this nursing value.

SIGNIFICANCE OF STUDY

Other studies and writings on laughter indicate a growing trend toward workshops and therapeutic programs using laughter for stress reduction (Bloch, Browning, & McGrath, 1983; Flynn, 1980). Indiscriminate programming for general populations, however, may have the opposite response for some unsuspecting hopefuls. As positive as laughter may be for some individuals, it seems irresponsible to develop programs on the assumption that such programs are unequivocally meaningful to all who attend. Conversations with countless people concur with the literature and attest to the fact that some shy away from programs that are designed to make one laugh uproariously, for reasons of culture or ethnicity, or experiences of war and/or family practices (Reeder & Malinski, 1988; Jackson & King, 1982; LeShan, 1977; Mindess, 1976; Potter & Goodman, 1983; Peter & Dana, 1982; Robinson, 1978). Again, few research studies have addressed the subject's perspective on the experience of laughter itself, nor on the experience of laughing at oneself; both appear to be necessary foundations for therapeutic practice.

Laughing at oneself appears to be an experience and orientation to life that does not carry the negative connotations of laughter in general cited in the literature. Also, the promise of laughter being an index of reserves for meeting unexpected events in the course of one's life cannot be assumed, but needs exploration. The long-range benefit this human strength may have on one's life orientation and life choices is a phenomena of significant interest to nursing as a practice discipline. Laughing at oneself is possibly another significant use of oneself as the primary instrument of healing, only recently recognized (or rediscovered) for its potential as a natural caring modality.

METHODOLOGY: HUSSERLIAN PHENOMENOLOGY

Descriptive study of the nature of nursing's concerns through phenomenological inquiry is not new. The study of laughing at oneself through Husserlian phenomenology (Husserl, 1970), rather than Heideggerian or derivatives of Merleau-Ponty, is promising because the eidetic features of Husserl's unique radical approach to gain access to the transcendent eidetic meanings of a phenomenon are congruent with the purpose of this study. A similar study on the meaning of laughing at oneself in the elderly is being carried out in another part of the country by a colleague using a different qualitative methodology. The findings of these two studies will be examined in a later article for purposes of illuminating the strengths and limitations of each approach for such an elusive phenomenon of interest. Husserlian phenomenology is not yet commonly used in nursing and needs greater exposure to discriminate its relevance for nursing science. Its congruence with Rogers' conceptual system has already been upheld (Reeder, 1984). Further theoretical relevance to natural caring modalities may be discovered in the phenomenon of expanding consciousness, common to the writings of nursing theorists such as Watson, Newman, and Rogers, as well as Husserl and Gurwitsch in phenomenology. Further, the phenomenon of laughing at oneself could serve as a clue to health as expanding consciousness.

The Research Process

The study design selected for this study was descriptive. Husserlian phenomenology, as interpreted by the researcher (Reeder, 1984), was used. Thematic generation and synthesis of meanings were obtained from transcribed unstructured interviews with 14 seniors living independently in their own homes. Significant statements were recognized through a series of perspectival variations and intuitive reflections during the interviews as well as during analysis of the transcripts. This integral research process, in which the researcher and participant are respected as sources of thematic generation through dialogue, gave evidence of meanings co-constituted, and ultimately synthesized essential themes belonging to this senior citizen sample.

Description of Sample

The sample of senior citizens was purposive and convenient, acquired by using a list of potential participants nominated by their peers as being leaders in their community. Some were publicly recognized as active contributors to their profession and/or society. Participants were those who were willing and able to articulate experiences of laughing at themselves as they lived them, from childhood to the present, and particularly to articulate the meaning these experiences have had for them in life.

Nearly all the subjects were English-speakers between the ages of 60 and 84. The natural settings provided 12 partners who were interviewed together. Four were married couples, and two were female friends living together. One of these women, age 40, was the exception in age. The last two participants interviewed were a man whose wife could not be present and a widow whose home aide was present but declined participation. Two were Hispanic and two were foreign born—one Norwegian, one Welsh. Two were of Jewish descent; the remaining caucasians were combinations of German, Irish, and English descent. The majority had attended college, some for four or more years; three were high school graduates.

Effort was made to satisfy the phenomenological requirement for coherent, full verbal descriptions of the lived experience of laughing at oneself as well as insights into the meaning of these experiences. Each participant reported that he or she had a high level of interest in the topic, which made the process enjoyable and effortless. Every participant completed the study.

Procedures

After obtaining approval from the university's human subjects review committee and written consent of participants to be audiotaped, the researcher made appointments by phone to conduct the interviews at a mutually agreeable time and place. Home was the location chosen by nearly all the participants.

The interview was initiated with a general overview of the purpose of the study, followed by an invitation for open dialogue in response to the opening question: "What is the meaning of the experience of laughing at oneself? Describe or elaborate on times in your life when you had this experience. Does it have any importance to you or not?"

A dialogue was thus set in motion. Descriptions of recent experiences and statements about what laughing at oneself meant in general to the participants occurred quite spontaneously. Attentive listening by the researcher was deliberately engaged in throughout the session, thereby generating new questions from the content, insights, and nature of the responses. Clarifying questions evoked further elaboration of meanings and experiences from childhood and even anticipations of future hopes associated with laughing at oneself. Raising questions in response to insights, memories, and anticipations verbalized by participants is a form of varying the possible perspectives germane to phenomenological awareness of one's life experiences. Also, attention to contrasting events spontaneously shared in the narrative, such as hardships, tragedies, or losses endured in life, provided rich descriptions associated with the importance laughing at oneself has had for each participant.

It became obvious that first level analysis had already taken place for some of the participants as they offered personal reflections on their experiences expressed as meaningful insights, rather than descriptions of events. For example, reflective insights were recognized in responses such as "laughing at oneself means being able to take criticism" and "laughing at oneself is being optimistic and seeing the positive side of life rather than the negative." First level analysis for the researcher is initiated in the interview process by the very act of attentive listening to responses. The purpose of posing new questions is based on a sense that full description and meanings are possible and forthcoming.

Phenomenological questioning and listening continued until participants gave some indication that self-disclosure on the topic was exhausted. The interview was closed when new questions ceased to be generated and the narratives were saturated with recurrent themes. Another contact date was scheduled with each participant to share the results of the study, and to return a transcript or copy of the study as they desired. The purpose of the sharing was not for validation of the findings as this is not required with the phenomenological method, which acknowledges the tentative nature of knowledge and the infinite unfolding of meaning co-constitued by both researcher and informants over time. Participants expressed their pleasure in participating in the study and said they were happy their meanings and insights would be published so others could benefit from them.

HUSSERLIAN FIELD OF CONSCIOUSING THE WORLD: CONTEXT FOR GENERATION ANALYSIS OF PHENOMENOLOGICAL THEMES

As previously stated, the first level of analysis for the researcher actually began during the interview through attentive, reflective listening. The posing of questions, evoking of responses, and generation of new questions was based on the premise that human beings are capable of learning and knowing the world. The researcher has made explicit Husserl's Principle of Intentionality (Figure 18-1) and the Multiple Modes of Awareness (Figure 18-2), which together are referred to here as the Husserlian Field of Consciousing the World (FCW) (Gurwitsch, 1966). Thus, FCW was recognized as being the context which made attentive listening, constituting of meanings, and synthesis of essential themes possible from the narratives shared by the participants.

Benefits of an Explicit Horizon of Meaning

The benefits of the FCW context to phenomenological analysis of narratives are particularly noticeable in three areas. First, the focus is shifted from preconceived notions about what to find in the interview (bracketing) to the actual narratives shared by the participants; second, there is an openness to attend to any and all possible and actual ways of relating to the world that the participants chose to include in their narratives; third, there is the fluency of attention to move from detailed events of the narratives to a reflective attitude, quite spontaneously and simultaneously.

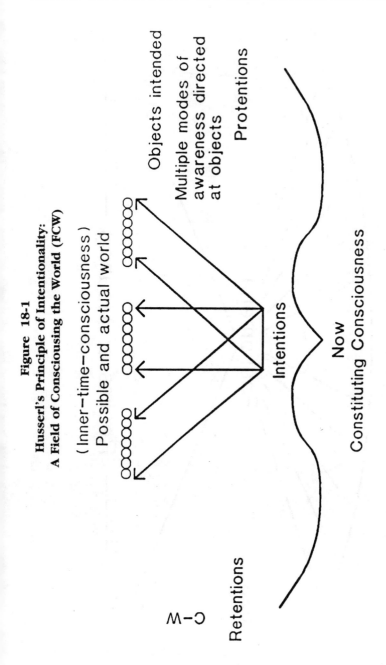

Figure 18-1
Husserl's Principle of Intentionality:
A Field of Consciousing the World (FCW)

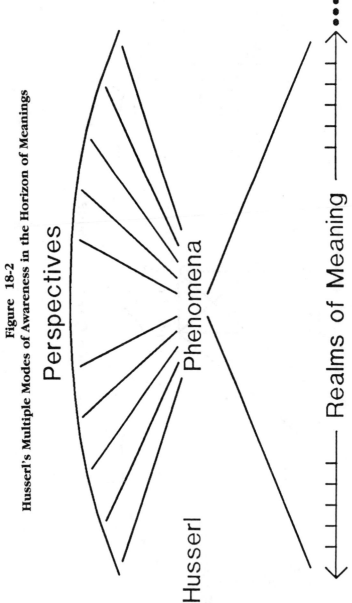

Figure 18-2
Husserl's Multiple Modes of Awareness in the Horizon of Meanings

All data are thus respected without premature judgment or closure (*epo-che*), while clarifying questions can seek extensive variation of perspectives from the participants. The skill of disciplined attention to the natural narratives of participants through this first-hand multiple dimensional hearing is accompanied by the researcher's first level, and then second level reflection on the stories as they unfold. These attitudes of listening (and reading later on) and hearing reflectively lead to exceptional penetration of the data and to sensitive recognition of the conscious and/or unconscious meanings held by participants.

The second and later level analyses, which focus on the transcripts after the interview is completed, use the same three attitudes and context. As analysis in this study continued, significant statements were noted reflectively, meanings were constituted through several readings, themes were recognized within each transcript, and unifying themes were synthesized. After each transcript was sufficiently analyzed, comparison across transcripts gave rise to the summative unity of meanings (universal ground) for this population.

FINDINGS

One unifying grounding theme was recognized in every narrative of the study: Recognition of the importance of knowing what to care about is foundational to balancing self-preservation activities and relational responsibilities.

The subthemes were recognized as insights and meanings expressed in the majority of narratives, and differed across transcripts only in their particularity and uniqueness. There were seven subthemes: (1) honesty and seeing oneself in perspective, (2) openness to spontaneity and surprise, (3) decisiveness, (4) self-respect and sense of self-preservation, (5) acceptance of incongruity as funny, (6) courage and silent strength, and (7) magnanimity.

The notion of a grounding theme means that actual everyday experiences and meanings of laughing at oneself will always be more than the sum of the above subthemes, but will always include the unifying grounding theme. All narratives are characterized by this enduring theme.

Laughing at oneself is not a simple or isolated event. It is manifest or experienced in conjunction with, as well as through, other phenomena, e.g., tragedy and comedy, pain and joy, frustration, unexpected events, incongruities of self-image and reality, adversity, survival, and serendipity. Laughing at oneself may occur anywhere and anytime in a person's life experience. One's perspective makes all the difference in whether or not life experience is transcending and/or transforming to the one involved.

The seven subthemes identified were found to hold true for the meaning of laughing at oneself for senior citizens in this study. In order to facilitate the understanding of the unifying grounding theme as well as subthemes, direct quotations from the participant's narratives are included as clarifying examples.

Instead of describing instances in which laughing at oneself occurred, participants frequently began by sharing insights into this experience; such as in a dynamic gestalt, aha, or realization of what motivates their actions and stances toward the world.

The following excerpts are spontaneous insights shared without any explicit attention to detail and represent the participants' own first level of analysis and reflection. Excerpts have been organized under the subthemes. The contexts in which subthemes were recognized are presented later to illuminate the relationships among the themes.

(1) *Honesty, seeing yourself in perspective.*

"Not taking yourself too seriously."

"Having no pretense about how we live, just being honest and laughing at ourselves."

"Being able to take criticism."

"Time really changes your perspective on your own importance, it's really funny."

"Knowing you can't always win."

"It's a matter of perspective, it includes some realism, that is laughing at oneself is different than frivolity; the image of our world corresponds to the real world whatever it is."

(2) *Openness to spontaneity and surprise.*

"Learning to laugh at oneself when your best self-image is different from what is really happening."

"Willing to see things the way others do."

"Thank you for helping me see with a new insight that I *do* laugh at myself."

"Being flexible and resourceful in response to challenges you didn't expect to happen."

"Being interested and enjoying oneself, not being bored."

(3) *Decisiveness.*

"Being flexible with unimportant differences yet remaining steadfast over very important issues."

"Letting go of obstacles in your way of no consequence."

"Not taking stupid, ridiculous behavior to heart but rather laughing at yourself instead of getting angry or embarrassed."

"Making up your mind about what is important to care about, choosing it, and not regretting or fretting over it afterwards."

"We raised our kids the best way we knew how, we may not have had

the most up-to-date knowledge, but they turned out pretty good."
(4) *Self-respect and sense of self-preservation.*
"If you respect yourself, then you can really laugh at yourself and the world, treating yourself with some importance is basic to laughing at oneself."
"I felt like I was invincible during the war and believed nothing would happen to me but I didn't volunteer for anything beyond my duty."
"I had to learn how to laugh at myself very early in life just to survive because short people aren't taken seriously very often. I introduced myself as the Hobbit, so other people would laugh with me instead of at me, and they could too, when they saw that I accepted myself for who I was."
(5) *Acceptance of incongruity as funny.*
"Being able to distinguish between essential and incidental things in your life."
"Noticing your best self-image is not the same as your body now looks, and seeing it as funny."
"When I drove the car through the garage door I just laughed and said well, I'm sure not going to let a car get me down but it sure is funny."
"When I realized how very tall I appeared to the little Japanese children who were pointing at and laughing at me, I thought how funny, and it became funny for me too."
(6) *Courage and silent strength.*
"Doing the best you can under the circumstances."
"Regaining inner space to move again and start over."
"Willing to make sacrifices for the good in the long run."
"We got along without it before, we can do without it again."
"When my handsome brother and beautiful sister and my mother called me 'Pokey Ha Ha' I used to kick and fight back; but then I learned to just sit there but I would go somewhere else in my mind."
"My mother laughed at herself and had a marvelous sense of humor. But as kids we saw her cry at night as she got everything ready for us to go to school the next day; my father was alcoholic and left the family for a long time. My mother had a silent strength, she needed a sense of humor to get through all that she had to deal with."
(7) *Magnanimity.*
"Choosing to live for purposes larger than your own self."
"Seeing the positive side instead of the negative in life."
"Having a sense of resilience in meeting challenges or even danger."
"Having an optimistic point of view on life, believing things will get better."
"Being at peace with yourself."
"It's your own philosophy of mind to laugh at yourself."

"Laughing at your own frailties and mistakes lets other people know they can make a mistake too."

"It helps others know how to adjust to a difficult situation and that it's OK."

"I survive long boring meetings by doodling; then at the end of the meeting share humorous poems at the conference that put everything in its context of absurdity and everyone enjoys laughing at themselves."

"Having a survivor attitude toward the big picture of life; not just coping day to day."

"Living with your life circumstances is not as burdensome or overwhelming when I laugh at myself but is contagious and helps other people discover their own joys."

"Sometimes when I think of things in my life and how everything has worked out, I have joy bubble up inside and I feel peaceful. I want to share it with other people who have a hard time finding any joy in their lives."

"Laughing at myself is very important to me; even more important for my future."

The above expressions illuminate the meanings near and dear to the participants' hearts. It was after sharing these initial insights that participants began to describe in greater detail situations of laughing at oneself as a child, young adult, or older adult, and in comparison to relatives whom they thought knew how to laugh at themselves. Expanded narratives including their actions, attitudes, feelings, and thoughts in the context of other life events began to unfold. Narratives expressed the variety of ways a multidimensional world was experienced in the lives of senior citizens. The following excerpts manifest several of the above themes in the fabric of their lived world.

Bob recalled an experience from his high school days:

> Looking back at our football scores and write-ups at high school reunion time, the funniest thing was that we sure weren't the athletes we thought we were back then; we got creamed about every game. Time has changed our perspective on our own importance. When you're that age though, things are real important . . . You are real serious playing on a team.

The themes here are honesty, change in perspective of self-importance, and incongruity experienced as being funny. The contrast between adolescent and adult perspectives provided a variation on the theme.

Elise shared an insight from the context of her ethnic background.

As Norwegians we were very serious. When I was a small child, my mother had a group of female friends over for a party and after awhile I heard my mother laugh uproariously; it was so out of character for her that I was embarrassed and must have shown it on my face! Everyone was having a little sherry and she must have had a little too much, but one of the women came over to comfort me and said, 'It's all right! Your mother is just having a good time.'

Elise says she had to learn to laugh at herself and recalled the specific time when she felt it the first time. The last year of college!

I had a distinct feeling of just sort of sloughing off a lot of constraints, I had a sense of just opening up and life was fun. . . . My perspective was changing. I was beginning to see that you could do things for their own sake and not just because they were goals to achieve. . . . I could do things because they were fun. There was more to life than accomplishing tasks. For example, later as a mother I could enjoy things such as changing diapers while at the same time was able to spend time with parenting groups on how to raise children to be peacemakers. One activity had large consequences and the other didn't. It was a matter of keeping the balance.

Gail, a widow living in her own home, considered herself to be independent, yet was receiving chemotherapy for cancer of the bone. She began by saying she didn't know if she really laughed at herself but thought she did better than some people.

I don't take things as seriously as I did when I was a child or during college days. I figure, well, things will work out some way. Because it doesn't do much good to do it otherwise. It makes you unhappy and you don't have to be unhappy if you don't want to be; but if its gonna help in the long run, why, you put up with it.

Gail is a person who has, at least within the context of the situation, particular interests and concerns. She is past president of the regional American Association of Retired Persons (AARP). At this time in her life she knew what to care about and trusted this inner wisdom as expressed in her actions and choices. She conveyed a sense of confidence, honesty about herself in the world, and even an air of free abandon.

New questions prompted by the participant's narratives led to further clarification. The following is an excerpt from Patricia's response to the question of how she usually responded to frustration. She described an incident which revealed earnestness of purpose, physical inability to fulfill a task, shift of insight followed by laughing at herself, resilience and resolve, decisiveness to do something else, and the reason.

> I wanted to learn how to pick chile. I went only about a half a row and that was it for me because I couldn't handle it. I think it was because I wasn't experienced in how to pick it and I was left behind. I didn't get angry: I gave up! Yes, I laughed at myself and I gave up! I said this is not for me. I'll just go to the store and buy it!

Thus, six perspectives were expressed in Patricia's narrative. The meaning of laughing at oneself emerged from these perspectives and indicated that she knew what to care about, trusted it, and acted by making a choice not to care about her original goal. A certain abandon and freedom characterized her next choice.

Kaye shared the meaning of laughing at oneself in the following narrative. "When I laugh at myself, it shows that most of the time you have done something not necessarily wrong but maybe foolish or stupid or silly, you don't laugh at yourself if you're having a heart attack." The appropriateness of laughing at oneself involves a sense of realism and seeing oneself in perspective.

Kenneth shared the following insight about laughing at oneself that expresses its link with self-respect and a sense of realism. "We should not treat ourselves frivolously. Frivolity is not laughing at oneself. I think there is a sense of realism in treating ourselves with some importance; that our image of the world corresponds with the real world whatever it is. If we respect ourselves then we can really laugh at ourselves and the world." Kenneth had the habit of doodling to survive boring meetings. His wife said that he has become famous for standing up at the end of a conference and reading a funny poem about what everybody has said (comical observations). He sort of turns everybody's ideas, accurately reflecting them, but putting them in their context of absurdity. These became ballads. Everyone could then laugh at themselves and put the whole conference into perspective. This included not giving too much importance to honors received. For example, after receiving an honorary degree from Cambridge, Kenneth spontaneously wrote the following verse:

> Contemplating works of Marx
> My inner mental watchdog barks

and even turns into a snarl
For Groucho's much more fun than Karl.

The verse was translated and read to everyone in Latin! Kenneth said the whole event "was hilarious!"

This example conveys the close relationship between laughing at oneself, self-respect, and realism. Magnanimity, spontaneity and surprise, acceptance of incongruity, and decisiveness were present in this slice of life.

Finally, the following narrative concludes with the entwined lives of two female friends who were mirror opposites of each other. Self-preservation was the common underlying theme expressed in their stories, but each chose different means to survive adversity in their lives. Laughing at oneself had very different meanings for them initially, but transformation of perspectives was observed within the interview itself.

Mary, an author esteemed in her discipline and now learning how to play the harp in her 70th year, related the childhood experience of "being laughed at by my handsome brother, beautiful sister, and mother who called me 'Pokey Ha Ha' because I was short, fat, and slow." Mary said

> I didn't laugh at myself because that would have been laughing with them at me; I would have joined them in their ridicule, discounting my own value; I couldn't, out of a sense of self-preservation. At first I would kick and fight back, but then I learned to just stay put bodily while I would go somewhere else in my mind.

The phrase laughing at oneself here distinguished between Mary's body and her very self-worth as a person. Ultimately, Mary's action was laughing with herself by shifting her attention away from the threatening laughter directed at her by her family. With silent strength she learned to preserve her self-worth, which was more important to her than the appearance and performance of her body. Adversity was met by shifting perspective according to a decision based on knowing what was important to care about.

Mary also experienced a transformation in the meaning of the phrase "laughing at oneself" as she listened to the story told by her partner. Andy described herself as being "four foot nothing" and reflected "Short people have a hard time being taken seriously. I needed to feel respected and not ignored or laughed at; so I would introduce myself as 'The Hobbit' and gave people the permission, so to speak, to laugh *with* me before they could laugh *at* me. It made them feel at ease because I felt at ease with my own shortness." Andy had learned to laugh at herself very early in life in order "to survive and get beyond my limitations to what life was all about." She knew what to care about: Herself, the "elf within the self." She was creative and resilient in her choices. Instead of relying on silent strength, Andy's inner wisdom led to reaching beyond herself with a confidence that enabled others to see her as she was. Yes, as incongruent physically, but as a person with self-worth. Andy was someone who was to be taken seriously. Her magnanimous personality was convincing to Mary who couldn't believe what had just happened in the interview process. With awe Mary turned to her partner and said "Thank you for that insight! I never saw myself this way before. Laughing at myself *has* always been an important part of my life."

DISCUSSION

Knowing what to care about in life is characteristic of senior citizens, who in this study shared stories about the importance laughing at oneself has had in their lives. Survival attitudes, lived through hardship and ruthless honesty about themselves and their place in the world, were generously described with a refreshing lightness of heart. A sense of contagious abandon accompanied their descriptions of choices and actions made during adverse life events inherent in such historical events as the Depression, First and Second World Wars, Korean conflict, loss of loved ones, catastrophic illnesses, and the like. The telling of these experiences was free of disguise or pretense, and actually conveyed a feeling of pride and personal strength for not simply "getting through" the event by a series of coping strategies, but by doing so with magnanimous foresight and creativity.

The benefits to the participants as they perceived them were of an enlarging, enduring quality; they were still reaping the benefits of having the ability to laugh at themselves. For example, confidence in their personal wisdom, and strength, and clarity of vision to size up situations and life events empowered them to put things in perspective and to make critical decisions. No guilt or regret about past decisions seemed to linger over into their present lives. Further, the importance of knowing what to care about in their own lives had more than personal benefit. The lives of the participants gave generous evidence of being full and purposeful. In the context of their lives each knew their own identity: who they were in the scheme of history. They did not give themselves excessive importance, but with self-respect laughed at the world while being able to take the world very seriously.

Recall that many participants in the study had been nominated by their peers as being leaders in the local community or publicly recognized in their professions or society. All were to some degree actively involved in organizations, social responsibilities, and daily recreational activities. Some included national and world travel on a regular basis.

CONCLUSIONS

Knowing what to care about is a type of wisdom that characterizes the survival and self-preservation choices people make, especially in a pattern of life heavily fraught with adversity and many years of unexpected losses and tragedies. Surprisingly, the clue to this wisdom was the phrase laughing at oneself and its meaning to persons with many years of experience living independently in their own homes.

Having a transcendent life perspective is characteristic of the senior citizens in this study. Memories recalled were from childhood, youth, and early adulthood. Meanings of their experiences in the present senior years were described, as well as anticipations of possibilities in the future. Together these perspectives were varied and evoked diverse, yet enduring, features in the meaning of laughing at oneself. The major summative theme derived from the study illuminated the presence of a remarkable wisdom: The meaning of laughing at oneself in persons with many years of experience is knowing what to care about in life and choosing to trust it and live by it, spontaneously and deliberately. Knowing what to care about is foundational to balancing self-preservation activities and relational responsibilities.

IMPLICATIONS FOR FUTURE RESEARCH AND NURSING PRACTICE

Health defined as knowing what to care about and making choices out of wisdom, especially over time from childhood to later adulthood, has salient implications for natural caring modalities, nursing practice of enhancing the use of self in healing, and the realization of human potential. The questions that remain for future research and theory development reach beyond what was expected.

For example, if life histories were included in health histories, much relevant information could be available for anticipatory guidance, sharing, and joint decision making between nurse and client. Specifically, a history of the ability to laugh at oneself in times of unexpected loss, tragedy, or illness, or in contrast, the ability to survive hardship in resourceful, resilient, and even magnanimous ways, can provide indices of personal strengths and health potential to forge ahead to meet similar life events now and in the future. Consistent with the findings of this study, future research is warranted on the influence of trust and optimism on patterns of survival. Is there reason to believe the wisdom of knowing what to care about is an enduring wisdom of embodiment that can be relied upon to meet ever new challenges in living, aging, and dying? What is the role of laughing at oneself in preserving life through all of its evolving forms?

A study of non-leaders in the community with the same design and methodology could illuminate the relevance of social responsibility to the development of the ability to laugh at oneself. Several narratives gave evidence that laughing at oneself could be learned, and suggestions were offered for teaching children how to laugh at themselves when they take themselves too seriously. Research on the learning experiences of persons who never learned to laugh at themselves compared to those who learned later in life to laugh at themselves could provide important knowledge for health enhancement programs. What is the origin and nurturance of laughing at oneself?

Laughing at oneself in persons living with chronic illness such as HIV or rheumatoid arthritis represent embodied situations of adversity requiring enormous personal strength. If self-preservation and survival attitudes are foundational to laughing at oneself in senior citizens, what is the potential resource available to survivors of tragic illnesses that can be fostered in communities of caring? Further qualitative research is recommended to address these relationships. Perhaps forecasting patterns of life choices through unexpected life events would be enhanced by using laughing at oneself as a clue.

Relative to theory development, can laughing at oneself be a manifestation of pattern-seeing in the midst of adversity and diversity of life events? The theory of change in Rogerian nursing science could be advanced by research on the nature of the "shift of focus", or perspective in life which is characteristic of laughing at oneself in this study. The significance of being able to recognize what is essential to one's life, while letting go of destructive fixations, seems promising based on the findings in this study which associate such an ability with survival skills through tragedy and personal loss of various intensities.

This study, which focused on the meaning of laughing at oneself in senior citizens, has presented some of the features of an oxymoron. Laughing at oneself, among other things, is a profound wisdom and ability with incredible worth.

REFERENCES

American Nurses' Association. (1980). *Social policy statement*. Kansas City, MO: Author.

Barrett, E. (1989). *Visions of Rogers' science-based nursing*. New York: National League for Nursing.

Bloch, S., Browning, S., & McGrath, G. (1983). Humour in group psychotherapy. *British Journal of Medical Psychology, 56*, 89–97.

Brady, P.F. (1986). Mental health of the aging. In B.S. Johnson (Ed.), *Psychiatric-mental health nursing: Adaptation and growth* (pp. 419–432). Philadelphia: Lippincott.

Chapman, A.J. (1983). Humor and laughter in social interaction and some implications for humor research. In P. McGhee & J.H. Goldstein (Eds.), *Handbook of Humor Research, Vol I, Basic Issues*. New York: Springer.

Clark, C.D. (1981). *Enhancing Wellness: A Guide for Self Care*. New York: Springer.

Coser, R.L. (1959). Some social functions of laughter: A study of humor in a hospital setting. *Human Relations, 12,*171–182.

Cousins, N. (1979). *Anatomy of an illness as perceived by the patient: Reflections on healing and regeneration*. New York: W.W. Norton.

Eastman, M. (1966). *Enjoyment of laughter*. New York: Harcourt.

Eble, K. (1966). *The perfect education*. New York: Macmillan.

Flynn, P.A.R. (1980). *Holistic health: The art and science of care*. Bowie, MD: Robert J. Brady Company.

Freud, S. (1960). Humor. In Strachey (Ed.), *The complete psychological works of Sigmund Freud* (161–166). London: Hogarth Press.

Fry, W. (1963). *Sweet madness: A study of humor*. Palo Alto: Pacific Books.

Fry, W. F., Jr. (1977). The respiratory components of mirthful laughter. *Journal of Biological Psychology, 19*(2),39–50.

Goldstein, J. H., & McGhee, P. E. (1956). *The psychology of humor. Theoretical perspectives and empirical issues*. New York: Intercontinental Medical Book Corporation.

Goodman, J. (1983). How to get more smileage out of your life: Making sense of humor, then serving it. In P.E. McGhee & J.H. Goldstein (Eds.), *Handbook of humor research*, Vol II (pp. 1–22). New York: Springer-Verlag.

Greig, J.Y.T. (1923). *The psychology of laughter and comedy*. London: Dodd, Mead & Co.

Grotjahn, M. (1957). *Beyond laughter*. New York: McGraw-Hill.

Gurwitsch, A. (1966). The phenomenological and the psychological approach to consciousness. In A. Gurwitsch (Ed.), *Studies in Phenomenology and Psychology*. Evanston, IL: Northwestern University Press.

Henry, B.M., Moody, L.E. (1985). Energize with laughter. *Nursing Success Today*, 2 (1):4–8, 36.

Hertzler, J. O. (1970). *Laughter: A socio-scientific analysis.* New York: Exposition Press.

Hill, L., Smith, N. (1985). *Self Care Nursing.* Englewood Cliffs, NJ: Prentice-Hall.

Holland, N.N. (1983). *Laughing: A psychology of humor.* Ithaca: Cornell University.

Hultsch, D.F., Deitsch, F. (1981). *Adult development and aging: A lifespan perspective.* New York: McGraw-Hill.

Husserl, E. (1970). *Crisis of european science* (D. Carr, Trans.). Evanston, IL: Northwestern University Press.

Jackson, H.J., & King, N.J. (1982). The therapeutic management of an autistic child's phobia using laughter as the anxiety inhibitor. *Behavioural Psychotherapy*, 10:364–369.

LeShan, L. (1977). *You can fight for your life: Emotional factors in the treatment of cancer.* New York: M. Evans & Co.

Lorenz, K. (1936). *On Aggression.* New York: Harcourt.

Luce, G. G. (1979). *Your second life: Vitality and growth in middle and later years.* New York: Dell.

McDougall, W. (1960). *Social psychology.* New York: Barnes & Noble.

McGhee, P.E., & Goldstein, J.H. (Eds.). (1983). *Handbook of humor research* (Vol. II). New York: Springer-Verlag.

Mindess, H. (1971a). *Laughter and liberty.* Los Angeles: Nash.

Mindess, H. (1971b). The sense in humor. *Saturday Review*, 10–12.

Mindess, H. (1976). The use and abuse of humor in psychotherapy. In A.J. Chapman & H.D. Foot (Eds.). *Humour and laughter: Theory, research, and applications* (331–341). New York: John Wiley & Sons.

Morreall, J. (1983). *Taking laughter seriously.* Albany: SUNY Press.

Newman, M. (1986). *Health as expanding consciousness.* St. Louis, MO: Mosby.

Paterson, J., & Zderad, L. (1971). *Humanistic nursing.* New York: John Wiley & Sons.

Paterson, R.D., & Abrahams, R.B. (1982). Providing services to the elderly. In H.D. Schulberg, & M. Killilea (Eds.), *The Modern Practice of Community Mental Health* (334–357). San Francisco: Jossey-Bass.

Peter, L.J., & Dana, B. (1982). *The laughter prescription.* New York: Ballantine.

Peterson, J.P., & Pollio, H.R. (1982). Therapeutic effectiveness of differentially targeted humorous remarks in group psychotherapy. *Group,* 6(4),39–50.

Piddington, R. (1963). *The psychology of laughter: A study in social adaptation.* New York: Gamut Press.

Plessner, H. (1970). *Laughing and crying.* Evanston: Northwestern University Press.

Potter, R. E., & Goodman, N.J. (1983). The implementation of laughter as a therapy facilitator with adult aphasics. *Journal of Communication Disorders, 16,*41–48.

Prerost, F.J. (1983). Locus of control and aggression inhibiting effects of aggressive humor appreciation. *Journal of Personality Assessment, 47,* 294–299.

Reeder, F. (1984). *Nursing research, holism, and philosophies of science: Points of congruence between M.E. Rogers and Edmund Husserl.* Dissertation No. 84–21466: New York University.

Reeder, F., & Malinski, V. (1988). *The meaning of the experience of laughing at oneself: State of the art in literature search.* Unpublished Manuscript, University of Colorado.

Robinson, V.M. (1978). Humor in nursing. In C.E. Carlson & B. Blackwell (Eds.), *Concepts and nursing intervention (2nd Ed.)* (pp. 191–210). Philadelphia: Lippincott.

Robinson, V.M. (1983). Humor and health. In P.E. McGhee & J.H. Goldstein (Eds.), *Handbook of Humor Research (Vol. II)* (pp. 109–128). New York: Springer-Verlag.

Rogers, M.E., (1970). *An introduction to the theoretical basis of nursing.* Philadelphia: F. A. Davis.

Schaier, A.H., & Cicirelli, V.G. (1976). Age differences in humor comprehension and appreciation in old age. *Journal of Gerontology, 31,* 577–582.

Scogin, F.R., & Merbaum, M. (1983). Humorous stimuli and depression: An examination of Beck's premise. *Journal of Clinical Psychology, 39,* 165–169.

Watson, J. (1985). *Nursing: Human science and human care.* Norwalk, CT: Appleton-Century-Crofts.

Ziv, A. (1984). *Personality and sense of humor.* New York: Springer.

19

Practice Or Perish:
A Faculty Practice Innovation

Sally A. Forsstrom and Joanne E. Gray

Nurses employed in tertiary education are familiar with the idea that in terms of academic development one must publish or perish (Joachim, 1988). In terms of demonstrating academic leadership in teaching and/or research, publication of work is vital for recognition by the discipline and recognition by the employer for promotion (Moore, 1989). With the recent development of clinical career structures in Australia, nurses employed in practice are also expected to conduct research and publish results for the benefit of the profession (Gaston, 1989). Nurse academics must "practice or perish" (Forsstrom & Gray, 1989). Practice is viewed as a means to facilitate the development of nursing theory, and hence contribute to the development of the discipline of nursing. Nurse academics must practice in order to explore the process of caring. "A science of caring seeks to understand how health and illness problems relate to human behavior and how human behaviors influence health-illness outcomes" (Watson, 1981, p. 61). Faculty practice will contribute to the development of the unique role of the nurse and will energize teaching and so contribute to the development of both the discipline and the profession. This paper explores a model for faculty practice developed at a university in a rural setting, demonstrating how faculty practice can integrate the many roles of an academic: theory development, teaching, research, professional commitment, and publication. It is argued that negotiating a faculty practice in a particular academic setting and a given context of health care delivery, allows for the development of a collegiality between nurses in both settings which facilitates collaborative research that will further develop nursing knowledge. Engaging in faculty practice has implications for many issues related to the development of an academic career, e.g., having practice recognized for promotion and progression within the university, developing nursing theory from practice, and developing the profession of nursing (Stainton, Rankin, & Calkin, 1989).

FACULTY PRACTICE: WHAT IS IT?

The nursing literature contains considerable debate on the nature of faculty practice. Algase (1986) argues that faculty practice refers to a particular role for the nurse academic that allows practice to be a scholarly activity. This practice demonstrates "a mature recognition of the accountability of the discipline to the profession of nursing; it is evidence of an understanding of our nature, purpose and destiny as a clinical discipline, a professional discipline and an applied discipline."

Faculty practice is a means of developing nursing theory grounded in the real world of nursing. Faculty practice is an expression of the critical paradigm where

> The theorist-practitioner aims at raising their own and others consciousness through collaboratively analysing and seeking understandings of the real situation, and to search out for alternative ways of seeing the situation. This paradigm involves a dialectic transaction between theory and practice and therefore welds the two together [Pearson, 1989].

The focus of faculty practice is the development of knowledge related to the caring process. Faculty practice is more than an opportunity for academics to maintain clinical competence, being defined as

> those functions performed by faculty in a service setting that have as their principal goal the continued advancement of the nursing care of clients, a goal congruent with the role of an academician in a professional discipline [Lambert & Lambert, 1988, p. 57].

The following literature review will analyze the various interpretations of the concept of faculty practice, emphasizing that practice is an integral part of academic activity. The discussion of the issues arising from faculty practice will identify that opposition to the concept of faculty practice arises from the continuing influence of the positivist paradigm, in which the theory development role of the academic is seen as appropriate to an academic setting and not a clinical one. In the positivist view, faculty practice is an added on, optional role, not an integral role of the academic.

LITERATURE REVIEW

Definition

A review of the Australian (Emden, 1986 & Crane, 1989) and international (Davis & Tomney, 1982; Hollingsworth 1989; Salvage, 1983; Stainton, Rankin, & Calkin 1989; Van Ort, 1985) nursing literature indicates that since the 1970s there has been increasing interest in the concept of faculty practice, yet there is a lack of agreement about the concept. Most writers have developed a definition from a literature review, or from surveying academics (Just, Adams, & De Young, 1989). Stainton et al. view the following as the hallmarks of faculty practice:

1. the approach to human experiences with actual or potential health problems reflects depth and breadth in current knowledge, clinical curiosity and salience.

2. it includes research both in application and research activity.

3. it generates published case studies, reports on intervention issues or problems resolved.

4. it generates changes in care delivery [1989, p. 24].

In reviewing this list, one might argue against Stainton et al. (1989) that faculty involved in clinical teaching are engaging in faculty practice and that, therefore, clinical teaching is a form of faculty practice (Collison & Parsons, 1980). Littlefield, Keenan, and Skillman (1988) have reported the difficulty of achieving the goals of faculty practice while concurrently teaching graduate students. Providing care for clients, without the responsibility of supervising student caring, was argued as an essential component of faculty practice.

To define a faculty practice, the following criteria proposed by Stainton et al. (1989) are useful: "operant with a formalized agreement; focused on care of clients; research activity as an outcome of caring for clients and teaching as an outcome of caring for clients."

In negotiating faculty practice with the nurses in the clinical area, the activity of caring for clients is viewed as the central activity, with all academic activities viewed as arising from this caring. This is consistent with the view of nursing as a caring process.

The goals of faculty practice defined in the literature include the following:

1. identifying tangible examples of excellence in nursing care [Littlefield et al., 1988];
2. generating nursing theory from practice (Denyes, O'Connor, Oakley, & Ferguson, 1989);
3. facilitating faculty research;
4. minimizing faculty and clinical costs (Littlefield et al., 1988);
5. giving credibility to the professional role of nursing in a medical center in which all other professionals conduct research or clinical practice in addition to teaching (Cook & Finelli, 1988);
6. improving the quality of student outcomes, e.g., education for nurses must meet emerging needs of clients; faculty practice should prevent serious gaps and deficits in care (Cook & Finelli, 1988);
7. demonstrating clinical practice as a credible criterion for progression and promotion in the university (Moore, 1989).

Models for Faculty Practice

Hollingsworth (1989) argues that a nurse who teaches nursing must be both a professional academic and a practitioner of nursing. Several models are analyzed, identifying the impact of faculty practice on the nursing profession, the consumer, and society.

Stainton et al. (1989) also describe several models of faculty practice, with minor variations from Hollingsworth: unification (practitioner-teacher), with joint administration of the clinical agency and school (Rush Presbyterian University, University of Rochester); collaboration (clinician-educator), with separate administration of the school and the clinical agency, but all faculty holding joint appointments (Case Western Reserve University, USA; McMaster University, Canada); integration (private practice), in which the school of nursing creates a non-traditional health care setting where faculty and students provide direct nursing care (Pennsylvania State University, University of Wisconsin–Milwaukee); private practice, where the faculty individually negotiate practice in an inpatient or outpatient setting (University of Tennessee); and the Calgary Model (University of Calgary), which focuses on faculty practice as scholarship. The negotiation model presented in this paper involves individual negotiation between the faculty member and the clinical area where the faculty will provide nursing care as part of his or her academic role. The literature strongly supports the individual negotiation of faculty practice.

Australian writers have identified joint appointments (Crane, 1989; Emden, 1986) and faculty practice days (Taylor, 1988), while British writers discuss similar initiatives in a variety of practice settings (Fasano, 1981; Piggott & Gough, 1989; Wright, 1988). The literature demonstrates a diversity of faculty practice models, demonstrating a strong trend toward faculty practice being considered essential for the continued growth of the discipline and the profession. This trend represents the changing view of nursing knowledge as described by Pearson (1989).

As identified by Stainton et al. (1989), faculty practice does not include: "volunteerism (or moonlighting; consultation only; conducting research in a clinical setting; or teaching of learners assigned to a clinical setting."

Volunteerism and moonlighting may result in scholarly work, but they lack the formalized commitment to a practice setting that can lead to collaboration with service staff in research and other activities to develop the discipline (Mills & Free, 1984). Consultation only may develop informally as an outcome of clinical teaching with students in a service setting (Johnson, 1980), or as an alternative to faculty practice where geographical constraints apply (Polifroni & Schmalenberg, 1985). As with moonlighting, scholarly work may arise from consultation with nursing practitioners in the clinical area. It is argued, however, that unless the faculty member is involved in direct patient care, the activity is not faculty practice. This argument will be explored further in a discussion of the issues arising from faculty practice.

Facilitating Faculty Practice

The literature identifies a number of issues that impede or facilitate faculty practice. Lambert and Lambert (1989) explore one of the impediments frequently mentioned in the literature: the role conflict many academics experience between the roles associated with teaching in a university and the roles associated with practice. Smith (1980) also identifies the issue of role conflict and argues that the institution must support faculty in practice activities. Without administrative support (both faculty and clinical), it is difficult for individual academics to engage in faculty practice. The beliefs about nursing held by faculty may impede faculty practice; for example, faculty members are unlikely to be supportive if the philosophy of nursing devalues practice. If one views nursing as a process of caring, however, then faculty practice is essential for the continued development of nursing knowledge.

In planning faculty practice using the negotiation model, it is imperative to gain the support of both the academic and clinical administration. Through negotiation, supportive mechanisms for the individual academic can be planned to facilitate practice. The belief that practice is a scholarly activity helps to integrate the roles of the academic in the practice area. Faculty practice is not just a way to maintain clinical competence, but a means of developing and evaluating nursing knowledge. Therefore, practice is more than maintaining clinical skills as identified by Kuhn (1982): "I began to wonder whether I could really give an IM, monitor central venous pressure, or start an IV."

If nursing faculty or practitioners view faculty practice as focusing on clinical skills only, their support for the initiative may be limited, as the practice is for the personal needs of the academic. Viewing faculty practice as scholarly activity with outcomes that may be beneficial to the profession as a whole invites other nurses, faculty and practitioners, to contribute to the initiative, therefore inviting supportive behavior. The negotiation model discussed in this paper develops a supportive environment, faculty and clinical, as part of the negotiation procedure, thus maximizing support for the faculty practice role and reducing the potential for role conflict.

Issues that facilitate faculty practice include recognition of faculty practice in criteria for academic progression and promotion (Kuhn, 1982). Free and Mills (1985) argue for a private practice model because the negotiation of the practice rests with the faculty member and so can facilitate consideration of activities that will meet the criteria of promotion committees. In this model, the practice generates income, which may influence the administration to view it as a valid use of faculty time. Maurin's (1986) study of nursing services provided by schools of nursing found that for 43 percent of the respondents, funding for the project was inadequate, with only 33 percent of projects funded by client fees and 18 percent through insurance reimbursement. In Australia, where it is far more difficult to obtain payment for independent nursing practitioner services, a private practice model would appear to be difficult to negotiate.

As argued by Stainton et al. (1989), university faculty are evaluated for their teaching, research, and community participation. Therefore, if faculty are involved in clinical teaching, this is evaluated in the area of the teaching mission of the school; consultation is evaluated in terms of community involvement; and research arising from faculty practice or generated from other sources is evaluated using research criteria. Faculty practice is expected to be consistent with advanced nursing practice (Calkin, 1984) and is related to the three broad missions of any university.

THE NEED FOR FACULTY PRACTICE

The perceived need for faculty practice at Charles Sturt University, Riverina has arisen from the following issues.

Teaching

The traditional role of nurse educators in Australia has changed since the move of nurse education into the tertiary sector. Prior to the move, nurse educators worked in a school that was located close to a clinical facility, and they had access to the clinical area to conduct research in teaching and to be involved in clinical teaching. Nurse educators are now physically isolated, in most cases, from the clinical area. Since teaching in a university is expected to be research based, there is a felt deficit in teaching nursing from the literature. By engaging in faculty practice, the faculty will focus on the nature of nursing and use reflective practice techniques to develop an understanding of nursing (Agan, 1987; Boud, Keough, & Walker, 1985; Clarke, 1986; Taylor, 1988, Thompson, 1987). It is believed that such a process will enrich teaching, just as initiatives such as those at McGill University have enriched the theoretical base of nursing using a practice-derived model (Gottleib & Rowat, 1987).

The quality of teaching has implications not only for meeting the mission of the university, but for meeting the teacher's obligation to the nursing students, who not only require experiences to develop a theoretical body of knowledge, but require preparation for professional practice. Following regular interaction in the clinical area, the teacher may implement the planned curriculum in a way that is cognizant of the current demands on the profession for the delivery of care. The influence of critical social theory in developing nursing knowledge (Speedy, 1989), and the work of Benner (1982, 1984) on intuitive knowing, have relevance to the way the student develops nursing knowledge that is relevant to the needs of the community (Hagell, 1989; McMurray, 1989; Webb, 1989). Perry (1985) questions whether nurses "think nursing," and argues that nurses should "begin to incorporate the three functional areas of nursing (teaching, research, and practice) into one nursing role so that gaps between these three sectors of the nursing knowledge system will cease to exist."

In nurse education in Australia, how many academics teach a view of nursing that has not been personally implemented in practice? Faculty practice has the potential for such integration of theory and practice. In Australia this has been achieved at the Deakin University School of Nursing, where the transformative curriculum requires collegiality among students, lecturers, and clinicians, who are all students of the discipline of nursing. Development of the discipline is seen as requiring "successful integration of theoretical thinking, research and creative practice" (Perry & Moss, 1988).

This approach requires a practicing faculty and underlies the benefits of faculty practice to the teaching role.

Criteria for Promotion and Progression
in the University

For promotion and progression in the university, it is important for nurse academics to not only research and publish, but also practice. The academic isolation that has occured with the move of nursing to the tertiary sector has seen many nursing faculties give only "lip-service" to the importance of clinical practice. Many faculties state that they feel recent clinical practice is essential, and should be undertaken by nurse academics, but how many faculties encourage and support nurse academics to undertake clinical practice? How many ensure that they only employ academics with credible clinical experience? How many consider that clinical experience is an important criterion for academic promotion? The authors argue that this negation of the importance of clinical practice for nurse academics represents the influence of the positivist paradigm in academic institutions (Pearson, 1989). It is argued that nurse academics have expended considerable energy in the development of the discipline of nursing according to positivist rules. Consequently, there has been little time and energy allocated for clinical practice.

Nurse academics are in a difficult position in Australia. Many have gone into tertiary institutions on lower salaries than their colleagues in other faculties because, on appointment, their years of clinical service in nursing were not considered as important as their academic qualifications. As academic qualifications in nursing were fairly scarce in Australia in the 1970s and 1980s (many nurses had only just begun a bachelors degree), nurse academics were placed at low levels of appointment with the criteria for promotion or progression being a higher degree, research, and publications (Robinson, 1990). Therefore, with most nurse academics having to meet these criteria, where is the time and energy for clinical practice? The argument of this paper is that clinical practice as a scholarly activity should form criteria for academic promotion and progression. According to the positivist rules, nurse academics could develop nursing knowledge from their university armchairs; however, with the acceptance of the critical paradigm by nursing academics, the focus for the development of nursing knowledge has return to the clinical area. An important need for the development of a faculty practice model is to demonstrate that an integrated faculty practice meets the criteria for academic promotion and progression.

Faculty practice is not an afterthought of nuisance value for a busy nurse academic, but a necessary means of keeping in touch with the reality of nursing to generate nursing knowledge that is meaningful to the profession.

Gender Issues

An important issue underlying the need for faculty practice is that nursing practice is viewed as "women's work," and as such, is undervalued by our technological society. From the positivist perspective, nursing is an extension of the role of women in the family caring for others. While this is a valued contribution to society, it does not have any recognition as a source of scientific knowledge. Nursing is a female-dominated profession in terms of numbers employed. The 1981 Australian census showed that 93 percent of nurses were female. Willis (1988) asserts that

> Historically, nursing has been viewed as women's work, and traditionally the skill which nurses applied has been defined in feminine terms. While nurses themselves have moved well beyond this, I think that there is a fairly widespread community perception along these lines [p. 71].

How does this perception of nursing as "women's work" affect the notion of nursing as a scholarly activity? Spender (Barclay, 1986) feels that:

> Having been initiated into a male dominated society, they (women) have been well instructed in the art of women devaluation, and if they have learnt their lessons well women will have emerged with their confidence undermined, their assurance dissolved and their sense of self debased [p. 125].

Willis gives some enlightenment of this topic by quoting Feelgood in *Australian Hospital* (May 1986):

> In those days, the good old days, a nurse knew her place, obedience was a religion and the doctor's word was final. You may call me old-fashioned, but I believe a good nurse is an obedient nurse, she should follow her instructions to the letter and should never question or challenge a doctor [Willis, 1988, p. 71].

From this history of the caring nurse in a subservient role to the male medical scientist, has arisen the dilemma of trying to establish oneself as a practitioner with equal merit. Thus, one of the challenges and one of the reasons there is a need for faculty practice is to demonstrate the unique role of the nurse as a carer in the provision of health services.

A FACULTY PRACTICE INNOVATION

Two faculty members of Charles Sturt University, Riverina designed a program that allowed faculty practice at a local base hospital for one day a week. This particular faculty practice is based on the negotiation model, since it was independently organized with academic and hospital administrators to fit both the development needs of the faculty members and the particular needs of the nursing practitioners at the hospital. It is similar to the private practice model as defined by Mills and Free (1984), but there is no reimbursement to the school and no negotiation for payment for service delivered during the course of faculty practice. Faculty have negotiated the right to engage in care for their personal and professional development, with the formal agreement of the service administration, but with no financial reimbursement. It is interesting to note that in the study by Maurin (1986) on nursing services developed by schools of nursing, that 42 percent of the projects were initiated by faculty, suggesting that faculty and service administrators may best facilitate faculty practice by supporting the initiatives of individual faculty members.

Whether faculty should receive payment for faculty practice is an issue that will be discussed below. However, requesting payment for services provided to the clinical institution in caring for clients may create an organizational block to faculty practice (Beattie, 1989), particularly in the Australian health care system, since nurses are rarely seen as a fee-for-service practitioner, rather as a service provider within an organizational framework.

Stainton et al. (1989) argue that faculty practice must be negotiated to develop: "a 'fit' between the growth of a faculty member's advanced practice focus, teaching and research requirements and that of service setting opportunities and needs." A regular evaluation is required to assess whether the needs of faculty and the service setting are met by the practice model.

DEFINING THE ISSUES RELATED TO FACULTY PRACTICE

Any implementation of faculty practice involves a consideration of the issues related to faculty development in general: industrial, economic, political, professional, and gender.

Industrial

As an employee, an academic has duties and responsibilities to the institutional employer, and the employer has responsibilities to the employee. Speedy (1987) describes an Australian study on the critical issues for consideration in the development of nursing faculty: socialization, faculty role delineation and development, career development, and gender, concluding that: "Heads of nursing programs confirmed the importance of socialization and faculty role delineation and development, but accorded less importance to career planning and development and gender."

Faculty practice has implications for socialization and faculty role delineation. The philosophy of the school of nursing will influence the value placed on faculty practice, as the beliefs about nursing and education will value practice, or value practice differently from research and/or scholarly publication.

Junior faculty will find it difficult to initiate faculty practice if it is undervalued in relation to the teaching or research mission of the university. Therefore, a nurse considering an academic appointment should obtain information about the school of nursing philosophy prior to the interview. If the administration of the nursing faculty delineates the academic's role as primarily a teacher and a researcher, and places more importance on these functions as discrete roles, rather than being incorporated in faculty practice, new faculty members with a clinical background may develop role conflict if they attempt to maintain discrete practice roles. This problem is identified by Lambert and Lambert (1989) in their review of research on role conflict in nurses involved in faculty practice. This paper argues that the employer has responsibilities to the employee to facilitate professional activities that will lead to the development of an academic career, not just to socialize new and ongoing faculty into the teaching role of the university. This responsibility involves developing a faculty practice model that represents faculty practice as scholarly activity, not as a means of maintaining clinical skills.

Workload is cited by many writers on faculty practice as the major institutional factor that acts as a barrier to faculty development activities. For example, in the study by Lane et al. (1981), workload was cited as the single most frequent barrier to participation for all categories of faculty development activities: "it deterred 73% of the respondents from participating in independent professional activities, such as research, consultation clinical practice, and preparing professional papers or presentations."

New faculty, unfamiliar with the academic work environment, can easily be in the situation of having a heavy workload. These faculty may find difficulty in initiating research, publication, and conference attendance, while attempting to meet their new teaching commitments.

In this faculty innovation, practice was undertaken during teaching preparation and research time. There was no reduction in the semester teaching load. One of the concerns of colleagues expressed during a recent academic staff seminar (Forsstrom & Gray, 1989) was that pursuing a faculty practice day without a reduction in the teaching load, will result in an excessive workload and fatigue. Mills and Free (1984) identify over-commitment and burn-out as two difficulties that may arise following faculty practice with high teaching and research loads, and Van Ort (1985) argues that time commitment is one factor that is cited as an argument against faculty practice. This factor has been considered by the faculty at Deakin University, where the faculty practice day is considered as 20 percent of the teaching load (Taylor, 1988).

Workload is a factor that must be considered in the evaluation of this innovation. However, Stainton et al. (1989) argue that:

> practising faculty are highly efficacious in their use of time and resources. Instead of experiencing dissonance and tension between research, teaching and service, perhaps even in different settings, practising faculty use the practice as their base and integrator of these activities [p. 25].

This issue also highlights the importance of negotiating for faculty practice to meet the particular context of academic activity. For the trial period, faculty members have nominated one day a week for faculty practice. On this day there are no scheduled teaching commitments or meetings. Students and faculty are aware that on the nominated faculty practice day, the faculty members will not be at the university. Similarly, the nurses in the clinical institution will not expect faculty to practice at times other than the nominated day.

By clearly stating the definition of faculty practice during the negotiation period, it is hoped that faculty and practitioners will understand the nature of the activity, and similarly value the concept of engaging in direct patient care to develop nursing knowledge. As identified by Joel (1985):

> The origins of the nursing profession are deeply embedded in service agencies. After a period of denying these roots, we are now beginning to see the benefits of mutual support. The schism created over the years is real, and resistance is predictable in all but the most ideal situations [p. 221].

The benefit of negotiation is to identify resistance in faculty or clinicians, and encourage dialogue to overcome blocks and develop support. The workload may be heavy, but the work will be productive if the issues are clearly identified and discussed before faculty practice begins.

One issue of concern to some academics is the effect of faculty practice on the employment opportunities of casual clinical staff. It seems important for any negotiation of faculty practice to include industrial union representation to allow for the exploration of any industrial implications of faculty practice. Representatives of the industrial unions have been supportive of the initiative, and argue that the nursing unit managers are responsible for adequate staffing of the unit, so any industrial issues must be addressed at unit level. For example, there is some concern that unit staff will be transferred to a second unit with inadequate staffing on the faculty practice day. The responsibility to control this practice it is argued, rests with the unit manager (personal communication, Murray, R., October 18, 1989).

The advantages of increased collegiality between clinical and academic nurses are not just in the development of the discipline and the profession, but in the benefit to students. The time spent in faculty practice can promote a supportive atmosphere for students placed in the clinical institution for practicum (Hollingsworth, 1989). Time spent in faculty practice is indirectly related to the teaching role as it facilitates a supportive atmosphere for students on clinical practicum.

Economic

Reimbursement for service provided during faculty practice is one way to validate the workload involved, for example, Smith (1980) argues for a faculty practice reimbursement plan, similar to a medical practice plan. However, this argument is for a private practice model as defined above, and is not relevant to the Australian health system where nurses do not have insurance reimbursement rights. Indeed, this is one of the barriers to independent nursing practice in Australia (Keane, 1989). However, the private practice model is worth considering as a long-term goal for Australian academics. Nichols (1985) clearly identifies the beneficial outcome for the practitioner when the service has financial status: "The process of setting prices for one's services, collecting fees, and paying physician consultants makes everyone connected with a nurse-managed faculty practice feel differently about that practice."

The issue of reimbursement and fee determination for independent nurse practitioners is an important one that must be considered if the nurse academic chooses independent practice. The health system in Australia, like others, depends on its financial resources. The Health Issues Centre (1988) argues that the health system in Australia is funded according to a medical model. This model precludes any notion of health promotion and prevention but rather focuses on the biomedical paradigm (Health Issues Centre, 1988). "It is a familiar criticism of medical services that they operate within a biomedical model which is individualistic, curative, and mechanistic in its understanding of how health problems occur."

Willis (1988) states that: "Medical dominance is a phenomenon which has state support through Medicare rebates in the form of subsidy, and other health occupations do not." It is extremely difficult for independent nurse practitioners to establish their services within a health system that only recognizes those services provided within a biomedical framework.

In discussion of an independent midwifery practice, Fagin (1977) supports the importance of nursing care and suggests that: "the evidence is clear that the positive outcomes of nurse-midwifery practice are staggeringly impressive." It can be seen then, that independent midwives provide a service that is an effective alternative to the traditional medical model of care provided within our health system.

Independent nurse practitioners in Australia are left in a difficult position. They are unable to receive Medicare rebates for their services and are, therefore, unable to provide services to a wide group of consumers. This has direct implications for the negotiation of faculty practice. Littlefield et al. (1988) describe a faculty practice in the United States where academics work as individual practitioners in women's health. The hospital clinic paid 20 percent of each faculty practitioner's salary and benefits to the university, hence reducing university costs. The hospital reduced costs by obtaining the additional income generated above the amount paid to the university. This practice was possible only because the nursing faculty were paid by the clients.

Nurses must be aware of the health system as a whole and make efforts to reshape the health system from one in which their services are viewed as unnecessary, and not able to receive reimbursement, to a system that recognizes their unique skills. As Austin (1978) states: "Nursing can expand roles, change names, and develop new settings in which to work. . . . Yet nursing will be of no value unless we also become politically active in changing our . . . health . . . systems. . . . "

Consumer groups such as the Health Issues Centre (1988) have taken on the role of challenging the current health system in Australia. The nurse must also join in this challenge so that consumers in this system achieve the changes that are paramount in the development of an improved health system. If a nurse academic then should choose individual practice, these are major economic issues that will need to be considered.

Other forms of reimbursement are discussed in the literature: e.g., Kuhn (1982) proposes to spend 20 percent of faculty time: "in service to the health care facility, in exchange for 20 percent of selected staff nurses' time spent serving as preceptors for students in the clinical area." This practice is another difference between the health care systems in Australia and in the United States. The nursing students of Charles Sturt University-Riverina work with registered nurse preceptors in the practicum for their final semester. The registered nurses perform this function as part of their role, without extra payment.

Performance Evaluation of Faculty

The evaluation of faculty is a political issue in Australia today with the restructuring of higher education by the Department of Employment,

Education and Training (DEET). DEET is demanding of the academic industry increased productivity, i.e., increased student loads and increased graduation rates, in return for academic pay increases. One would, therefore, expect access to comprehensive faculty development activities to be facilitated by the institutional employer to develop the teaching skills of academics in order to meet the requirements of DEET. The issue becomes contentious, however, when it is implied that all academic staff will develop the same educational philosophies and consequent teaching methods, and that all academic staff will be assessed by an institutional authority without regard for these differences in philosophical approach. Should nurse academics be assessed in the same manner as academics from other disciplines (Crawford, 1988)? Should an academic in nursing be concerned with the graduation rate, or with the ability of the graduate to provide a service to the consumer in the health care system?

One of the arguments for faculty practice is the opportunity provided for the academic to take responsibility to influence nursing practice and the delivery of that practice (Kramer, Polifroni, & Organek, 1986). This argument may not be acceptable to an employer concerned only with the graduation rate, even though a commitment to the community served by the university is a stated mission of the institution. However, for adherents to the view of nursing as caring as expressed, there is no doubt that an academic must be concerned with the role of education in developing nurses able to meet the health care needs of the consumer. Faculty practice allows the academic to not only provide advanced nursing care to clients of the local health care system, but also facilitate change in the curriculum to allow students to develop the knowledge and skills relevant to the community's needs. Therefore, it is argued that faculty practice must be seen as a scholastic activity and as part of the role of an academic in nursing. One significant way to achieve this outcome with the employer in the higher education system is to generate publications from faculty practice (de Tornyay, 1988).

The concern with the graduation rate has implications for nurses in clinical practice concerned with nursing staff shortages. Current research (Battersby et al., 1989), however, suggests that the new graduates are staying in the health care system; it is the experienced nurses who are resigning. Therefore, it seems that a nursing staff shortage is not a valid reason to increase nursing graduation rates without concern for the preparation of the graduate to meet the challenges of health care in the 1990s.

An important issue for nurses following an academic career is the notion of academic promotion and progression. As noted above, one criterion is the extent of publication in the discipline. The literature states that faculty practice can be a scholarly activity, resulting in publication. It remains to be seen whether the academic progression and promotion committee at Charles Sturt University-Riverina will view faculty practice as a professional academic activity. Moore (1989), in a study of academic reward structures in six universities in the United States, identified that achievement criteria for promotion were not confined to teaching, but included research, quality and quantity of publication, and success in obtaining research grants. The challenge remains with practicing faculty to demonstrate the manner in which faculty practice meets the mission of the university in teaching, research, and commitment to the discipline (Stainton et al., 1989).

Gender Issues

Career planning is a gender issue well recognized by the unions representing academics in Australia; e.g., level of appointment of females in institutions of higher education is usually lower than males, and females are unaware of the importance of negotiating employment opportunities for career development (such as research and scholarly publication) (Drakeford, 1987). Lane et al. (1989) identify that the traditional academic model of faculty development has focused on male-dominated disciplines, therefore, gender receives priority in discussions of nursing faculty development: " . . . it is reasonable to expect that career patterns and faculty development needs in nursing—a predominantly female profession—will differ from those in male-dominated groups and that factors which act as barriers to ongoing faculty development will also differ."

Therefore, when planning for faculty practice, a long-term goal is to have this activity recognized as a vital part of faculty development, to be considered as a criteria for academic progression and promotion. Faculty practice as defined by Stainton et al. (1989) is scholarly practice, therefore, it may be included in the evaluation of faculty activity for promotion. This recognition must be won, however, in a male-dominated view of academic scholarship.

CONCLUSION

The rationale for faculty practice is well supported by the nursing literature. The negotiation model of faculty practice is one that may facilitate the integration of teaching, research, and practice in a manner that is congruent with a particular academic and clinical context. It is an exciting time in nursing with the literature giving scholarly credibility to the knowledge that can be developed from clinical practice. It is hoped that faculty practice as proposed in this paper will enrich the learning process for students in a way that will facilitate the critical, creative thinking required to provide nursing services to meet current health care challenges. For the academics who engage in faculty practice, it is believed that this activity is not only scholarly, but essential for the development of the discipline and the profession of nursing.

REFERENCES

Agan, R.D. (1987). Intuitive knowing as a dimension of nursing. *Advances in Nursing Science, 10*(1), 63–70.

Algase, D. (1986). Faculty practice: A means to advance the discipline of nursing. *Journal of Nurse Education, 25*(74), 74–76.

Austin, R. (1978). The nurse practitioner in health care. *International Nursing Review, 25*(3), 82–88.

Barclay, L. (1986). Midwifery: A case of misleading packaging? *Australian Journal of Advanced Nursing, 3*(3), 121–126.

Battersby, D., Kermode, S., van der Wal, J., Boylan, C., Kerr, R., & King, B. (1989). Nursing staff turnover in New South Wales hospitals. *Nursing Research Unit Monograph 1.* Wagga Wagga: Charles Sturt University-Riverina.

Benner, P. (1982, March) From novice to expert. *American Journal of Nursing, 402*–407.

Benner, P. (1984). *From novice to expert: Excellence and power in clinical nursing practice.* Menlo Park: Addison-Wesley.

Boud, D., Keogh, R., & Walker, D. (Eds.). (1985). *Reflection: Turning experience into learning.* London: Kogan Page.

Calkin, J.D. (1984). A model for advanced nursing practice. *The Journal of Nursing Administration, 14*(1), 24–30.

Clarke, M. (1986). Action and reflection: Practice and theory in nursing. *Journal of Advanced Nursing, 11*, 13–11.

Collison, C.R., & Parsons, M.A. (1980). Is practice a viable faculty role? *Nursing Outlook, 28*(11), 677–679.

Cook, S.S., & Finelli, L. (1988). Faculty practice: A new perspective on academic competence. *Journal of Professional Nursing, 4*, 24.

Crane, S. (1989). Joint appointments: The Deakin experience. *The Australian Journal of Advanced Nursing, 6*(3), 31–25.

Crawford, L.A. (1988). Peer evaluation: A component of faculty performance appraisal. *Journal of Nursing Education, 27*(8), 377–379.

Davis, L., & Tomney, P. (1982). The best of two worlds: An appraising look at joint appointments in Canada today. *The Canadian Nurse, 78*(8), 34–37.

Denyes, M.J., O'Connor, N.A., Oakley, D., & Ferguson, S. (1989). Integrating nursing theory, practice and research through collaborative research. *Journal of Advanced Nursing, 14*(2), 141–145.

de Tornyay, R. (1988). What constitutes scholarly activities? *Journal of Nursing Education, 27*(6), 245.

Drakeford, V.N. (1987). *EEO in higher education: Myth or reality?* Unpublished study, Kuring-gai College of Advanced Education, Lindfield, NSW, Australia.

Emden, C. (1986). Joint appointment: An Australian study illuminates world views. *The Australian Journal of Advanced Nursing, 3*(4), 30–41.

Fagin, C. (1977). Nursing as an alternative to high cost care. *American Journal of Nursing, 77*(11), 1799–1803.

Fasano, N. (1981). Joint appointments: Challenge for nursing. *Nursing Forum. 20*(1), 72–85.

Forsstrom, S., & Gray, J. (1989, November). *Practice or Perish.* Paper presented at academic seminar, School of Education, Charles Sturt University, Riverina, Wagga Wagga.

Free, T., & Mills, B.C. (1985). Faculty practice in primary care. *Nursing Outlook, 33*(4), 192–194.

Gaston, C. (1989). Inservice education: Career develoment for South Australian nurses. *The Australian Journal of Advanced Nursing, 6*(4), 5–9.

Gottlieb, L., & Rowat, K. (1987). The McGill model of nursing: A practice-derived model. *Advances in Nursing Science, 9*(4), 51–61.

Hagell, E.I. (1989). Nursing knowledge: Women's knowledge. A sociological perspective. *Journal of Advanced Nursing, 14*(3), 226–233.

Health Issues Centre. (1988). *What's wrong with the health system?* Melbourne: Health Issues Centre.

Hollingsworth, A.O. (1989). The evolvement of faculty practice. In C.E. Lambert & V.A. Lambert, (Eds.), *Perspectives in nursing: The impacts on the nurse, the consumer and society.* East Norwalk: Appleton and Lange.

Joachim, G. (1988). Faculty practice: Dilemmas and solutions. *Journal of Advanced Nursing, 13*, 410–415.

Joel, L. (1985). The Rutgers experience: One perspective on service-education collaboration. *Nursing Outlook, 33*(5), 220–224.

Johnson, J. (1980). The education/service split: Who loses? *Nursing Outlook, 28*(7), 412–515.

Just, G., Adams, E., & DeYoung, S. (1989). Faculty practice: Nurse educators' views and proposed models. *Journal of Nursing Education, 28*(4), 161–168.

Keane, B. (1989). Independent nurse consultants: The lateral leap. In G. Gray & R. Pratt (Eds.), *Issues in Australian nursing 2.* Melbourne: Churchill Livingstone.

Kramer, M., Polifroni, E.C., & Organek, N. (1986). Effects of faculty practice on student learning outcomes. *Journal of Professional Nursing, 2*(5), 289–301.

Kuhn, J.K. (1982). An experience with a joint appointment. *American Journal of Nursing, 82*(10), 1570–1571.

Lambert, C.E., & Lambert, V.A. (1988) A review and synthesis of the research on role conflict and its impact on nurses involved in faculty practice programs. *Journal of Nursing Education, 27*(2), 54–60.

Lane, E.B., Lagodna, G.E., Brooks, B.R., Long, N.J., Parsons, M.A., Fox, M.R., & Strickland, O.R. (1981). Faculty development activities. *Nursing Outlook, 29*(2), 112–118.

Littlefield, V.M., Keenan, C., & Skillman, L. (1988). Academically based practice: Seizing opportunities, enhancing outcomes. *Journal of Professional Nursing, 4*(5), 329–338.

Maurin, J.T. (1986). An exploratory study of nursing services provided by schools of nursing. *Journal of Professional Nursing, 2*(5), 277–281.

McMurray, A. (1989). Time to extend the 'process'? *The Australian Journal of Advanced Nursing, 6*(4), 40–43.

Mills, B.C., & Free, T.A. (1984, May-June) Nursing faculty practice. *Pediatric Nursing,* 212–214.

Moore, M. (1989). Tenure and the university reward structure. *Nursing Research, 38*(2), 111–116.

Nichols, C.W. (1985). The Yale nurse-midwifery practice: Addressing the outcomes. *Journal of Nurse-Midwifery, 30*(3), 159–165.

Pearson, A. (1989, July). Translating rhetoric into practice: Theory in action. In Koch, T. (Ed.), *Theory and practice: An evolving relationship.* School of Nursing Studies, Sturt. South Australia College of Advanced Education.

Perry, J. (1985). Has the discipline of nursing developed to the stage where nurses do 'think nursing'? *Journal of Advanced Nursing, 10,* 31–37.

Perry, J., & Moss, C. (1988). Generating alternatives in nursing: Turning curriculum into a living process. *The Australian Journal of Advanced Nursing, 6*(2), 35–40.

Piggott, M., & Gough, P. (1989). Job swap. *Nursing Times, 85*(18), 36–38.

Polifroni, E.C., & Schmalenberg, C. (1985). Faculty practice that works: Two examples. *Nursing Outlook, 33*(5), 227.

Robinson, P. (1990, January 17). Shot in the arm lifts nursing outlook. *The Australian*, p. 34.

Salvage, J. (1983). Joint appointments 1: Building bridges. *Nursing Times, 74*(41), 49–51.

Smith, G.R. (1980). Compensating faculty for their clinical practice. *Nursing Outlook, 28*(11), 673–676.

Speedy, S. (1987). Critical issues in tertiary nursing faculty development. *The Australian Journal of Advanced Nursing, 4*(4), 39–50.

Speedy, S. (1989). Theory-practice debate: Setting the scene. *The Australian Journal of Advanced Nursing, 6*(3), 12–20.

Stainton, M.C., Rankin, J.A., & Calkin, J.D. (1989). The development of a practicing nursing faculty. *Journal of Advanced Nursing, 14*(1), 20–26.

Taylor, B. (1988, September). Dreaming and awake: Reflection on and in clinical practice. Paper presented at the Australian Nurse Teachers' Society (NSW), *3rd Annual Conference: "I have a Dream"*, Sydney.

Thompson, J.L. (1987). Critical scholarship: The critique of domination in nursing. *Advances in Nursing Science, 10*(1), 27–38.

Van Ort, S.R. (1985). Faculty role issues. In S.R. Van Ort, & A.M. Putt (Eds.), *Teaching in Collegiate Schools of Nursing.* Boston: Little, Brown.

Watson, J. (1981). Some issues related to a science of caring. In M. Leininger (Ed.), *Caring: An essential human need.* New York: Slack Inc.

Webb, C. (1989). Action research: Philosophy, methods and personal experiences. *Journal of Advanced Nursing, 14*(5), 403–410.

Willis, E. (1988). *Shaping nursing theory and practice: The Australian context. Monograph 1.* Melbourne: La Trobe University.

Wright, S. (1988). Joint appointments: Handle with care. *Nursing Times, 84*(1), 32–33.

BIBLIOGRAPHY

Benner, P., & Wrubel, J. (1989). *The primacy of caring: stress and coping in health and illness.* Menlo Park: Addison-Wesley.

Bishop, B.E. (1981). A case for collaboration. *Nursing Outlook, 29*(2), 110–111.

Carnevali, D.L., Mitchell, P.H., Woods N.F., & Tanner C.A. (1984). *Diagnostic reasoning in nursing.* Philadelphia: J.B. Lippincott.

Chaska, N.L. (Ed.). (1983). *The nursing profession: A time to speak.* New York: McGraw-Hill.

Chenitz, W.C., & Swanson, J.M. (1986). *From practice to grounded theory: Qualitative research in nursing.* Menlo Park: Addison-Wesley.

Colavecchio, R. (1982). Direct patient care: A viable career choice? *The Journal of Nursing Administration, 12,* 17–22.

Fenton, M.V., Rounds, L., & Wise, D. (1988). Strategies for faculty practice. *Nurse Practitioner, 13,* 56–60.

Gardner, H. (Ed.). (1989). *The politics of health: The Australian experience.* Melbourne: Churchill Livingstone.

Gray, G., & Pratt, R. (Eds.). (1989). *Issues in Australian nursing 2.* Melbourne: Churchill Livingstone.

Heaphy, K.M. (1987). Nurse-Midwifery practice and undergraduate nursing education: A unique model. *Journal of Nurse-Midwifery, 32*(2), 98–100.

Jennings, B.M., & Meleis, A.I. (1988). Nursing theory and administrative practice: Agenda for the 1990s. *Advances in Nursing Science, 10*(3), 56–59.

Kleinknecht, M.K., & Hefferin, E.A. (1982). Assisting nurses toward professional growth: A career development model. *The Journal of Nursing Administration, 12,* 30–36.

Koch, T. (Ed.). (1989). *Theory and Practice: An Evolving Relationship.* Adelaide: School of Nursing Studies, Sturt.

Lambert, C.E., & Lambert, V.A. (Eds.). (1989). *Perspectives in nursing: The impacts on the nurse, the consumer and society.* East Norwalk: Appleton and Lange.

Lambert, C.E., & Lambert, V.A. (1988). Faculty practice: Unifier of nursing education and nursing service? *Journal of Professional Nursing, 4*(5), 345–355.

Lambert, C.E., & Lambert, V.A. (1988). The economic relevance of nursing faculty practice programs. *Nursing Economics, 6*(6), 291–296.

Leddy, S., & Pepper, J.M. (1989). *Conceptual bases of professional nursing* (2nd ed.). Philadelphia: J.B. Lippincott.

Mason, D.J., & Talbot, S.W. (Eds.). (1985). *Political action handbook for nurses.* Menlo Park: Addison-Wesley.

Miller, A. (1985). The relationship between nursing theory and nursing practice. *Journal of Advanced Nursing, 10,* 417–424.

O'Neill, E. (1985). It falls short of nirvana, but . . .. *Nursing Outlook, 33*(5), 229–230.

Owen, G.M. (1985). Janforum: Innovation in nursing—The role of higher education in relation to nursing practice. *Journal of Advanced Nursing, 10,* 179-183.

Quinn, C.A., & Smith, M.D. (1987). *The professional commitment: Issues and ethics in nursing.* Philadelphia: W. B. Saunders.

Simpson, K. (1989). Community psychiatric nursing—A research-based profession? *Journal of Advanced Nursing, 14,* 274–280.

Williams, C.A. (1988). Faculty practice and knowledge development: Will there be a linkage? *Journal of Professional Nursing, 4*(5), 317.

20

A Methodological Review and Evaluation of Research on Nurse–Patient Touch

Joan L. Bottorff

Although nurses have traditionally held caring as an important aspect of nursing practice, the importance of using systematic investigation to identify the nature and qualities of caring practices has only recently been recognized. One nursing action, nurse–patient touch, has frequently been linked to caring (Bailey, 1984; Boyd, 1986; Farrah, 1971; Gadow, 1985; Hernandez, 1988; Leininger, 1981; McCoy, 1977): it is an aspect of practice that is universal and basic to the nurse–patient relationship. In the past, relatively little was known about nurses' use of touch as an intervention, but recently, attention has become increasingly focused on clarifying this component of practice (Burnside, 1981; Gentner, 1980; Ingham, 1989; Weiss, 1988). Thus far, the research literature has been characterized by considerable variation in approach and methodological rigor (Weiss, 1988). This review, which concentrates on methodological issues, was undertaken to provide an evaluative and orientative overview of previous research and provide direction for future studies.

In preparing this review, published and unpublished studies in which the phenomenon of nurse–patient touch was of either major or minor

The author acknowledges the comments of Dr. Janice Morse on earlier drafts of this paper. This work was supported by the National Health Research and Development Program through a Doctoral Fellowship Award.

interest were examined. Although most of this research was conducted by nurses, studies by non-nurses were also included. Studies of touch that did not directly involve nurse–patient touch (e.g., mother–infant touch) and studies related to therapeutic touch (as described by Krieger, 1975) were generally excluded; however, therapeutic touch studies that involved "ordinary" touch between nurses and patients were considered. This review is based on 27 unpublished and 56 published research reports (covering the 30-year period from 1959–1989) located through computer searches (Medline, Psychology, and Sociology Abstracts) and follow-up of citations from reference lists.

DEFINITIONS OF NURSE–PATIENT TOUCH

Most researchers have defined touch in relation to the physical contact or tactile stimulation it encompasses and its communicative role. For example, Weiss' (1979) conceptualization of touch has been influential in the study of nurse–patient touch. With a focus on describing the physical qualities of the act of touch, she suggests that these qualities, along with the intent of the caregiver, may be useful in differentiating between different types of touch. The four qualities given primary importance are location (the part of the patient's body that is touched), intensity (extent of indentation or pressure of the touch), action (the specific gesture or movement used in touching), and duration (the temporal length of the touch). For Weiss (1979), these "tactile symbols" form a language of communication and shared meaning. From this perspective, touch is viewed as a channel of communication that can function independently of others and, consequently, can be studied in isolation from other forms of verbal or nonverbal communication. As such, when other verbal or nonverbal behaviors have been considered in addition to skin-to-skin contact, they have not been considered as part of the touch itself. Rather, they have been considered as factors influencing the effectiveness of touch (Chen, 1986/1987), as accompaniments to touch (Pepler, 1984; Schoenhofer, 1989), or as measures of the effectiveness of touch (El-Kafass, 1982/1983; Knable, 1981; Langland & Panicucci, 1982; McCorkle, 1974).

There are indications in the literature, however, that a broader concept of touch may be necessary. For example, when Estabrooks (1987a, 1989) interviewed nurses about the kinds of touch they used in practice, the nurses had difficulty defining touch, yet they could describe various dimensions that, in addition to skin-to-skin contact, included voice, posture, affect, emotional contact, and context. The examples nurses gave of touch clearly showed that touch meant more to them than mere physical contact. In trying to interpret these findings, Estabrooks used Weiss' (1979) conceptualization of touch as a complex gestalt, suggesting that touch could not be entirely understood by identifying its components or dimensions. These notions of touch are not entirely new. In the descriptive literature, nurses (Gadow, 1984; Kelly, 1984; Paulen, 1984; Ujehly, 1979) and others (Heylings, 1973; Montague, 1986) have referred to other forms of touch that extend beyond the relatively narrow focus of most researchers. For example, Montague (1986) includes eye contact as a form of touch: "Seeing is a form of touching at a distance" (p. 124). Paulen (1984) discusses "touching the spirit of another human being" (p. 201). From this literature review it is clear that researchers have tended to address a single dimension of nurse–patient touch within a fairly narrow context. The use of a broader concept of touch would lead to the formulation of different questions, the use of different designs and methods of data collection, and the consideration of the interactive nature of a larger number of variables.

DESCRIPTION AND MEASUREMENT OF NURSE–PATIENT TOUCH

Two methods—self-report and observational—have been used to describe and measure the various dimensions of nurse–patient touch. Developments in the use of these data collection strategies will be traced, the underlying methodological assumptions will be examined, and areas in which the current literature can suggest future directions for research will be discussed. While it is recognized that psychological instruments and physiological indices have been used to study nurse–patient touch, this discussion will focus on methods that have been developed for the specific purpose of measuring aspects of nurse–patient touch.

Self-Report Approaches

Three types of self-report techniques—projective, questionnaires or survey, and interviews—have been used to elicit and measure the various dimensions of nurse–patient touch (Table 20-1).

Projective Techniques. Projective techniques, which include a variety of ambiguous stimuli that allow free response, are based on the assumption that interpretation of, and reaction to, such stimuli reflect an individual's needs, attitudes, values, and personality characteristics (Waltz, Strickland, & Lenz, 1984). These techniques have been used to describe both the patient's and the nurse's perceptions of or responses to touch. Day (1973) and DeWever (1977) studied perceptions of touch by analyzing the responses of patients to slides and photographs involving different nurse–patient touching situations. Similarly, Trowbridge (1967)

Table 20-1
Research Studies Using Self-Report Approaches to Describe Nurse–Patient Touch

Author (Year)	Type of Self–Report	Subjects (Number)	Dimensions of Touch Described/Measured	Reliability/ Validity
De Augustinis et al. (1963)	Q—Open-ended questions	Nurses (9), psychiatric patients (9)	Frequency, patterns of use, types of touch gestures, meanings of touch	Not addressed.
Trowbridge (1967)	PM—Seven pictures of nurse touch	Nurses (30), patients (30)	Interpretations of touch, similarity between patients and nurses	Not addressed.
Farrah (1971)	Q—Vignettes with forced–choice alternatives and open–ended questions	Medical/surgical nurses (49)	Frequency, patterns of use, meanings of touch	Not addressed.
Durr (1971)	I—Not described	Medical/surgical patients (13)	Meaning of touch, attitudes toward touch	Not addressed.
Day (1973)	PM—Eight slides of nurse touch	Medical/surgical patients (20)	Attitudes toward touch	Not addressed.
Allekian (1973)	Q—27 statements with forced–choice response format	Adult patients (76)	Feelings in response to intrusion	Not addressed.
McCorkle (1974)	Q—Four open-ended questions	Critically ill patients (60)	Recollections of touch and nurse who used touch	Not addressed.
Burkhardt (1975)	Q—Attitude scale	Nurses (38), nursing students (55)	Attitudes toward touch	Reliability: .30.
Miller (1976)	Q—20 statements with forced–choice response format	Nurses (24)	Awareness and perception of touch	Content validity.
Stolte (1976/77); Penny (1979)	I—Structured	Obstetric patients (150)	Patterns, types, and meanings of touch; attitudes toward touch	Content validity.

Q—Questionnaire.
PM—Projective Measure.
I—Interview.

(continued on next page)

Author (Year)	Type of Self–Report	Subjects (Number)	Dimensions of Touch Described/Measured	Reliability/ Validity
DeWever (1977)	PM—Photo- graphs of affective touch	Elderly patients (99)	Attitudes toward touch	Reliability: .70–.98; construct validity using factor analysis
Ellis et al. (1979)	Q—Not described	Nursing students (100)	Attitudes toward touch	Not addressed.
Tobiason (1981)	Q—Open–ended questions	Nursing students (69 pretest and 52 post–test)	Attitudes toward touch	Not addressed.
Lorensen (1983)	Q—10 forced–choice and one open–ended question	Obstetric patients (12)	Patient perceptions of experience during labor with two questions directly related to use of touch by nurses	Not addressed.
Morse (1983)	I—Open–ended; ethnographic	Mothers (2), nurses (2)	Patterns of use of touch	Reliability and validity: intra– and inter–subject agreement.
Pratt & Mason (1984)	Q—28 statements with 10 response categories provided	Lay participants (30) and health practitioners (46, including 9 nurses)	Meanings of touch	Not addressed.
Pepler (1984)	Q—Touch Message Scale	Nurse aides (25), elderly patients (41)	Relational messages of touches	Reliability: .64–.94; construct validity using item correlations.
Torres (1985)	Q—Attitude and feeling survey	Nursing students (25)	Attitudes and feelings related to touch and interaction in close proximity	Test–retest reliability: .86.

(continued)

Table 20-1 *(continued)*

Author (Year)	Type of Self–Report	Subjects (Number)	Dimensions of Touch Described/Measured	Reliability/ Validity
Birch (1986)	I—Structured	Obstetric patients (30)	Patterns of use, types, and meanings of touch; attitude toward touch; context of touch	Not addressed.
Redfern & Le May (1987)	PM—Eight pairs of photographs	Elderly patients (86), nurses (133)	Preferences for touching and being touched	Not addressed.
Estabrooks (1987a, 1989)	I—Open–ended; ethnographic	ICU nurses (8)	Frequency, patterns of use, types, and meanings of touch; attitudes toward touch; context of touch	Reliability: documentation of decision trail; validity—criterion of adequacy, meaningfulness to audience.
Lane (1989)	Q—Territory/ Inter-personal space questionnaire	Nurses (80), surgical patients (80)	Feelings in response to intrusion	Reliability: .64–.85; construct validity using factor analysis.
Fisher & Joseph (1989)	Q—Attitude scale (15 items)	Medical/surgical patients (52)	Attitudes about nonprocedural touch	Reliability: .68; construct validity using factor analysis.

used photographs to compare nurses' and patients' interpretations of touch, while Le May and Redfern (1987) used eight pairs of photographs to determine nurses' and patients' preferences for touching and being touched. (The photographs within each pair were similar, except that in one of each pair the nurse is touching the patient.) Although Day (1973) argues that subjects may respond more freely to these techniques than to a more direct method (e.g., questionnaire), others criticize the use of this approach in touch research. For example, Knapp (1983) contends that it is invalid to assume that subjects responding to photographs or videos would have the same motivation and involvement as people making judgments in face-to-face encounters in high-information contexts.

Questionnaires. Systematic self-report measures, in the form of questionnaires and attitude scales, have been used to describe and assess the following: meanings or messages associated with nurse–patient touch

(De Augustinis, Isani, & Kumler, 1963; Pepler, 1984; Pratt & Mason, 1984); nurses' attitudes toward touching (Burkhardt, 1975; Ellis, Taylor, & Walts, 1979; Farrah, 1971; Tobiason, 1981); nurses' awareness and perceptions of touch (Miller, 1976); patients' feelings as a result of intrusion into personal space which in part is associated with a nurse's touch (Allekian, 1973; Lane, 1989); patients' recollection of touch (McCorkle, 1974); patient attitudes toward nonprocedural touch (Fisher & Joseph, 1989); and patients' perceptions of their experiences during labor, including the nurse's use of touch (Lorenson, 1983). Questionnaires have become progressively more structured as researchers have moved from using open-ended questions related to a variety of issues associated with nurse–patient touch (e.g., De Augustinis, Isani, & Kumler, 1963) to using more narrowly focused questionnaires characterized by statements with forced–choice response formats (e.g., Lane, 1989; Pratt & Mason, 1984). However, relatively little progress in measuring aspects of nurse–patient touch has been made using self-report measures. Many of these instruments lack a sound conceptual basis; in addition, the tendency to use investigator-developed, unvalidated measures has made it impossible to compare studies. Only one instrument has been developed and tested in more than one investigation (Allekian, 1973; Lane, 1989). Those who have assessed the reliability and validity of newly developed instruments (Burkhardt, 1975; Fisher & Joseph, 1989; Lane, 1989; Pepler, 1984) have found the results to be informative, although not always favorable. For example, Burkhardt (1975) reports a low reliability (Cronbach's alpha = .3078) for a 24-item questionnaire used to measure nurses' attitudes toward non-necessary touch, i.e., touch that is primarily affective. Pepler's (1984) evaluation of the Touch Message Scale led to the conclusion that the instrument's reliability and validity were questionable when used as a self-report measure, although its use as an observational tool was supported. These results illustrate the need to rigorously develop new instruments.

The need to move beyond this initial stage in the measurement of nurse–patient touch toward the development of more refined measures (as researchers who are interested in touch outside the nursing context have done) is urgent. Instruments such as the Touch Avoidance Measure (Andersen & Leibowitz, 1978) and the Same Sex Touching Scale (Larsen & LeRoux, 1984) are an improvement over earlier methods of measurement because they have been developed from conceptual definitions or empirical findings and because their psychometric properties are more fully established; however, those who developed these instruments recognize that further evaluation is needed. For example, Andersen, Andersen, and Lustig (1987) raise questions concerning the relationship between attitude scores and actual patterns of touching and the degree to which attitude scales can be used to predict the tactile behavior of individuals in different kinds of relationships. Because researchers involved in instrument development outside of nursing have, for the most part, employed strangers and university students, these instruments may not be suitable for measuring any aspect of nurse–patient touch with specific clinical populations and the nurses who work with them. The development of sound instruments is fundamental to the advancement of knowledge related to nurse–patient touch, and this development depends on a commitment to further conceptual work in this field and the systematic evaluation of measures.

Interviews. Although interviews provide an in-depth method of obtaining information on complex processes such as touch, this approach has not been used as extensively as other self-report techniques in studying nurse–patient touch. In early studies detailed descriptions of interviewing techniques used were often not included (e.g., Durr, 1971). More recent reports have included both data analysis strategies and more detail with regard to interviewing techniques. Stolte (1976/1977) and Birch (1986) used similarly structured interviews to describe patients' perceptions of touch during labor, while Estabrooks (1987a, 1989) and Morse (1983) used an open-ended style of interviewing to support the inductive nature of their studies of nurses' descriptions of touch and comfort (of which touch was viewed as an important aspect). By using interviews, researchers have been able to provide detailed descriptions of a broad range of dimensions involved in nurse–patient touch, and this important descriptive and conceptual information is needed to guide future quantitative studies. The use of interview techniques, however, depends on the ability of respondents to be insightful about their touch behaviors and responses to touch and their willingness to share this information. If some dimensions of nurse–patient touch are too personal or private to be explored by direct questioning (or observation), the use of questionnaires may be preferable.

Methodological Assumptions and Implications. Three major assumptions have direct implications for the use of structured or semi-structured self-report techniques in studying nurse–patient touch. First, it is assumed that investigators understand tactile codes, meanings, and behaviors well enough to identify relevant factors and ask appropriate questions (Jones & Yarbrough, 1985). Yet the incomplete understanding of the concept of touch in nursing (Estabrooks, 1987a, 1987b; Weiss, 1979, 1986) and problems achieving respectable estimates of reliability and validity (when this has been attempted) make this assumption tenuous. By using open-ended interviews and qualitative methods, Estabrooks (1987a, 1989) and Morse (1983) were able to make important contributions to the description and conceptualization of touch. Further inductive research is needed to provide detailed descriptions of a broad range of dimensions of nurse–patient touch on which the development of structured measuring instruments and experimental studies can be based.

Second, by using questionnaires, certain researchers (e.g., Pratt and Mason, 1984) have assumed that touch gestures can be meaningfully interpreted when respondents are provided with statements that describe unambiguous situations involving touch. However, Knapp (1983) argues that it is unrealistic to assume that the intents or meanings attributed to statements describing touch behaviors are the same as the intents or meanings that would be attributed in similar real-life situations where touches are experienced in the context of other nonverbal behaviors, interpersonal relationships, and situational and historical factors. For example, Pepler (1984) found that multiple factors were involved in interpreting the relational messages represented in touch gestures between nursing aides and elderly nursing home residents. It also appears that several incompatible interpretations related to intimacy and status can be ascribed to any particular touch gesture (Major, 1981); that specific touch gestures do not have universal meanings, even within the same culture or context (De Augustinis et al., 1963); and that contextual factors are critical to the meaning attributed to touch (Jones & Yarbrough, 1985). The characteristic ambiguity of the meanings associated with touch may limit the precision to which they can be described, at least with the structured forced-choice response formats that are currently available. Development of innovative ways to measure nurse–patient touch is needed.

Finally, the use of direct methods of questioning to examine nurse–patient touch is based on the assumption that individuals are sufficiently aware of experiences with touch to recall and report them accurately (Jones & Yarbrough, 1985). Individuals may not be sufficiently aware of their experiences with touch to recall and report the details needed to describe many aspects of complex behavioral interactions (Benner, 1984; Brannigan & Humphries, 1972; Burnside, 1977). For example, can nurses be expected to remember how many times they had eye contact while touching a patient or precisely what stimuli evoked the touching behavior? If such behavioral sequences and interactions are seen as important, and if nurse–patient touch is believed to be sufficiently complex to require detailed analysis, total reliance on direct questioning using either an interview or questionnaire may lead to disappointing results. At the same time, it must be recognized that the private dimension of the experience of touching and being touched (Pratt & Mason, 1981) may only be accessible through self-report of some kind.

Observational Approaches

Twenty-one studies that used observational approaches to desribe spontaneous nurse–patient touch were examined (Table 20-2). In all instances observations were carried out in hospital wards, with a few researchers (Blackburn & Barnard, 1985; Pepler, 1984; Watson, 1972/1973, 1975) making their observations using videotaped recordings of touch interactions. Observational strategies included the simple recording of frequency and

Table 20-2
Research Studies Using Observational Approaches to Describe Nurse-Patient Touch

Author (Year)	Type of Touch Observed	Mode of Observation/ Setting	Sampling Methods	Observational Outcomes	Reliability
Charlton (1959)	Any physical contact	Live/ psychiatric	Sequence sampling (?S)[a]	Observed 24 sequences involving patient or nurse– initiated touch	Not reported.
De Augustinis et al. (1963)	Any physical contact	Live/ psychiatric	Sequence sampling (CS)[b]	Six 1-hour observation and interviewing periods yielding 22 nurse– initiated touches	Not reported.
Marshall (1969)	Any physical contact	Live/labor and delivery	Focal subject (CS) all–occurrence sampling	Varied lengths of observation periods with five primigravidas yielding 794 touches	Not reported.
Barnett (1972)	Non- necessary touch	Live/nine hospital wards	All–occurrence sampling with random selection of time and place to conduct observations	180 30–minute observation periods yielding 452 occurrences of non–necessary touch	Not reported.
Watson (1972/1973, 1975, 1979–80)	Any physical contact	Video/ geriatric institutional setting (two wards)	Sequence sampling with random selection of time periods to conduct observations	839 behavioral unit sequences yielding 187 interactions involving touch	74–80% agreement.
Griffin (1978)	Any contact that is in addition to procedural contact	Live/ emergency room	Focal subject (CS) one-zero sampling with randomly selected periods of time and area for observations	Observed 88 nurse–patient encounters, 43 of which were touch encounters	Not reported.

[a]Use of random or convenience sampling not reported.
[b]Convenience sampling.
[c]Random sampling.

Author (Year)	Type of Touch Observed	Mode of Observation/ Setting	Sampling Methods	Observational Outcomes	Reliability
Copstead (1980)	Any physical contact	Live/nursing home	Focal subject (RS)[c] all–occurrence sampling during administration of medications	33 observation periods with 33 subjects, of whom 22 experienced touch	81% agreement (total instrument).
El-Kafass (1982/1983)	Expressive touch	Live/four ICUs	Focal subject all–occurrence sampling with random selection of observation times	60 1-hour observation periods yielding 175 expressive touches	95.7–96% agreement.
Clement (1983)	Any physical contact	Live/ICU	Focal subject (RS) all–occurrence sampling	225 20-minute observations with 75 patients yielding 9.0 touches/hour	66–100% agreement.
Dahill (1984)	Instrumental and expressive touch	Live/three pediatric units	Focal subject (CS) all–occurrence sampling	20 patients observed for one or two 30–minute periods yielding 112 touches	88–100% agreement.
Pepler (1984)	Any physical contact	Video/three nursing homes	Focal subject (CS) all–occurrence sampling during transfers or assistance with other daily activities	41 patients observed being cared for by 25 nurse aids yielding 512 touch events of which 202 were randomly selected for analysis	Tactile Indication Indicator: percent agreement "high levels;" Touch Message Scale: $r = .67-.94$.
Probrislo (1984)	Comforting touch	Live/labor and delivery	Focal subject (CS) all–occurrence sampling	1200 30–second observation periods with 10 patients (one hour each) yielding 1701 touches	90% or more agreement in all areas.

(continued)

313

Table 20-2 *(continued)*

Author (Year)	Type of Touch Observed	Mode of Observation/ Setting	Sampling Methods	Observational Outcomes	Reliability
Johnson (1984)	Nonprocedural touch	Live/pediatric ICU	Focal subject (CS) all–occurrence sampling	47 4-hour observation periods with 13 patients yielding a mean of 6.95 nurse touches per observation period	90% agreement.
Wagnild & Manning (1985)	Procedural and non-procedural touch	Live/eight long–term care settings	Focal subject (RS) all–occurrence sampling during bathing procedure	42 5- to 8-minute observation periods with 42 patients yielding 42 nonprocedural touches; number of procedural touches not reported	Not reported.
Tulman (1985)	Touch involved in handling infant	Live/newborn nursery	Focal subject (CS) one-zero sampling	1620 5-second observations of 36 nursing student/infant dyads; touching patterns described	.82–.90 inter-rater reliability.
Mitchell et al. (1985)	Procedural and non-procedural touch	Live/pediatric ICU	Focal subject (CS) all–occurrence sampling	1-10 observational periods per child, length of observational periods not reported; observations of 13 children resulted in mean nurse nonprocedural touch of 6.73 and procedural touch of 6.8 per observation period	90% agreement for categorizing touch.
Blackburn & Barnard (1985)	Caregiving activity	Video/ preterm nursery	Focal subject (CS) one–zero sampling	1140 1–minute epochs with 102 infants; care-- giving activities occurred 14.4% of 24–hour period	Above .80 intra-and inter-rater reliability.

Author (Year)	Type of Touch Observed	Mode of Observation/ Setting	Sampling Methods	Observational Outcomes	Reliability
Porter et al. (1986)	Any physical contact	Live/setting not reported	Focal subject (RS) all–occurrence sampling	72 40-minute observation periods with two patients; number of touches not reported	Kappa .23–.72; r=.98 (duration of touch).
Le May & Redfern (1987)	Any physical contact	Live/four geriatric care wards	Focal subject (?S) all–occurrence sampling	318 interactions observed with 30 patients, yielding 1402 touches; length of observation periods not reported	Kappa .25–.98; 52–99% agreement.
Redfern & Le May (1987)	Any physical contact	Live/10 geriatric care wards	Focal subject (?S) all–occurrence sampling	86 14.25-hour observation periods with 86 patientes yielding 2590 touches	Kappa ≥ .60 for seven of the schedule compo- nents; remaining three unreliable.
Schoenhofer (1989)	Affectional touch	Live/three ICUs	Focal subject (CS) all–occurrence sequence sampling	30 1-hour observation periods with 30 nurse–patient dyads yielding 84 affectional touches	50–100% agreement.

location of touch (Barnett, 1972), ethnographic descriptive levels of observation (De Augustinis et al., 1963), and, more recently, the use of more
rigorous and complex observational schedules in which patterns of touch
were coded for information on touch quality, as well as for nurse and
patient characteristics and context variables (Le May & Redfern, 1987;
Pepler, 1984; Porter, Redfern, Wilson-Barnett, & Le May, 1986; Redfern &
Le May, 1987; Schoenhofer, 1989). The results are difficult to compare
because researchers observed touch in a variety of settings with different
kinds of subjects; focused on different types of touch; and used different
sampling strategies, coding schemes, and data collection tools. In addition,

researchers have paid little attention to describing the context in which the touching took place or to the effects of observation on the variables being studied (Weiss, 1988).

Observations in these studies have focused on various dimensions of touch. In relation to the "quality of touch," several researchers have tried to use Weiss' (1979) framework to guide their observations. The number of qualities used has varied, as have the coding and precision of observations. For example, the duration of touch has been coded as "long or short" (Schoenhofer, 1989), rated with two different four-point scales (Clement, 1983; Porter et al., 1986; Redfern & Le May, 1987), and measured in seconds (Pepler, 1984). The purpose or meaning of the touch was interpreted by the observers in six of the studies; for the most part, interpretation involved classifying touch into broad categories (e.g., instrumental and expressive). Although it is suggested in the literature that the types of touch may not be as separate as was first thought (Estabrooks, 1989; Watson, 1975; Weiss, 1986), observations suggest that these categories were viewed as quite distinct. Even if it is possible to observe both the expressive and instrumental significance of any particular touch, given the level of specificity of observations in these studies, it is probably impossible to obtain the fine discrimination that may be needed to study the expressive features of an instrumental touch or vice versa.

Some studies have included observation of specific nonverbal behaviors other than touch that were exhibited by both nurses and patients. These observations have varied in terms of the number and type of nonverbal behaviors taken into account and the level of coding used. Using a checklist of common positions, Le May and Redfern (1987) recorded the body position of both the nurse and patient in each touch episode. Schoenhofer (in 1989a) recorded other supplemental behaviors (e.g., eye contact and vocalization) of the person delivering the touch, as well as the verbal and nonverbal behavior of the patient prior to the touch behavior (coded as direct or indirect). Observers who rated patient response to touch used broad interpretive coding categories (e.g., positive, negative, neutral), with one exception. Pepler (1984) did not include this as part of the observation tool; instead, patients rated their own comfort with the touch on a five-point scale after viewing videotapes of selected touch episodes in which they had been involved. While the inclusion of nonverbal behaviors as a part of the touch gesture is important, the use of broad interpretive coding strategies and lack of attention to the complete range of behaviors in nurse–patient interactions in any one study limits the descriptions provided by these researchers. Data showing the physiological and psychological reactions (e.g., changes in anxiety) associated with touch gestures used by nurses in the natural context of their work were not included in any of these studies.

For the most part, description of the context in which touch occurs has been limited to demographic variables (nurse and patient), patient diagnosis or condition, and type of ward. Only a few researchers have attempted to describe context in greater detail. Pepler (1984) recorded the presence of other people, the availability of clothing and furniture, whether a radio or television was on, and the relationship between the patient and the nurse (by identifying the length of time the nurse and patient had known each other), the verbal behavior of the nurse, and so on. Le May and Redfern (1987) included observations related to the task being performed when touch occurred, the timing of the touch during the nurse–patient interaction (approach, interface, or separation), and the duration of the nurse–patient interaction. Greater attention should be given to context, timing, and sequence of behaviors in relation to both nurse and patient in order to increase understanding of touch as a dyadic interaction. A touch from a nurse to a patient does not convey the same message in all circumstances, and simple tabulations of frequencies of the occurrence of touch reveal very little. Lamb (1979) explains that when attempting to answer sophisticated questions about social interaction "it is necessary to take into account the behavior of all the participants, and analyze the actions of every one in the context of each others' behavior" (p. 7). Thus, to determine the differences between positive and negative touch experiences and other important aspects of nurse–patient touch, all components of the touch situation must be examined. To date, the variables involved in nurse–patient touch have not been systematically examined.

Sampling strategies. One problem of observational research involves maximizing the chance of actually observing the behavior of interest in sequences that are representative of the subjects being studied (Sackett, 1978). When short-duration, infrequent behaviors such as expressive touch behaviors are of interest, relatively long-time samples have been used to observe these behaviors (Johnson, 1984, Schoenhofer, 1989). Shorter sampling periods have been used effectively to capture frequent or longer types of touches (Probrislo, 1984; Tulman, 1985). In the majority of investigations (12 out of 21 studies), researchers studying nurse–patient touch used a combination of focal subject and all-occurrence sampling methods, varying the number and length of observational periods to meet their purposes. Although the combination of more than one sampling method enhances the efficiency of data collection (Lehner, 1979), some sampling problems are evident in this research. Unbiased sampling was enhanced by investigators who were able to randomly select subjects, times for observation, place of observation, and/or touches. Nevertheless, much less confidence can be placed in results obtained when the number or length of observations per subject was varied with small convenient samples (e.g., Mitchell, Habermann-Little, Johnson, VanInwegen-Scott, &

Tyler, 1985) or when sampling strategies were not fully reported (e.g., Charlton, 1959; Redfern & Le May, 1987). While truly random sampling is difficult to achieve in field research, attempts should be made to equalize the number and temporal distribution of observations among individuals when the purpose is to describe normative patterns of touch. Furthermore, if the purpose is to describe specific characteristics of touch, attempts should be made to maximize observation of the number of touch episodes of interest during the observational period. In this case, it is important to note that the number of patients or number of hours of observation do not constitute the sample, but rather the sample is the number of touch episodes that are observed. One-zero sampling (often referred to as time sampling) was used effectively in two investigations of handling and caring for infants (Blackburn & Barnard, 1985; Tulman, 1985). When used with a sample period that is sufficiently short in relation to the duration of and interval between behaviors of interest, this method can provide data on frequency, duration, and patterns or sequencing of behaviors. However, when this approach is used with relatively long sample periods (such as those used in Griffin, 1978), a large amoung of data on frequency and duration is lost. The fact that few researchers used sequence sampling methods probably accounts for the current focus on describing the touch behaviors themselves, rather than the process of touching.

Reliability and Validity. Reliability has been either unreported (especially in early studies) or inconsistently reported. For the most part, researchers have relied on percentage agreement as an estimate of reliability for the nominal data collected to describe nurse–patient touch. However, estimates were sometimes obtained inappropriately. In some cases, estimates were based only on touches seen by both observers (e.g., touches observed by only one of the observers were excluded [Le May & Redfern, 1987]); in other instances, estimates were made from data collected in circumstances that were different from those used in the actual study (e.g., using staged simulations [Schoenhofer, 1989]). In a third case, two observers were involved in estimating inter-rater reliability when three observers were actually involved in data collection (e.g., El-Kafass, 1982/1983). Intra-rater reliability was estimated in only one study (Blackburn & Barnard, 1985).

The use of percentage agreement has been criticized because estimates can be affected by how agreements are defined (i.e., if agreement on nonoccurrence is included), and because it does not correct for chance agreements (Topf, 1986). In addition, percentage agreement reported on its own (as in the majority of the studies reported here) is not an estimate of reliability unless it is compared with an established standard since all observers could be consistently applying the same incorrect behavioral definitions (Hollenbeck, 1978). The consensus among some behavioral scientists suggests that 70 percent agreement is necessary, 80 percent is adequate, and 90 percent is good (Topf, 1986). However, Topf points out that these values are harder to achieve using occurrence agreement than other percentage agreement formulas. Kappa, a correlational measure of agreement that controls for chance, was used in one series of studies (Le May & Redfern, 1987; Porter et al., 1986; Redfern & Le May, 1987).

The validity of observational tools has received little attention. Researchers have used the literature or have arbitrarily selected variables to guide the development of their observation schedules and, in some cases, have used panels of judges to establish content validity.[*] When using a deductive approach to develop an observational schedule, however, researchers create the risk of focusing on insignificant behavioral sequences or missing a significant phenomenon altogether, thereby presenting a serious threat to validity (Morse & Bottorff, 1990).

Methodological Assumptions and Implications. Observational methods used in the study of touch are based on three assumptions that have direct implications for the study of nurse–patient touch. First, it is assumed that the relative importance of all behaviors is known. However, it is clear that, to date, researchers have tended to overlook subtle behavioral changes during touch episodes or the complexity of the behavioral patterns in which touch episodes are embedded in the following ways: by restricting their observations to isolated touch behaviors, disregarding changes in other nonverbal behaviors (except to make gross evaluations), ignoring aspects of sequencing, and using general rather than detailed behavior coding schemes. In other disciplines, researchers studying nonverbal behavior have recognized the need to use a more refined approach to analysis (Knapp, 1983) and to move away from focusing on a single channel of nonverbal behavior (Harrison, 1984; Patterson, 1984; Siegman & Feldstein, 1987). As Patterson and Edinger (1987) explain, examining isolated behaviors may be helpful in building knowledge of nonverbal social behavior, but it contributes little to understanding the coordinated multichannel reactions that occur in real-life situations.

It has also been assumed that the best level at which to code behaviors is known. Although the types of behaviors to be recorded may vary from study to study, the question of how fine or gross data units should be remains important. For example, in studying nurse–patient interactions involving touch, should one distinguish between a "half smile," "full smile," or "bright-face," or record all of these as instances of a "positive nonverbal behavior"? As Lamb (1979) suggests, either decision carries a

---

[*]One exception to this is the Touch Message Scale (Pepler, 1984), which evolved through an inductive process of grounded theory development.

risk. By recording nonverbal behavior in relation to a few gross categories, important patterns of interaction can be completely obscured. On the other hand, adopting a highly refined inventory can lead to the identification of a number of distinct behaviors that may be perceived as semantically similar by the participants in the interaction. In addition, it may be difficult to identify a consistent response to behaviors such as "raises eyebrows," where as, if "raises eyebrows," "face brightens," and "raises corners of mouth" are treated as one unit—a smile—the respondent's reactions may be more apparent. Lamb (1979) suggests that behavioral units should be roughly equivalent to the unit of meaning; however, this presupposes that the researcher already knows which behaviors are important to the participants in a touching interaction. Considering the lack of systematic research in relation to nurse–patient touch, this assumption is tenuous at best.

Ethology, which facilitates the systematic observation and analysis of behavior under natural conditions, has been used to study certain aspects of human and animal behavior (Eibl-Eibesfeldt, 1989; Lehner, 1979). Although ethological methods have been used in studies of maternal-infant interaction (Klaus & Kennell, 1976), child behavior (Jones, 1972), and facial expression (Ekman, Sorenson, & Friesen, 1969), they have not been used to study nurse–patient behaviors or interactions. Ethological methods allow the study of complex behavior patterns at fine levels of detail, characteristically beginning with an inductive descriptive phase to establish "what there is to explain in real-life occurrences" (Jones, 1972, p. 11). On the basis of this foundation, decisions are made about the significance of behaviors that may answer the research questions of interest. The use of ethological methods to study nurse–patient touch would allow researchers to identify which behaviors are significant and should be observed in touch episodes; observe a wide range of nonverbal behaviors simultaneously, including touch behaviors; capture aspects of timing, sequencing, or other features of the organization of behavior that may be important in understanding nurse–patient touch; and identify subtle or rapid changes in behavior associated with touch and touching. By replacing less refined approaches to the study of nurse–patient touch with more sophisticated levels of analysis, it may be possible, for example, to describe the difference between an instrumental touch that is flavored with expressive touch, and one that is not. Despite this, it may not be necessary or beneficial to conduct all research related to nurse–patient touch by examining molecular units of behavior. Hartup (1979) suggests that the understanding of any social activity can be enhanced by simultaneous study at different levels of analysis. This approach may be fruitful in the development of knowledge on nurse–patient touch.

If more refined approaches to observing nurse–patient touch are pursued, the ability of the observer to record important behaviors reliably must also be considered. Using videotapes, nurse–patient touch episodes can be rerun and examined at length. Despite the obvious advantages of this approach in observing fleeting touches and the nonverbal behaviors associated with them, Redfern and Le May (1987) caution that the detrimental effects of intrusion and altered behavior in the observed subjects must be considered, as must the loss of depth perception. Less intrusive methods of videotaping, such as mounting cameras on the wall and using remote control monitoring devices, should be explored in order to increase the ease of recording data. Presently, Redfern and Oliver (Redfern, personal communication, October 1987) are testing the feasibility and reliability of the touch observation schedule (Porter et al., 1986) using a portable lap computer programmed as an event recorder.

Finally, the use of observational approaches includes the assumption that touching interactions are reflected in and can be adequately described by attention to observable behaviors. While many of the behaviors that comprise touching gestures may be observable, the experience of touch and touching is essentially a private one that is influenced by extraneous and interpersonal factors as well as by cultures and systems of thinking; thus, each act of touch is a unique event that reflects the personal experience and judgment of both practitioners and patients (Pratt & Mason, 1981). Consequently, it may not be possible to study touch objectively solely by using an observational approach. Although it has been shown that inferences relating to the emotional or affective states can be made with some degree of certainty from observational data (i.e., facial expressions and other nonverbal behaviors [Ekman & Friesen, 1969; Mehrabian, 1972, 1981; Patterson, 1983]), some aspects of touch and touching, such as understanding the meaning shared by nurses and patients as they experience touch, may not be observable. Following Pepler's (1984) example, it may be necessary to use other qualitative methods (e.g., open-ended interviews) in conjunction with observational methods in order to gain a more complete understanding of touch, that is, if nurses and patients are able and willing to share their experiences.

EVALUATING THE EFFECTS OF NURSE–PATIENT TOUCH

A number of researchers have attempted to identify the effects of nurse–patient touch encounters, some of which included primarily tactile interventions such as back rubs (Table 20-3). It is important to recognize, however, that the literature is biased toward the positive effects of nurse–patient touch. This bias has operated in two ways. First, most investigations have been conducted with populations that would benefit from increased tactile contact rather than with those that might be harmed by it

Table 20-3
Research Describing the Effect of Nurse–Patient Touch

Author (Year)	Type of Touch	Design	Sample	Outcomes Evaluated	Findings
INFANT/CHILD STUDIES					
Hasselmeyer (1963)	Handling of infant	Experimental	Preterm infants (1500–2000 g)	Behavioral and physiological measures, feeding patterns	Group receiving high amount of handling in state of "quiescent being" more frequently; passed less feces than control group.
Solkoff et al. (1969)	Gentle rubbing of back, neck, and arms	Experimental	10 low-birth-weight infants (1190–1590 g)	Activity, weight, temperature, startle response crying, elimination patterns, physical development	Infants who received treatment more active, regained birth weight faster, and described as physically healthier compared to controls.
Scarr-Salapatek & Williams (1973)	Special visual, tactile, and kinesthetic stimulation	Experimental (demonstration project)	30 low-birth-weight infants (1300–1800 g)	Infant development, major caretaker characteristics, living conditions	Infants who received treatment showed greater developmental progress at four weeks and greater weight gain than controls.
Solkoff & Matuszak (1975)	Stroking	Experimental	11 low-birth-weight infants (978–1871 g)	Neonatal Behavioral Assessment Scale (NBSA); weight	Subjects showed more positive changes on NBSA subscales than controls; no difference in weight gain.
White & Labarba (1976)	Rubbing body and gentle flexing	Experimental	Eight low-birth-weight infants (1500–2000 g)	Physiological data, feeding information, weight	Subjects gained weight at a significantly greater rate; ingested more formula than controls.
Kramer et al. (1975)	Gentle non-rhythmic stroking of greatest part of infant's body	Experimental	14 "normal-for date" premature infants (1800 g or less)	Physical and social development; ability to tolerate stress, weight	Infants who received treatment showed more rapid rate of social development from six weeks after transfer to crib to three months after this transfer, and greater degree of motor skill development at time of transfer to crib than controls.

Author (Year)	Type of Touch	Design	Sample	Outcomes Evaluated	Findings
INFANT/CHILD STUDIES *continued*					
Triplett & Arneson (1979)	Patting, stroking, holding, rocking to soothe or comfort child	Exploratory, with random assignment to two groups	100 interventions with 63 infants/children	Observation of response to verbal and tactile comforting measures	Verbal and tactile measures more successful in quieting more subjects than use of verbal measures alone.
Rausch (1981)	Rubbing with gentle stroke procedure to all areas of body; gentle flexing	Quasi-experimental	40 premature infants (1000–2000 g)	Weight, stooling, caloric intake	Infants who received treatment showed increased stooling frequency on days 5–10 and increased feeding intake on days 6–10; gained increasingly more weight but not significantly so.
Jay (1982)	Gentle skin to skin contact to head and abdomen of infant	Quasi-experimental	26 mechanically ventilated, short–gestation infants	Physiological and behavioral data	Decreased oxygen requirements and higher hematocrit levels were shown for intervention group; infants became more relaxed during touch periods over last five days of intervention.
Johnson (1984)	Hand-holding, stroking of chest and face	Experimental	Four patients in pediatric ICU	Intracranial pressure (ICP)	Mixed results; no ICP changes outside child's resting variability.
Blackburn & Barnard (1985)	Caretaking activities, including social stroking	Descriptive	102 premature infants (mean birth weight 1309 g)	Motor activity, type of caretaking activity	Infant activity level higher than baseline levels prior to diapering/feeding and out-of-incubator events; remaining high after some procedures; social stroking showed no relationship to activity levels.

(continued)

Table 20-3 *(continued)*

Author (Year)	Type of Touch	Design	Sample	Outcomes Evaluated	Findings
INFANT/CHILD STUDIES *continued*					
Mitchell et al. (1985)	Spontaneous touch and investigator touch (deliberate stroking to body and face without talking)	Descriptive	13 children with intracranial tension (seven months–seven years); six of the children received investigator touch	Intracranial pressure, arterial blood pressure	Intracranial pressure did not increase or decrease outside range of resting variability of any individual; arterial blood pressure and heart rate remained stable.
CHILD/ADULT STUDIES					
Ellis et al. (1979)	Pulse taking, patting hand or arm	Quasi-experimental	45 patients (18 months to 82 years)	Facial expression, body movement, eye contact, general response	Trend for more positive responses in touch group compared to control.
ADULT STUDIES					
Charlton (1959)	Any physical contact	Descriptive	Psychiatric patients involved in 23 nurse–patient interactions	Description of patient response to physical contact (move toward, away, against nurse)	Patterns of patient movement described in relation to context of nurse–initiated touch.
Saltenis (1962)	Low and high degree of physical contact	Quasi-experimental	21 primigravida mothers in first stage labor (three–six cm)	Mother's reactions to contractions; BP, pulse	Patients' ability to work effectively with their contractions increased with high degree of physical contact and dropped when touch withheld; systolic BP and pulse dropped with introduction of touch.
Kaufmann (1964)	Back rub	Quasi-experimental	36 medical patients	Galvanic skin response, BP, pulse, brief interview	Although patient reaction positive, no significant changes in autonomic activity demonstrated.
Aguilera (1967)	Simple appropriate touch gestures	Quasi-experimental	36 psychiatric patients, six nurses	Changes in verbal interaction, patient attitude toward nurse, nurse's attitudes toward subjects	Touch increased verbal interactions, rapport, and approach behavior beginning on eighth day.

Author (Year)	Type of Touch	Design	Sample	Outcomes Evaluated	Findings
ADULT STUDIES *continued*					
Greenberg (1972)	Stroking, clasping, and embracing	Experimental	10 elderly female psychotic patients	Psychotic behavior	No significant differences.
Slone (1973)	Low (procedural touch) and high touch (procedural touch supplemented with other contacts)	Pilot study, experimental	Eight obstetrical patients	Vocal/non-verbal and physical activity, control of breathing, expressed attitude toward contraction, BP, pulse rate	Only in terms of vocal activity were significant differences found; diastolic BP decreased and pulse rate increased in response to high touch.
McCorkle (1974)	Gentle touch on wrist	Experimental	60 seriously ill patients	Verbal and non-verbal behavior, postinteractive questionnaire, electrocardiograph (ECG)	Touch increased positive responses as measured by facial expression and verbal response.
Lynch et al. (1974a)	Pulse palpation and holding hand or touching arm with verbal comforting	Case study	Four curarized patients in shock–trauma unit	ECG	Heart rate changes observed during human contact.
Lynch et al. (1974b)	Pulse palpation; measuring BP	Case study	Three critical care unit (CCU) patients	ECG	Heart rate, heart rhythm, and frequency of ectopic beats influenced by human contact.
Thomas et al. (1975)	Interactions with nurse, most of which involved physical contact	Case study	One CCU patient	ECG	Heart rate, ectopic beats influenced by routine interactions that occur in CCU.
Mills et al. (1976)	Pulse palpation	Quasi–experimental	62 CCU patients	ECG	Frequency of ectopic beats increased significantly when pulse taken on patients with low incidence of baseline arrhythmia; no change in average heart rate.

Table 20-3 *(continued)*

Author (Year)	Type of Touch	Design	Sample	Outcomes Evaluated	Findings
ADULT STUDIES *continued*					
Lynch et al. (1977)	Pulse palpation	Quasi–experimental	225 CCU patients	ECG	Significant reduction in ventricular arrhythmias following pulse palpitation in high arrhythmia group; no change in heart rate.
McCoy (1977)	Touch on wrist/arm during assessment interview in emergency department	Quasi–experimental	40 adult patients	Observation of verbal and non-verbal behavior; short interview	Patients who were touched showed positive response and saw nurse as caring.
Whitcher & Fisher (1979)	Touching hand and arm during preoperative teaching	Experimental	48 elective surgery patients	Affective, evaluative, behavioral, physiological indices	Female subjects who were touched experienced more favorable affective, behavioral, and physiological response than control group; male subjects reacted more negatively than controls.
Copstead (1980)	Any physical contact	Correlational	33 elderly, institutionalized patients	Self-appraisal (Second/Jourard Self Cathexis Scale)	Frequency of touch correlated positively with positive self-appraisal.
Sommer (1979/1980)	Reassuring touch in response to expressions of anxiety (touch to arm, forehead, or hand)	Experimental	90 obstetrical subjects (transition phase of labor)	Anxiety (BP, verbal expressions by subject, self-report questionnaire)	Experimental group less anxious on all three measures than control group.
Heidt (1981)	Casual/known touch (pulse-taking) and therapeutic touch	Experimental	90 cardiovascular patients	Anxiety (STAI; patient interview)	Casual touch and no–touch group not significantly different in post–treatment anxiety.

Author (Year)	Type of Touch	Design	Sample	Outcomes Evaluated	Findings
ADULT STUDIES *continued*					
Knable (1981)	Hand-holding	Case study	15 ICU patients; 12 nurses	Physiological response, nonverbal behaviors	Positive responses observed in facial expression, body movement, and eye contact during hand-holding; changes in vital signs also observed.
Walleck (1982)	Stroking face and back of hand	Experimental	30 patients with intracranial monitoring device in place	ICP, arterial blood pressure, pulse	Touch lowered ICP in 25 of 30 patients; no significant difference between touching face or hand.
Langland & Panicucci (1982)	Touch on forearm with verbal request	Experimental	32 elderly, confused female nursing home patients	Attention, verbal response, appropriate action gesture	Increased attention when touch used.
Longworth (1982)	Slow stroke back massage	Exploratory (with repeated measures)	32 healthy female subjects	Anxiety state–trait anxiety inventory (STAI), generalized muscle tension, heart rate, BP, GSR, finger temperature	Significant decrease in STAI; 3–minute massage produced significant increase in systolic BP and 6–minute massage showed a significant increase in mean heart rate.
Lorensen (1983)	High and low degree of physical touch	Pilot study, experimental	12 obstetrical patients	Patient's experience during labor, patient satisfaction, length of labor	Treatment group considered touch to be important during labor, while controls identified nurse talk as important and were more likely to believe that nothing seemed to relieve their discomfort; labor shorter for treatment group.
McCormick (1984)	Back rub using slow strokes	Experimental	30 neuro–otologic surgical patients in intensive care	Anxiety (STAI)	Back rub effective in reducing anxiety for patients with Meniere's disease (chronic) but not for other acute conditions.

(continued)

Table 20-3 *(continued)*

Author (Year)	Type of Touch	Design	Sample	Outcomes Evaluated	Findings
ADULT STUDIES *continued*					
Bailey (1984)	"Caring touch" (touches exceeding five seconds to hand, arm, shoulder, etc.)	Field experiment	28 adult patients being treated in emergency	Patient evaluation of nurse	No significant differences in groups on attitudes toward nurse; attitudes not related to number of touch encounters.
Bramble (1985)	Stationary touch used with routine hospital admission questions	Experimental	50 adult patients	Anxiety (STAI, BP, pulse)	No significant differences although in the touch group a greater number of subjects had a decrease in STAI than in no-touch group.
Guerrero (1985)	Casual touch (taking pulses) and therapeutic touch	Experimental	30 oncology patients	Anxiety (STAI)	Patients in casual touch and therapeutic touch groups showed significantly lower levels of anxiety from baseline mean of trait and state anxiety to post-intervention state anxiety.
Curry (1985)	Intentional nonprocedural touch and procedural touch associated with health examination	Experimental (double-blind)	24 well adult women participating in health maintenance examination	Anxiety (STAI, BP, finger temperature)	No treatment effect (i.e., use of nonprocedural touch) demonstrated.
Birch (1986)	Any physical contact	Descriptive	30 obstetrical patients	Patient perceptions of effects of touch during labor	Touch identified as therapeutic was perceived to have a comforting effect and assisted coping efforts; effects of nontherapeutic touch described as irritating/annoying.
Hollinger (1986)	"Hands-on-top-of-hands" touch during interview	Experimental (using partial counter-balancing)	Eight female, elderly, hospitalized patients	Duration and frequency of verbal response, length of silence	Touch increased duration and frequency of verbal responses during the time period that touch was applied.

Author (Year)	Type of Touch	Design	Sample	Outcomes Evaluated	Findings
ADULT STUDIES *continued*					
Glick (1986)	Procedural touch (taking vital signs) and caring touch (holding patient's hand)	Quasi–experimental	33 acute myocardial infarction (MI) patients	State anxiety (STAI)	No significant differences.
Chen (1986/1987)	Expressive (hand-shake) and instrument-al touch (pulse–taking)	Experimental (double blind)	45 CCU patients	Psychological effect of touch, heart rate, ECG	Expressive touch significantly reduced anxiety levels.
Norberg et al. (1986)	Circular, stroking movements to face, neck, shoulders, back, arms, hands, lower legs, and feet	Case study	Two female Alzheimer patients	Verbal and nonverbal behaviors, heart rate, respirations	No specific behavioral response to touch observed.
Fakouri & Jones (1987)	Slow stroke back massage	Quasi–experimental	18 nursing home patients	Heart rate, skin temperature, BP	Significant changes in physiological indicators of relaxation.
Bauer & Dracup (1987)	Slow stroke back massage	Quasi–experimental	25 coronary ICU patients	Heart rate, BP, muscle tension, skin conductance, skin temperature	No significant differences on any of the dependent variables.
Redfern & Le May (1987)	Any physical contact	Descriptive	66 elderly patients	Patient response to touch (verbal/nonverbal); well-being	No relationship between amount or type of touch and well-being.
Henneman (1989)	Holding hand with verbal interaction	Experimental	26 adult patients being weaned from ventilation	Stress (heart rate, BP, respirations)	No significant difference in stress response; respiratory rate increased five minutes after weaning for both groups.

(continued)

Table 20-3 *(continued)*

Author (Year)	Type of Touch	Design	Sample	Outcomes Evaluated	Findings
ADULT STUDIES *continued*					
Tough (1989)	Slow stroke back massage	Experimental	21 elderly patients in extended care facility	Anxiety (STAI, pulse, BP, electromyogram readings	No significant differences between back massage group and conversation group on dependent variables.
Marx, Werner & Cohen–Mansfield (1989)	Any physical contact	Descriptive	24 agitated and cognitively impaired nursing home residents	Number and kind of agitated behaviors	Aggressive behaviors were manifest more often when residents were touched. Nonaggressive behaviors (e.g., repetitious mannerisms) were manifest less frequently when residents were touched.

(Weiss, 1986). Second, researchers have tended to look for the positive effects of touch (e.g., decreased anxiety, increased patient satisfaction with care), and their choice of dependent variables and data collection techniques reflects this bias. In studies in which the investigator not only applied the touch intervention, but also later interviewed the patients to determine their response to the touch (McCoy, 1977), the results were biased toward the positive effects of touch because it is unlikely that patients would be willing to give any negative feedback under these circumstances. Yet it is evident from at least one study (Birch, 1986) that patients may find some touches annoying or irritating.

In studying the effects of nurse–patient touch, investigators have examined developmental responses of infants to tactile stimulation, interpersonal responses of patients to interactions involving touch, psychological responses (including self-image and indices of arousal) to a variety of types of touch, and the influence of touch on well-being and progress in labor. Dependent variables have been measured by a number of means, including investigator-developed questionnaires, standardized questionnaires, interviews, observational measures, and physiological indices. Yet methodological problems associated with a lack of clear or consistent touch interventions, small sample sizes, inadequate attention to the reliability and validity of measurements, and lack of adequate control of extraneous variables, in addition to the use of a wide variety of settings, patients, and dependent measures, make it difficult to identify areas of coherence among the findings.

One area, the effects of nurse–patienttouch on anxiety, has received a substantial amount of attention; nevertheless, the findings are conflicting. The use of diverse (and often multiple) methods of measurement across a variety of settings has provided evidence that touch can produce anxiety (Whitcher & Fisher, 1979), decrease anxiety (Chen, 1986/1987; Fakouri & Jones, 1987; Guerrero, 1985; McCormick, 1984; Sommer, 1979/1980), or have no effect at all (Bauer & Dracup, 1987; Bramble, 1985; Curry, 1985; Glick, 1986; Heidt, 1981; Kaufmann, 1964; Tough, 1989). Even investigators that have used similar physiological measures (Knable, 1981; Lynch, Flaherty, Emrich, Mills, & Katcher, 1974; Lynch, Thomas, Mills, Malinow, & Katcher, 1974; Lynch, Thomas, Paskewitz, Katcher, & Weir, 1977; Mills, Thomas, Lynch, & Katcher, 1976) have reported inconclusive results or no effects (Henneman, 1989; Whitcher & Fisher, 1979). While identifiable differences in anxiety may be diminished as a result of the large variability in physiological indicators that exists both between and within individuals (Tough, 1989), other factors must be considered. The meaning of touch may change when it is used in different contexts, which may explain the variation in responses reflected in these findings and negate the underlying assumption made by investigators that all types of touch have similar meanings (Weiss, 1988). In addition, the mere presence of a supportive individual may relieve symptoms of anxiety and decrease arousal (Sivadon, 1969). In most studies, touch was administered while conversing with the patient. Thus, the results of these investigations of nurse–patient touch may be confounded by the effect of simply having someone to talk to (or someone close by); this extraneous variable was controlled by only two investigators (Chen, 1986/1987; Tough, 1989).

Inadequate control of other forms of communication that may be part of or associated with the touch gesture (e.g., eye contact, tone of voice, body position, purpose of the interaction) may influence outcomes and explain inconclusive findings. In many instances, the investigator presented the touch gesture and interacted with the control group. Thus, it may be incorrect to conclude that differences between the outcomes of experimental and control groups are the result of the touch intervention. For example, in replicating a study by Boderman, Freed, and Kinnucan (1972), Breed and Ricci (1973) showed that, when the accomplice's behavior and touch gestures were controlled, no effect was created by touch. Preference for future interaction with the accomplice was significantly affected by the accomplice's behavior (i.e., being "warm" or "cold") rather than by the use of touch. The possibility that a researcher who has a vested interest in the positive effects of touch may be more warm and friendly in touch conditions than in the no-touch conditions has been ignored by those investigating nurse–patient touch. Future research would profit by controlling for the influence of important nonverbal behaviors and different types of touch (e.g., interested versus disinterested).

The majority of researchers who have studied the effects of nurse–patient touch have used deductive approaches and thus have assumed that the effects of touch can be predicted and measured on the basis of existing theory. This assumption has been challenged by those who believe that the poor understanding of the concept of touch is one of the most salient problems associated with this approach to research (Estabrooks, 1987a; Jones & Yarbrough, 1985; Weiss, 1979, 1986). Estabrooks (1987a) suggests that most investigators have designed studies without critically reflecting on the question, "What is touch?" If the most important aspects of touch have been predetermined on the basis of previous work done in different contexts, it is not surprising that the resulting research has not contributed meaningfully to our understanding of nurse–patient touch. In addition, the use of experimental designs is based on the assumption that contrived touch interventions (which were often brief, almost unnoticeable touches) initiated by a nurse in a controlled fashion will increase the understanding of the effects of touch. The use of such designs fails to consider the interactive, reciprocal nature of interpersonal communication, and the continuous feedback and readjustment that characterize dyadic communication, including communication through the use of touch. When a stranger (who for the most part has been the researcher) enacts the touch intervention, touching gestures and the associated effects that are characteristic of relationships at various stages of intimacy are not addressed.

Descriptions of nurse–patienttouch in the context in which it occurs, including descriptions of hitherto unnoticed but associated nonverbal and verbal behavior patterns, would help to show which aspects of touching behavior determine impressions of the meaning of touch and would increase our ability to test interpretations and examine behavior (Jones & Woodson, 1979). In addition, paying more attention to the perceptions of those who touch and are touched may assist in determining which effects of touch should be addressed. Therefore, if researchers are willing to accept the trade-off between maintaining a certain level of control and choosing a method that is appropriate to the model under investigation (Seigman & Feldstein, 1987), the use of descriptive, naturalistic methods may help capture the interactive nature of touching behaviors and their effect.

In summary, while nurses' clinical reports of the effects of touch in practice suggest that touch may be a powerful therapeutic tool (Amacher,

1973; Bean, 1980; Bledsoe, 1984; Burnside, 1973; De Thomaso, 1971; Preston, 1973; Seaman, 1982; Waddell, 1979; Zefron, 1975), and patients' accounts of the need for and effects of touch are often dramatic (Colton, 1983; Huss, 1977; McGuire, 1983; Older, 1982; Pratt & Mason, 1981), systematic investigation has yet to demonstrate these effects with any degree of consistency.

CONCLUSION

This review of the literature reinforces the fact that little is known with certainty about nurse–patient touch. The lack of definitive findings in this field is due to the influence of unsubstantiated *a priori* assumptions that underlie the predominantly deductive approaches used to investigate touch, the lack of attention to the context in which touch occurs (which is central to the understanding of touch), methodological problems, and problems associated with the definition of touch. Because understanding and documentation of the effects of therapeutic interventions are vital to improvements in caring in nursing practice, changes are needed in the approaches used in the research of touch; in particular, increased use of the inductive approach is crucial to development of a more complex understanding of touch. Such approaches would help to identify the nurses' and patients' behaviors that may be important for study (rather than deciding this *a priori*), permit exploration of the experience of touching and being touched from the perspective of the nurse and the patient, and allow consideration of the important factors of context and relationship. The findings of inductive research on these and other dimensions of touch could contribute significantly to the development of the adequate theoretical and operational definitions of nurse–patient touch that are needed to provide a basis for more productive deductive work.

REFERENCES

Aguilera, D.C. (1967). Relationship between physical contact and verbal interaction between nurses and patients. *Journal of Psychiatric Nursing, 5,* 5–21.

Allekian, C.I. (1973). Intrusions of territory and personal space: An anxiety-producing factor for hospitalized patients—an exploratory study. *Nursing Research, 22,* 236–241.

Amacher, N.J. (1973). Touch is a way of caring. *American Journal of Nursing, 73,* 852–854.

Andersen, J.F., Andersen, P.A., & Lustig, M.W. (1987). Opposite sex touch avoidance: A national replication and extension. *Journal of Nonverbal Behavior, 11*(2), 89–109.

Andersen, P.A., & Leibowitz, K. (1978). The development and nature of the construct touch avoidance. *Environmental Psychology and Nonverbal Behavior, 3,* 89–106.

Bailey, J.R.S. (1984). *Touch and patients' perceptions of the nurse as a caring person in the emergency room.* Unpublished master's thesis, Texas Women's University, Denton.

Barnett, K.A. (1972). A survey of the current utilization of touch by health team personnel with hospitalized patients. *International Journal of Nursing Studies, 9,* 195–209.

Bauer, W.C., & Dracup, K.A. (1987). Physiological effects of back massage in patients with acute myocardial infarction. *Focus on Critical Care, 14*(6), 42–46.

Bean, C. (1980). The importance of touch in patient care. *Imprint, 27*(5), 46, 71.

Benner, P. (1984). *From novice to expert: Excellence and power in clinical nursing practice.* Don Mills, Ontario: Addison-Wesley.

Birch, E.R. (1986). The experience of touch received during labor. Post-partum perceptions of therapeutic value. *Journal of Nurse-Midwifery, 31,* 270–276.

Blackburn, S.T., & Barnard, K.E. (1985). Analysis of caregiving events relating to preterm infants in the special care unit. In A.W. Gottfried & J.L. Gaiter (Eds.), *Infant stress under intensive care* (pp. 113–129). Baltimore, MD: University Park Press.

Bledsoe, A. (1984). The importance of touch in nursing care. *Imprint, 13*(4), 58–59.

Boderman, A., Freed, D.W., & Kinnucan, M.T. (1972). "Touch me, like me": Testing an encounter group assumption. *Journal of Applied Behavioral Science, 8,* 527–533.

Boyd, C. (1986). Nursing journal recruitment advertisements: Symbolic indicators of care. *Journal of Nursing Administration, 16,* 27–28.

Bramble, B. (1985). The effect of one touch modality on state anxiety during a hospital admission procedure (Doctoral dissertation, Texas Women's University, 1985). *Dissertation Abstracts International, 46,* 1867B. (University Microfilms No. 85–16713).

Brannigan, C.R., & Humphries, D.A. (1972). Human non-verbal behaviour, a means of communication. In N.B. Jones (Ed.), *Ethological studies of child behaviour* (pp. 37–64). Cambridge, England: Cambridge University Press.

Breed, G., & Ricci, J.S. (1973). "Touch me, like me": Artifact? *Proceedings of the 81st Annual Convention of the American Psychological Association, 8,* Part 1, 153–154.

Burkhardt, M.A. (1975). *Nurses' attitudes toward non-necessary touching with patients.* Unpublished master's thesis, University of Rochester, Rochester, NY. (University Microfilms No. 15000–NU).

Burnside, I.M. (1973). Touching is talking. *American Journal of Nursing, 73,* 2060–2063.

Burnside, I.M. (1977). The therapeutic use of touch with the elderly. In H. Shore & M. Ernst (Eds.), *Sensory processes and aging* (pp. 75–90). Dallas, TX: Dallas Geriatric Research Institute.

Burnside, I.M. (1981). The therapeutic use of touch. In I.M. Burnside (Ed.), *Nursing and the aged* (pp. 503–518). Toronto, Ontario: McGraw-Hill.

Charlton, A. (1959). *Identification of reciprocal influences of nurse and patient initiated physical contact in the psychiatric setting.* Unpublished master's thesis, University of Maryland, Baltimore.

Chen, G.L. (1987). Effects of touch on anxiety levels in coronary care patients (Doctoral dissertation, Texas Women's University, 1986). *Dissertation Abstracts International, 48*(4), 1002. (University Microfilm No. 87–15027).

Clement, J.M. (1983). A descriptive study of the use of touch by nurses with patients in the critical care unit (Doctoral dissertation, The University of Texas at Austin, 1983). *Dissertation Abstracts International, 43,* 1060B. (University Microfilms No. 83–19577).

Colton, H. (1983). *The gift of touch.* New York: Seaview/Putman.

Copstead, L.C. (1980). Effects of touch on self-appraisal and interaction appraisal for permanently institutionalized older adults. *Journal of Gerontological Nursing, 6,* 747–752.

Curry, R.L. (1985). *Effect of touch on client anxiety during health maintenance examinations.* Unpublished master's thesis, University of Florida, Gainesville. (University Microfilms No. 13–27301).

Dahill, C. (1984). *The use of touch with hospitalized children.* Unpublished master's thesis, University of Washington, Seattle.

Day, F.A. (1973). The patient's perception of touch. In E.H. Anderson, B.S. Bergersen, M. Duffy, M. Lohr, & M.H. Rose (Eds.), *Current concepts in clinical nursing* (Vol. 4, pp. 266–275). St. Louis, MO: C.V. Mosby.

De Augustinis, J., Isani, R.S., & Kumler, F.R. (1963). Ward study: The meaning of touch in interpersonal communication. In S.E. Bard & M.A. Marshall (Eds.), *Some clinical approaches to psychiatric nursing* (pp. 271–306). London: Macmillan.

De Thomaso, M.T. (1971). Touch power and the screen of loneliness. *Perspectives in Psychiatric Care, 9,* 112–118.

DeWever, M.K. (1977). Nursing home patients perception of nurses' affective touching. *The Journal of Psychology, 96,* 163–171.

Durr, C.A. (1971). Hands that help but how? *Nursing Forum, 10,* 392–400.

Eibl-Eibesfeldt, I. (1989). *Human ethology.* New York: Aldine de Gruyter.

Ekman, P., & Friesen, W.V. (1969). The repertoire of nonverbal behavior: Categories, origins, usage, and coding. *Semiotica, 1,* 49–98.

Ekman, P., Sorenson, E.R., & Friesen, W.V. (1969). Pan-cultural elements in facial displays of emotions. *Science, 164,* 86–88.

El-Kafass, A.A.R. (1983). A study of the expressive touch behaviors by nursing personnel with patients in critical care units (Doctoral dissertation, The Catholic University of America, 1982). *Dissertation Abstracts International, 43,* 3187B. (University Microfilms No. 83–04646).

Ellis, L., Taylor, J., & Walts, N. (1979). Personal awareness. Reach out and touch. *The Journal of Nursing Care, 12,* 19–21.

Estabrooks, C.A. (1987a). *Touching behaviors of intensive care nurses.* Unpublished master's thesis, University of Alberta, Edmonton.

Estabrooks, C.A. (1987b). Touch in nursing practice: A historical perspective. *Journal of Nursing History, 2* (2), 33–49.

Estabrooks, C.A. (1989). Touch: A nursing strategy in the intensive care unit. *Heart & Lung, 18,* 392–401.

Fakouri, C., & Jones, P. (1987). Relaxation Rx: Slow stroke back rub. *Journal of Gerontological Nursing, 13*(2), 32–35.

Farrah, S. (1971). The nurse—the patient—and touch. In M. Duffey, E.H. Anderson, B.S. Bergersen, M. Lehr, & M.H. Rose (Eds.), *Current concepts in clinical nursing* (Vol. 3, pp. 247–259). St. Louis, MO: C.V. Mosby.

Fisher, L.M., & Joseph, D.H. (1989). A scale to measure attitudes about nonprocedural touch. *Canadian Journal of Nursing Research, 21*(2), 5–14.

Gadow, S. (1984). Touch and technology: Two paradigms of patient care. *Journal of Religion and Health, 23,* 63–69.

Gadow, S.A. (1985). Nurse and patient: The caring relationship. In A.H. Bishop & J.R. Scudder (Eds.), *Caring, curing, coping: Nurse, physician, patient relationships* (pp. 31–43). Tuscaloosa, AL: University of Alabama Press.

Gentner, L. (1980). Touch: A review of the literature. *Baylor Nursing Education, 2,* 15–22.

Glick, M.S. (1986). Caring touch and anxiety in myocardial infarction patients in the intermediate cardiac care unit. *Intensive Care Nursing, 2*, 61–66.

Greenberg, B.M. (1972). *Therapeutic effects of touch on alteration of psychotic behavior in institutionalized elderly patients.* Unpublished master's thesis, Duke University, Durham, NC.

Griffin, M. (1978). *Frequency of touch communication as used by emergency room nurses.* Unpublished master's thesis, Texas Women's University, Denton.

Guerrero, M.A. (1985). *The effects of therapeutic touch on state-trait anxiety level of oncology patients.* Unpublished master's thesis, The University of Texas Medical Branch, Galveston. (University of Microfilms No. 13–26756).

Harrison, R.P. (1984). Nonverbal communication: Advances and anomalies. In B. Dervin & M.J. Voigt (Eds.), *Progress in communication sciences* (Vol. 5, pp. 255–274). Norwood, NJ: Ablex.

Hartup, W.W. (1979). Levels of analysis in the study of social interaction: An historical perspective. In M.I. Lamb, S.J. Suomi, & G.R. Stephenson (Eds.), *Social interaction analysis* (pp. 11–32). Madison, WI: The University of Wisconsin Press.

Hasselmeyer, E.G. (1963). Handling and premature infant behavior: An experimental study of the relationship between handling and selected physiological, pathological and behavioral indices related to body functioning among a group of prematurely born infants who weighed between 1,501 and 2,000 grams at birth and were between the ages of seven and twenty eight days of life. Doctoral dissertation, New York University, 1963). *Dissertation Abstracts International, 24*, 2874–2875. (University Microfilms No. 64–257).

Heidt, P. (1981). Effect of therapeutic touch on anxiety level of hospitalized patients. *Nursing Research, 30*, 32–37.

Henneman, E.A. (1989). Effect of nursing contact on the stress response of patients being weaned from mechanical ventilation. *Heart & Lung, 18*, 483–489.

Hernandez, C.G. (1988). A phenomenologic investigation of the concept of the lived experience of caring in professional nurses. In *Caring and nursing exploration in the feminist perspectives* (pp. 122–152). Denver, CO: School of Nursing, University of Colorado Health Sciences Center.

Heylings, P.N.K. (1973). Personal view. The no touching epidemic—an English disease. *British Medical Journal, 2*, 111.

Hollenbeck, A.R. (1978). Problems of reliability in observational research. In G.P. Sackett (Ed.), *Observing Behavior, Vol. 2, Data collection and analysis methods* (pp. 79–98). Baltimore, MD: University Park Press.

Hollinger, L.M. (1986). Communicating with the elderly. *Journal of Gerontological Nursing, 12*(3), 9–13.

Huss, A.J. (1977). Touch with care or a caring touch? *American Journal of Occupational Therapy, 31*, 11–18.

Ingham, A. (1989). A review of the literature relating to touch and its use in intensive care. *Intensive Care Nursing, 5*, 65–75.

Jay, S.S. (1982). The effects of gentle human touch on mechanically ventilated very-short-gestation infants [Monograph 12]. *Maternal-Child Nursing Journal, 11*, 199–256.

Johnson, F. (1984). *The effects of touch on intracranial pressure in children.* Unpublished master's thesis, University of Washington, Seattle.

Jones, N.B. (1972). Characteristics of ethological studies of human behaviour. In N.B. Jones (Ed.), *Ethological studies of child behaviour* (pp. 3–33). Cambridge, England: Cambridge University Press.

Jones, N.B. & Woodson, R.H. (1979). Describing behavior: The ethologists' perspective. In I.M. Lamb, S.J. Suomi, & G.R. Stephenson (Eds.), *Social instructional analysis* (pp. 97–117). Madison, WI: University of Wisconsin Press.

Jones, S. E., & Yarbrough, A.E. (1985). A naturalistic study of the meanings of touch. *Communication Monographs, 52*, 19–56.

Kaufmann, M.A. (1964). Autonomic responses as related to nursing comfort measures. *Nursing Research, 13*, 45–55.

Kelly, L.S. (1984). High tech/high touch—now more than ever [Editorial]. *Nursing Outlook, 32*(1), 15.

Klaus, M., & Kennell, J. (1976). Parent-to-infant attachment. In D. Hull (Ed.), *Recent advances in pediatrics* (pp. 129–152). Edinburgh: Churchill Livingstone.

Knable, J. (1981). Handholding: One means of transcending barriers of communication. *Heart & Lung, 10*, 1106–1110.

Knapp, M.L. (1983). Dyadic relationship development. In J. Wiemann & R.P. Harrison (Eds.), *Nonverbal interaction* (pp. 179–207). Beverly Hills, CA: Sage.

Kramer, M., Chamorro, I., Green, D., & Krudtson, F. (1975). Extra tactile stimulation of the premature infant. *Nursing Research, 24*, 324–334.

Krieger, D. (1975). Therapeutic touch: Imprimature of nursing. *American Journal of Nursing, 75*, 784–787.

Lamb, M.I. (1979). Issues in the study of social interaction: An introduction. In M.I. Lamb, S.J. Suomi, & G.R. Stephenson (Eds.), *Social interaction analysis* (pp. 1–10). Madison, WI: The University of Wisconsin Press.

Lane, P. (1989). Nurse-client perceptions: The double standard of touch. *Issues in Mental Health Nursing, 10*, 1–13.

Langland, R.M., & Panicucci, C.L. (1982). Effects of touch on communication with elderly confused patients. *Journal of Gerontological Nursing, 8*, 152–155.

Larsen, K.S., & LeRoux, J. (1984). A study of same sex touching attitudes: Scale development and personality predictors. *Journal of Sex Research, 20*, 264–278.

Lehner, P.H. (1979). *Handbook of ethological methods*. New York: Garland STPM Press.

Leininger, M.L. (1981). The phenomenon of caring: Importance, research questions and theoretical considerations. In M.L. Leininger (Ed.), *Caring: An essential human need* (pp. 3–15). Thorofare, NJ: Charles B. Slack.

Le May, A.C., & Redfern, S.J. (1987). A study of non-verbal communication between nurses and elderly patients. In P. Fielding (Ed.), *Research in the nursing care of elderly people* (pp. 171–189). Chichester, England: John Wiley & Sons.

Longworth, J.C.D. (1982). Psychophysiological effects of slow stroke back massage in normotensive females. *Advances in Nursing Science, 4*(4), 44–61.

Lorensen, M. (1983). Effects of touch in patients during a crisis situation in hospital. In J. Wilson–Barnett (Ed.), *Nursing research. Ten studies in patient care* (pp. 179–193). Chichester, England: John Wiley & Sons.

Lynch, J.J., Flaherty, L., Emrich, C., Mills, M.E., & Katcher, A.H. (1974). Effects of human contact on the heart activity of curarized patients in a shock-trauma unit. *American Heart Journal, 88*, 160–169.

Lynch, J.J., Thomas, S.A., Mills, M.E., Malinow, K., & Katcher, A.H. (1974). The effects of human contact on the cardiac arrhythmia in coronary care patients. *The Journal of Nervous and Mental Disease, 158*, 88–99.

Lynch, J.J., Thomas, S.A., Paskewitz, D.A., Katcher, A.H., & Weir, L.O. (1977). Human contact and cardiac arrhythmias in a coronary care unit. *Psychosomatic Medicine, 39*, 188–191.

Major, B. (1981). Gender patterns in touching behavior. In C. Mayo & N.M. Henley (Eds.), *Gender and nonverbal behavior* (pp. 15–37). New York: Springer/Verlag.

Marshall, M.H. (1969). *An exploratory study of tactile contact utilized by nurses caring for five primigravida patients in labor.* Unpublished master's thesis, University of Washington, Seattle.

Marx, M.S., Werner, P., & Cohen-Mansfield, J. (1989). Agitation and touch in the nursing home. *Psychological Reports, 64*(3), Part 2, 1019–1026.

McCorkle, R. (1974). Effects of touch on seriously ill patients. *Nursing Research, 23,* 125–132.

McCormick, S.L. (1984). *The effect of back rubs on anxiety in the surgical patient.* Unpublished master's thesis, California State University, Long Beach. (University Microfilms No. 13–24742).

McCoy, P. (1977). Further proof that touch speaks louder than words. *R.N., 40*(11), 43–46.

McGuire, M.A. (1983). A touch in the dark. *Critical Care Nurse, 3,* 53–56.

Mehrabian, A. (1972). *Nonverbal communication.* New York: Aldine.

Mehrabian, A. (1981). *Silent messages: Implicit communication of emotions and attitudes* (2nd ed.). Belmont, CA: Wadsworth.

Miller, N.M. (1976). *An analysis of the awareness of touch as a communicative process.* Unpublished master's thesis, Texas Women's University, Denton.

Mills, M.E., Thomas, S.A., Lynch, J.J., & Katcher, A.H. (1976). Effect of pulse palpation on cardiac arrhythmia in coronary care patients. *Nursing Research, 25,* 378–382.

Mitchell, P.H., Habermann-Little, B., Johnson, F., VanInwegen-Scott, D., & Tyler, D. (1985). Critically ill children: The importance of touch in a high-technology environment. *Nursing Administration Quarterly, 9,* 38–46.

Montague, A. (1986). *Touching: The human significance of the skin* (3rd ed.). New York: Harper & Row.

Morse, J.M. (1983). An ethnoscientific analysis of comfort: A preliminary investigation. *Nursing Papers, 15,* 6–19.

Morse, J.M., & Bottorff, J.L. (1990). The use of ethology in clinical nursing research. *Advances in Nursing Science, 12*(3), 53–64.

Norberg, A., Melin, E., & Asplund, K. (1986). Reactions to music, touch and object presentation in the final stage of dementia. An exploratory study. *International Journal of Nursing Studies, 23,* 315–323.

Older, J. (1982). *Touching is healing.* New York: Stein and Day.

Patterson, M.L. (1983). *Nonverbal behavior. A functional perspective.* New York: Springer/Verlag.

Patterson, M.L. (1984). Nonverbal exchange: Past, present and future. *Journal of Nonverbal Behavior, 8,* 350–359.

Patterson, M.L., & Edinger, J.A. (1987). A functional analysis of space in social interaction. In A.W. Siegman & S. Feldstein (Eds.), *Nonverbal behavior and communication* (2nd ed.) (pp. 523–562). Hillsdale, NJ: Lawrence Erlbaum.

Paulen, A. (1984). High touch in a high tech environment [Editorial]. *Cancer Nursing, 7,* 201.

Penny, K.S. (1979). Postpartum perceptions of touch received during labor. *Research in Nursing and Health, 2,* 9–16.

Pepler, C.J. (1984). Congruence in relational messages communicated to nursing home residents through nurse aid touch behaviors (Doctoral dissertation, University of Michigan, 1984). *Dissertation Abstracts International, 45,* 2106B. (University Microfilms No. 84–22312).

Porter, L., Redfern, S.J., Wilson-Barnett, J., & Le May, A. (1986). The development of an observation schedule for measuring nurse-patient touch, using an ergonomic approach. *International Journal of Nursing Studies, 23,* 11–20.

Pratt, J.W., & Mason, A. (1981). *The caring touch.* London: Heydon.

Pratt, J.W., & Mason, A. (1984). The meaning of touch in care practice. *Social Science Medicine, 18,* 1081–1088.

Preston, T. (1973). When words fail. *American Journal of Nursing, 73,* 2064–2066.

Probrislo, J.M. (1984). *Comforting-touch behaviors in childbirth.* Unpublished master's thesis, University of Arizona, Tucson. (University Microfilms No. 13–24585).

Rausch, P.B. (1981). Effects of tactile and kinesthetic stimulation on premature infants. *Journal of Obstetric, Gynecologic and Neonatal Nursing, 10,* 34–37.

Redfern, S.J., & Le May, A.C. (1987, September). *Communicating through touch with the elderly.* Paper presented at the "Ageing and Well" Conference, Brighton, UK.

Sackett, G.P. (1978). Measurement in observational research. In G.P. Sackett (Ed.), *Observing behavior, Vol. 2, Data collection and analysis methods* (pp. 25–43). Baltimore, MD: University Park Press.

Saltenis, I.J. (1962). *Physical touch and nursing support in labor.* Unpublished master's thesis, Yale School of Nursing, New Haven, CT.

Scarr-Salapatek, S., & Williams, M.L. (1973). The effects of early stimulation on low-birth-weight infants. *Child Development, 44,* 94–101.

Schoenhofer, S.O. (1989). Affectional touch in critical care nursing: A descriptive study. *Heart & Lung, 18,* 146–154.

Seaman, L. (1982). Affective nursing touch. *Geriatric Nursing, 3,* 162–164.

Siegman, A.W., & Feldstein, S. (1987). Introduction. In A.W. Siegman & S. Feldstein (Eds.), *Nonverbal behavior and communication* (2nd ed.) (pp. 1–18). Hillsdale, NJ: Lawrence Erlbaum.

Sivadon, P. (1969). Social and milieu therapy. In M.H. Lader (Ed.), *Studies of anxiety* (pp. 131–134). London: Headley Brothers.

Slone, K. (1973). *A study of the effects of touch in nursing support in labor.* Unpublished master's thesis, Yale University, New Haven, CT.

Solkoff, N., & Matuszak, D. (1975). Tactile stimulation and behavioral development among low–birthweight infants. *Child Psychiatry and Human Development, 6,* 33–37.

Solkoff, N., Yaffe, S., Weintraub, D., & Blase, B. (1969). Effects of handling on the subsequent developments of premature infants. *Developmental Psychology, 1,* 765–768.

Sommer, P.A. (1980). Obstetrical patients' anxiety during transition of labor and the nursing intervention of touch (Doctoral dissertation, Texas Women's University, 1979). *Dissertation Abstracts International, 40,* 5610B.

Stolte, K.M. (1977). An exploratory study of patients' perceptions of touch they received during labor (Doctoral dissertation, University of Kansas, 1976). *Dissertation Abstracts International, 37,* 4708A.

Thomas, S.A., Lynch, J.J., & Mills, M.E. (1975). Psychosocial influences on heart arrhythmias in a coronary-care unit. *Heart & Lung, 4,* 746–750.

Tobiason, S.J.B. (1981). Touching is for everyone. *American Journal of Nursing, 81,* 728–730.

Topf, M. (1986). Three estimates of inter-rater reliability for nominal data. *Nursing Research, 35,* 253–255.

Torres, L.S. (1985). *The relationship between student nurses' feelings and attitudes about touch and their success in clinical nursing.* Unpublished master's thesis, California State University, Long Beach. (University Microfilms No. 13–25795).

Tough, J.H. (1989). *The psychophysiological effects of back massage in elderly institutionalized patients.* Unpublished master's thesis, University of Alberta, Edmonton.

Triplett, J.L., & Arneson, S.W. (1979). The use of verbal and tactile comfort to alleviate distress in young hospitalized children. *Research in Nursing and Health, 2,* 17–23.

Trowbridge, J. (1967). *Nurse-patient interpretations of nurse's touch.* Unpublished master's thesis, Loma Linda University, Loma Linda, CA.

Tulman, L.J. (1985). Mothers' and unrelated persons' initial handling of newborn infants. *Nursing Research, 34,* 205–210.

Ujehly, G.B. (1979). Touch: Reflections and perceptions. *Nursing Forum, 18*(1), 18–32.

Waddell, E. (1979). Quality touching to communicate caring. *Nursing Forum, 18,* 288–292.

Wagnild, G., & Manning, R.W. (1985). Convey respect during bathing procedures. *Journal of Gerontological Nursing, 11*(12), 6–11.

Walleck, C.A. (1982). *The effect of purposeful touch on intracranial pressure.* Unpublished master's thesis, University of Maryland, Baltimore.

Waltz, C.F., Strickland, P.L., & Lenz, E.R. (1984). *Measurement in nursing research.* Philadelphia, PA: F.A. Davis.

Watson, W.H. (1973). Body idiom in social interaction. A field study of geriatric nursing (Doctoral dissertation, University of Pennsylvania, 1972). *Dissertation Abstracts International, 33,* 3778A.

Watson, W.H. (1975). The meanings of touch: Geriatric nursing. *Journal of Communication, 25,* 104–112.

Watson, W.H. (1979-80). Resistances to naturalistic observation in a geriatric setting. *International Journal of Aging and Human Development, 10*(1), 35–45.

Weiss, S.J. (1979). The language of touch. *Nursing Research, 28,* 76–80.

Weiss, S.J. (1986). Psychophysiological effects of caregiver touch on incidence of cardiac dysrhythmia. *Heart & Lung, 15,* 495–505.

Weiss, S.J. (1988). Touch. In J.J. Fitzpatrick, R.L. Taunton, & J.Q. Benoliel (Eds.), *Annual review of nursing research* (Vol. 6, pp. 3–27). New York: Springer/Verlag.

Whitcher, S.J., & Fisher, J.D. (1979). Multi-dimensional reaction to therapeutic touch in a hospital setting. *Journal of Personality and Social Psychology, 37,* 87–96.

White, J.L., & Labarba, R.C. (1976). The effects of tactile and kinesthetic stimulation on neonatal development in the premature infant. *Developmental Psychobiology, 9,* 569–577.

Zefron, L.J. (1975). The history of the laying-on of hands in nursing. *Nursing Forum, 14,* 350–363.

21

Restlessness in the Elderly: A Concept Analysis

Ann M. Kolanowski

Restlessness is a universal phenomenon which health practitioners often encounter in the clinical area (Thomas, 1988). Despite the reported prevalence of this behavior, very little has been written about it in the geriatric nursing literature. The etiology of restless behavior remains unclear and its management continues to be problematic (Cohen-Mansfield, 1986). In current nursing practice, the use of restraints and medications is a major focus of care (Zimmer, Watson, & Treat, 1984). The ineffectiveness of these methods and their side effects point to the need for a better understanding of restlessness and more appropriate nursing interventions.

Improvement in the care of patients who experience restlessness can occur only when this concept is clearly defined and placed within a theoretical framework. It is then that propositions may be scientifically tested and support generated for alternative interventions.

The purpose of this paper is to explore restlessness in the elderly using Walker and Avant's (1983) strategy for concept analysis. Review of pertinent literature on theory and research will be followed by defining attributes, antecedents and consequences, and empirical referents.

REVIEW OF LITERATURE

Theoretical Background

Norris (1975) was one of the first to analyze restlessness from a nursing perspective. She defines this concept as " . . . a discontinuous animal behavior evidenced by non-specific, repetitive, unorganized, diffuse, apparently non-purposeful motor activity that is subject to limited control" (Norris, 1975, p. 107). Norris (1986) notes that while this behavior is generally thought of as negative, its real purpose is to prepare the organism to cope with change, challenge, or threat. In this sense, restlessness is conceptualized as a disturbance in rhythmicity and is related to changes or stimuli in a person's environment which are perceived by that person as arousing. In systematizing restlessness, Norris (1978) points out that this behavior occurs along a continuum: first as small muscle activity, then as gross muscle activity, and then as total body involvement. Each stage expresses greater discomfort or tension. From this perspective, restlessness may be defined as a feeling of increased arousal accompanied by an increase in motor activity.

Research has documented a relationship between arousal or level of activation, and motor activity. The conceptual basis for this approach is derived from Activation Theory.

The term activation has been used to refer to the sleep-waking-excitement continuum—a state of arousal or level of drive (Malmo, 1959). More recently, the concept has been defined as a phenomenological awareness of general bodily energy state (Thayer, 1967). The concept of restlessness may be defined within the framework of Activation Theory. Historically, a good deal of work has been done to develop this perspective.

Using a neurophysiological approach, Lindsley (1951) developed an "Activation Theory of Emotion." He demonstrated that changes in alertness are associated with electroencephalogram (EEG) changes and suggested that a brain mechanism is responsible for this state of arousal.

Hebb (1955) and Malmo (1959) built on this work and held that one's level of activation is a function of cortical stimulation of the reticular activating system. This system can be externally stimulated by sights and sounds, or internally stimulated by such things as thought processes. The system, in turn, stimulates other areas of the brain and leads to increased arousal, psychological and motor activity, and information processing (Kroeber-Riel, 1979).

Berlyne (1960) expanded on this notion by suggesting that when environmental stimulation deviates in either an upward or downward direction from an optimum influx, it becomes drive inducing or aversive. He defines the arousal potential of a stimulus as the degree to which the stimulus can disturb or alert the organism and dominate behavior over the claims of competing stimuli (Berlyne, 1971). The specific determinants of arousal potential include intensity, size, color, sensory modality, novelty, complexity, degree of change, suddenness of change, incongruity, and uncertainty.

Fiske and Maddi (1961) elaborated on the function of motor activity and its relation to activation. According to their theory, when cortical arousal or activation is low, the individual will actively increase internal stimulation by becoming restless, that is by moving about to increase sensory inflow, or by seeking external sources of stimulation.

Research on Restless Behavior

Research has supported a relationship between level of activation and motor activity. Both high and low levels of arousal have been associated with an increase in motor activity. Several intervening variables, notably personality traits and age of subjects, tend to mediate the motor response to varying levels of arousal.

For example, Hocking and Robertson (1969), using a quasi-experimental design, compared 15 male undergraduates who scored high on the Zuckerman Sensation Seeking Scale (SSS) to 15 male undergraduates who scored low, during a three–hour sensory restriction experiment. They found that subjects who scored high on the SSS demonstrated a significantly ($p < .001$) greater need to move about than those subjects who scored low. Work by Zuckerman, Persky, Hopkins, Murtaugh, Basu, and Shilling (1966) and Lambert and Levy (1972) substantiate these findings in that both studies documented significantly more restlessness in high–sensation seekers in situations of sensory deprivation or low arousal.

There is also evidence for a relationship between an increase in cortical arousal and an increase in motor activity. Barry's (1974) research lends support to this proposition. The investigator found that both introverts and extroverts demonstrated high levels of motor activity when presented with confusing auditory input. This suggests that as sensory overload or arousal increases, motor activity increases in a similar fashion.

In a related investigation, Falco (1976) studied 56 female subjects between 18 and 30 years of age, who were confined to bed rest for one hour, and found a significant relationship between higher degrees of field dependence as measured by the Portable Rod-and-Frame test and the embedded figures test and gross motor activity of the nondominant limb. In addition, gross motor activity was found to be triggered by the visual environment; that is, those individuals who were tested under conditions of visual sensory deprivation and those who were exposed to a tension-producing five-minute silent movie, demonstrated greater motor activity.

No studies were found which addressed restlessness in the aged and environmental stimulation, but it has been shown that the elderly have lower sensation–seeking scores (Zuckerman, Eysenck, & Eysenck, 1978; Zuckerman & Neeb, 1980) and tend to be more field dependent (Schwartz

& Karp, 1967) than younger people. On the basis of these findings, one might hypothesize that the elderly would be more aroused and restless under conditions of increased stimulation as opposed to decreased stimulation. Welford (1965) suggests that the aged are in a chronic state of under-arousal, but when presented with novel or intense stimuli may become phasically over-aroused. This over-activation results in tension, anxiety, and heightened activity or restlessness.

Research on Restlessness in the Elderly

Restlessness in the elderly has not been widely researched, but similar behavior, such as agitation and wandering, has been described (Cohen-Mansfield, 1986; Cornbleth, 1977; Dawson & Reid, 1987; Monsour & Robb, 1982; Snyder, 1978; Struble & Sivertsen, 1987). For example, motor restlessness has been addressed as one behavior or manifestation of agitation. Cohen-Mansfield and Billig (1986), in an attempt to clarify the concept of agitation, define this behavior as " . . . inappropriate verbal, vocal, or motor activity that is not explained by needs or confusion per se" (p. 712). It includes behaviors such as aimless wandering, pacing, cursing, screaming, biting, and fighting.

As an initial effort to understand the phenomenon of agitation from a behavioral perspective, Cohen-Mansfield (1986) studied 66 nursing home residents from two nursing units for agitated, cognitively deteriorated elderly people. The frequency of agitated behaviors was documented by nursing home staff using a seven-point rating scale. Results indicated that the most frequent agitated behaviors reported were general restlessness, $(x = 3.7)$, constant unwarranted request for attention $(x = 3.91)$, complaining and negativism $(x = 2.86)$, and pacing or wandering $(x = 3.4)$. Pearson correlations between the agitated behaviors demonstrated significant relationships $(p < .05)$ between restlessness and pacing $(r = .75)$, dressing inappropriately $(r = .31)$, constant requests for attention $(r = .46)$, and trying to get to a different place $(r = .33)$. The concept of agitation seemed to emerge as a construct with interrelated behaviors, including restlessness. Finally, staff were asked what they felt precipitated these behaviors in patients. Staff reported frustration, invasion of one's territory or personal space, behavior of other residents, confusion, loneliness and need for attention, depression, past issues, phase of the moon, constipation, deafness, and restraints.

Several other studies have addressed wandering, a repetitive motor behavior. Cornbleth (1977) compared the differential effect of a protected ward area on wandering and nonwandering geriatric patients in terms of their physical, cognitive, and psychosocial functioning. Thirty wanderers and 18 nonwanderers served as subjects. The multivariate analysis for the physical variables was significant, with wanderers showing greater range of motion off the ward. The multivariate group effect for the psychosocial variables (social behavior, morale, mental status, and social desirability) was also significant, with wanderers showing less improvement than non-wanderers.

Dawson and Reid (1987), in their study of the behavioral dimensions of wandering patients, identified two factors which differentiated wanderers from nonwanderers—cognitive deficits and hyperactivity. The 59 wanderers were significantly more likely to have underlying cognitive impairments and a higher level of mobility than the 41 nonwanderers.

Snyder (1978) compared eight wanderers with eight nonwanderers. Despite the small numbers, findings indicated that wanderers engaged more often in nonsocial behavior (a finding supported by Cohen-Mansfield [1986]) and had lower mental status scores. Using a retrospective record audit, Snyder identified three psychosocial factors that may have influenced subjects' tendency to wander: activity as a lifelong pattern of coping with stress, previous work roles, and search for security.

Monsour and Robb (1982) explored the notion advanced by Snyder (1978), that the tendency to wander is consistent with life-long psychosocial patterns, in their study of 22 pairs of wanderers and nonwanderers ranging in age from 53 to 89 years. They conducted personally structured interviews with each subject's closest significant other to obtain data related to the life-style of each subject. Using paired t-tests it was determined that (1) before their illness, wanderers engaged in a higher level of social and leisure activities than did nonwanderers ($t = 3.36$, $p = .003$), (2) before their illness, wanderers experienced more stressful life events than did nonwanderers ($t = 4.88$, $p = .000$), (3) wanderers showed motor reactions to stress in their earlier years ($t = 6.79$, $p = .000$); and (4) wanderers demonstrated more motor behavioral styles in their earlier years ($t = 5.69$, $p = .000$).

While the foregoing research is limited by the fact that much of it is *ex-post facto* and involves cognitively impaired or small numbers of subjects, there is the suggestion that restless behavior in the elderly is a coping strategy and is related to environmental stimuli which are perceived as arousing. These findings support the notion of restlessness as conceptualized in Activation Theory, as well as Norris' analysis of restlessness as a reaction to change, challenge, or threat.

Using this perspective, research can be designed to ferret out those environmental factors, both internal and external, which are related to, or precipitate the behavior in the elderly. Nursing interventions which are philosophically congruent with this perspective would, in all likelihood, focus on reducing the environmental challenge rather than directly suppressing the behavior. These interventions might include noise reduction, temperature control, use of calming color schemes, soft indirect lighting patterns, and other environmental manipulations to reduce arousal.

Defining Attributes

The critical attributes of the concept of restlessness that emerge from the literature seem to be these: (1) diffuse motor activity that is prompted by, or is in response to, changes in the environment and (2) perception of these changes as arousing or challenging.

Antecedents and Consequences

Norris (1975) has identified a number of antecedents of restlessness: seasonal and meteorological changes, anticipation of challenge, joy and happiness, boredom, strangeness, fatigue, anxiety and fear, labor, illness, pain, increased intracranial pressure, hemorrhage, shock, mania, thyrotoxicosis, drug reactions, loneliness, alienation, rage, and impending death. Empirical findings suggest the following antecedents: stimulus deprivation (Hocking & Robertson, 1969; Zuckerman, Persky, & Hoskins, 1966; Lambert & Levy, 1972), bright fluorescent lighting (Fenton & Penney, 1985; Miller, 1985), coded auditory stimuli (Barry, 1974), visual stimulation (Falco, 1976), tension and stress (Monsour & Robb, 1982), and cognitive deficits (Dawson & Reid, 1987).

Clinically, the consequences of restlessness are varied. On one hand, restlessness may lead to release of tension (Jacobsen, 1967). On the other hand, perpetual motor activity that does not lead to tension release may result in fatigue. If restlessness occurs in an institutional setting and is perceived as annoying by staff or other patients, pharmacological interventions or physical restraints may be used (Zimmer, Watson, & Treat, 1984).

Empirical Referents

A variety of methods exist for the measurement of restlessness as defined above. Several investigators (Barry, 1974; Falco, 1976) have used actometers to measure gross motor activity. This instrument, when applied to an extremity, measures acceleration and deceleration of movement in the plane of the actometer.

Downs and Fitzpatrick (1976) report on the development of the Motor Activity Rating Scale (MARS). This tool was designed to measure gross motor activity and the intensity of that activity, and has been used both with children and the aged. Reliability and validity have been substantiated by high correlations between actometer scores (.88 and .86) and the tool.

The use of videotapes in conjunction with actometer instrumentation, as well as the MARS, may prove to be a more valid and reliable method than a single measure of motor activity.

Level of activation, or arousal, has been measured using physiological measures such as skin conductance, EEG, blood pressure, and heart rate (Thayer, 1967). Hoskins (1978) has done much work on self-report measures of levels of activation. Her twelve alternate forms of Thayer's Activation-Deactivation Adjective Checklist have been used in research involving older subjects (Kolanowski, 1990; Mason, 1987).

SUMMARY

The concept of restlessness has been explored and a definition proposed. The behavior has been described within the framework of Activation Theory, and several approaches to measurement have been suggested. It remains for nursing researchers to test the adequacy of this analysis, to support or reject the antecedents, and to propose interventions which are philosophically congruent.

REFERENCES

Barry, M.J. (1974). The relation between introversion-extraversion, auditory input, and motor activity in bed-confined individuals. (Doctoral dissertation, New York University, 1974). *Dissertation Abstracts International*, 35/10B, p. 4962.

Berlyne, D. (1960). *Conflict arousal and curiosity*. New York: McGraw-Hill.

Berlyne, D. (1971). *Aesthetics and psychobiology*. Englewood Cliffs, NJ: Prentice–Hall.

Cohen-Mansfield, J. (1986). Agitated behaviors in the elderly: II. Preliminary results in the cognitively deteriorated. *Journal of the American Geriatrics Society, 34* (10), 722–727.

Cohen-Mansfield, J. & Billig, N. (1986). Agitated behaviors in the elderly: I. A conceptual review. *Journal of the American Geriatrics Society, 34* (10), 711–721.

Cornbleth, T. (1977). Effects of a protected hospital ward area on wandering and nonwandering geriatric patients. *Journal of Gerontology, 32,* 573–577.

Dawson, P., & Reid, D. (1987). Behavioral dimensions of patients at risk of wandering. *The Gerontologist, 27*(1), 104–107.

APA

Downs, F., & Fitzpatrick, J. (1976). Preliminary investigation of the reliability and validity of a tool for the assessment of body position and motor activity. *Nursing Research, 25*(6), 404–408.

Falco, S.M. (1976). The relationship between field dependence, visual input, and gross motor activity in individuals confined to bed. (Doctoral dissertation, New York University). *Dissertation Abstracts International, 37/02B*, p. 697.

Fenton, D., & Penney, R. (1985). The effects of fluorescent and incandescent lighting on the repetitive behaviors of autistic and intellectually handicapped children. *Australia and New Zealand Journal of Developmental Disabilities, II* (3), 137–141.

Fiske, D., & Maddi, S. (1961). *Functions of varied experience.* Homewood, IL: Dorsey Press.

Hebb, D. (1955). Drives and the CNS (conceptual nervous system). *Psychological Review, 62*, 243–254.

Hocking, J., & Robertson, M. (1969). The Sensation-Seeking Scale as a predictor of need for stimulation during sensory restriction. *Journal of Consulting and Clinical Psychology, 33*, 367–369.

Hoskins, C. (1978). A study of the relationship between level of activation, body temperature and interpersonal conflict in family relationships. (Doctoral dissertation, New York University). *Dissertation Abstracts International, 39/04B*, p. 1702.

Jacobsen, E. (1967). *Biology of emotions.* Springfield: Charles C. Thomas.

Kolanowski, A. (1990). Restlessness in the elderly: The effect of artificial lighting. *Nursing Research, 39*(3), 181–183.

Kroeber-Riel, W. (1979). Activation research: Psychobiological approaches in consumer research. *Journal of Consumer Research, 5*, 240–250.

Lambert, W., & Levy, L. (1972). Sensation-seeking and short term sensory isolation. *Journal of Personality and Social Psychology, 24*, 46–52.

Lindsley, D.B. (1951). Emotion. In S.S. Stevens (Ed.), *Handbook of Experimental Psychology,* (pp. 473–516). New York: John Wiley and Sons.

Malmo, R.B. (1959). Activation: A neurological dimension. *Psychological Review, 66*(6), 367–386.

Mason, D. (1987). Circadian body temperature and activation rhythms and the well-being of independent older women. (Doctoral dissertation, New York University). *Dissertation Abstracts International, 48/06B*, p. 1641.

Miller, J. (1985, November). *Environmental influences on agitated confusion in Alzheimer's disease.* Paper presented at 38th Annual Scientific Meeting of the Gerontological Society of America, New Orleans.

Monsour, N., & Robb, S. (1982). Wandering behavior in old age: A psychosocial study. *Social Work, 9*, 411–416.

Norris, C. (1975). Restlessness: A nursing phenomena in search of meaning. *Nursing Outlook, 23*(2), 103–107.

Norris, C. (1978). Restlessness. In C. Carlson & B. Blackwell (Eds.), *Behavioral concepts and nursing intervention* (pp. 141–153). New York: J. B. Lippincott Co.

Norris, C. (1986). Restlessness: A disturbance in rhythmicity. *Geriatric Nursing, 7*(6), 302–306.

Schwartz, D.W., & Karp, S.A. (1967). Field dependence in a geriatric population. *Perceptual and Motor Skills, 24*, 495–504.

Snyder, L.H. (1978). Wandering. *Gerontologist, 18*, 272–280.

Struble, L. & Sivertsen, L. (1987). Agitation: Behaviors in confused elderly patients. *Journal of Gerontological Nursing, 13* (11), 40–44.

Thayer, R. (1967). Measurement of activation through self report. *Psychological Reports, 20*, 663–678.

Thomas, D. (1988). Assessment and management of agitation in the elderly. *Geriatrics, 43*(6), 45–50.

Walker, L., & Avant, K. (1983). *Strategies for theory construction in nursing.* Norwalk: Appleton-Century-Crofts.

Welford, A. (1965). Performance, biological mechanisms and age: A theoretical sketch. In A. Welford & J. Birren (Eds.), *Behavior, aging and the nervous system.* Springfield, IL: Charles C. Thomas.

Zimmer, J., Watson, N., & Treat, A. (1984). Behavioral problems among patients in skilled nursing facilities. *American Journal of Public Health, 74* (10), 1118–1121.

Zuckerman, M., Eysenck, S., & Eysenck, H. (1978). Sensation-seeking in England and America: Cross-cultural, age and sex comparisons. *Journal of Consulting and Clinical Psychology, 46*, 139–149.

Zuckerman, M., & Neeb, M. (1980). Demographic influences in sensation-seeking and expressions of sensation-seeking in religion, smoking and driving habits. *Personality and Individual Differences, 1*, 197–206.

Zuckerman, M., Persky, H., Hopkins, T., Murtaugh, T., Basu, G., & Shilling, M. (1966). Comparison of stress effects of perceptual and social isolation. *Archives of General Psychiatry, 14*, 356–365.